T4-BAH-047

THE OLD HERB DOCTOR

HARMONY THERAPIES, D.B.A
PAMELA K. SILLS-GRABOWSKI
407B W. 81st Ave.
Merrillville, IN 46410
(219) 736-1620

OTHER BOOKS AVAILABLE FROM THE PUBLISHER

By Joseph E. Meyer
THE HERBALIST, Revised & Updated

By Clarence Meyer
AMERICAN FOLK MEDICINE

FIFTY YEARS OF THE HERBALIST ALMANAC,
   Anthology

HERBAL RECIPES: For Hair; Salves & Liniments;
   Medicinal Wines & Vinegars; Plant Ash Uses

VEGETARIAN MEDICINES

THE OLD HERB DOCTOR

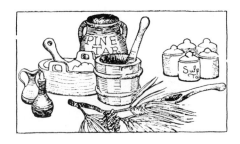

Compiled & Edited by
JOSEPH E. MEYER

With Illustrations by
CLARENCE MEYER

Second Edition, Revised

MEYERBOOKS
Glenwood, Illinois

9th printing, 1999

Copyright © 1941 by Hammond Book Company, founded
in 1910 by Joseph E. Meyer.

Index, illustrations and revisions appearing in this second
(revised) edition copyright © 1984 by David C. Meyer.

Published by Meyerbooks
P.O. Box 427
235 West Main Street
Glenwood, Illinois 60425

ISBN 0-916638-08-1

PREFACE TO THE SECOND EDITION

When first published, THE OLD HERB DOCTOR was essentially a book of testimonials recommending the medicinal virtues of herbs. My grandfather, Joseph E. Meyer, collected material for the book through the "Recipes Wanted" column of his annual publication, *The Herbalist Almanac*. Dried herbs, herbal compound teas and other health products from nature were advertised by means of this almanac. Customers who purchased herbs often wrote back when reordering to advise my grandfather of how they were using the herbs and how the herbs had helped them. Letters were often simply addressed to "The Herbalist" or "Herb Doctor," Hammond, Indiana, and in time these titles became second names for Joseph Meyer.

THE OLD HERB DOCTOR was compiled for the purpose of letting customers know how other customers had used herbs and the good results they had obtained from them. Recipes and testimonials shared space with advertisements for proprietary products which my grand-father marketed. For the benefit of the present-day reader, all of the outdated advertising has been removed, although an occasional reference to a 25¢ box of herbs (circa 1930) may still be found in the text. Also to be found, here and there, are blank spaces where advertising has been removed but no suitable text found to replace it.

THE OLD HERB DOCTOR sought to instill in the reader the virtues of "getting back to nature" to reclaim one's health. Native botanicals, including those used by American Indians, were extolled. To help convey this message of a "natural" and "native" means to health, the illustrations drawn for the book by my father tended to be less often medical and more often picturesque.

If any medical book can be said to possess a quaint charm, perhaps this one does.

David C. Meyer

PUBLISHER'S NOTE

The recipes contained in this book were collected in the 1920's and 30's — a time when self-treatment was commonly practiced and often necessary due to economic conditions or the scarcity of professional medical help. In some instances people who submitted recipes may have claimed cures for conditions which were self-diagnosed. While home treatment may be beneficial for minor conditions, it is important to have professional advice and services for treating serious ailments. For the above reasons, neither the editors nor the publisher can vouch for any claims made in this book.

ORGANIC SUBSTANCE OF PLANTS

Inorganic substances disturb the proper functioning of the organs of assimilation and elimination. They are considered unfriendly and in most cases dangerous and injurious, and very difficult to assimilate. Organic substances, however, such as are found only in plants, are easily and quickly assimilated and do not disturb the system.

The following plants contain such organic salts as Lime, Potassium, Sodium, Silicate, Manganese, Iron, Iodine, Bromine, Nitrous Acid, Sodium Carbonate, etc., the absence of which is very often the prime cause of many of our chronic ailments. By supplying these organic substances in a food form as in our herb teas—our resistance is built up and our natural forces of repair and recuperation bring relief.

Directions for Use—The Roots and Herbs listed here are absolutely harmless. They may be used in any combination. For an example, let us assume you desire a general tonic containing Iron, Iodine and Calcium. You could take one or two herbs listed under Iron—one or two listed under Iodine and one or two listed under Calcium. Take equal parts of these herbs and mix them; then take a heaping teaspoonful of the mixture into a cup of boiling water—let it stand until cool and drink one to two cupfuls of the tea a day. A very good tonic of this kind would be equal parts of Yellow Dock Root, Irish Moss and Horsetail Grass.

Iron—Is absolutely essential for the formation of rich red blood. Lack of Iron in food results in anemia, headaches, pallor of the face and lips, loss of weight, weakness and faintness and many other ills. Plants containing iron:

Yellow Dock	Burdock
Strawberry Leaves	Toad Flax
Stinging Nettle	Meadow Sweet
Silver Weed	Devil's-bit
Rest Harrow	Mullein Leaves
Salep	

Iodine—Deficiency of this element in food results in enlargement of the thyroid gland and develops into the ailment called "goitre." In children it results in arrested or impaired development, mental and physical. Plants containing Iodine:

Irish Moss	Sarsaparilla
Iceland Moss	

Calcium—This element in the form of carbonate, phosphate, silicate and fluoride is essential for the formation or growth of teeth and bones. It is especially essential in growing children. Plants containing Calcium:

Horsetail Grass	Plantain
Toad Flax	Silver Weed
Cleavers	Shepherd's-purse
Meadow Sweet	Mistletoe
Coltsfoot	Rest Harrow
Pimpernel	Chamomile
Dandelion	

Sulphur—Is essential to balance such other elements as Phosphorous, the dissipation of which it appears to retard: Plants containing this element are given below and are therefore indicated in Rheumatism, Gout, Anemia, Scrofula and to relieve phlegm of the respiratory organs:

Silver Weed	Rest Harrow
Stinging Nettle	Pimpernel
Fennel Seed	Shepherd's-purse
Coltsfoot	Eyebright
Calamus	Plantain Leaves
Waywort	Scouring Rush
Broom Tops	Meadow Sweet
Mullein	

Phosphorus—Is present in the nucleus of practically every cell of the body, but more abundantly in the brain and nerve tissue. Lack of this element may cause mental fatigue, listlessness, loss of memory, nervousness and a large number of ills. Plants containing Phosphorus:

Calamus	Meadow Sweet
Caraway Seed	Marigold Flowers
Chickweed	Licorice Root

Potassium—A very important element in the process of metabolism. Deficiency of this element checks growth. It is found in the blood corpuscles and soft tissues in the form of chloride and phosphate. Plants containing Potassium have a tendency to increase the flow of urine. They are as follows:

Walnut Leaves	Nettle Leaves
Mistletoe	Borage
Chamomile Flowers (German)	Couch Grass
	Primrose Flowers
Waywort	Dandelion
Calamus	Yarrow
Plantain Leaves	Mullein
Coltsfoot	Comfrey
American Centaury	Fennel Seed
Eyebright	Sanicle
Summer Savory	Oak Bark
Birch Bark	Carrot Leaves

Silicon—Is a constituent of the hair, nails and teeth. The amount required is very small—but this amount the body must have. Absorption takes place with the alkaline secretions of the intestines. Silicon is found in all plants but in Horsetail Grass in particular.

Magnesium—Not much is known of the action of this element, but that it is essential is certain. It is found in the bones and teeth. Plants containing Magnesium:

Meadow Sweet	Toad Flax
Rest Harrow	Silver Weed
Devil's-bit	Carrot Leaves
Black Willow Bark	Mullein Leaves
Walnut Leaves	
	Primrose

Chlorine—Has long been known to be essential to life. It is found in almost every tissue of the body—but more so in the blood chiefly as Sodium Chloride. It occurs in combination with Calcium, Potassium and Sodium. All plants contain more or less Chlorine in the form of Sodium Chloride.

Sodium—Occurs in the body chiefly as Chloride (table salt). The inorganic sodium chloride (table salt) should be used very sparingly. Excessive consumption of salt impairs the action of the kidneys and raises the blood pressure. Sodium is found as a carbonate in the blood where it is essential in contributing to the alkalinity of the blood.

Plants containing organic sodium are indicated in Liver, Gall Bladder, Kidney Troubles, Rheumatism, Gout and Chronic Swellings. The following are but a few:

Waywort	Stinging Nettle
Fennel Seed	Mistletoe
Black Willow	Meadow Sweet
Rest Harrow	Devil's-bit
Cleavers	Shepherd's-purse

For Brain Workers—Any occupation requiring much brain and nerve force, requires food containing phosphorus. Apples contain more phosphorus than any other fruit. The following herbs also contain phosphorus and they are entirely harmless:

Sweet Flag	House Leek
Licorice Root	Chickweed
Caraway Seed	Marigold

We can't seem to fight our common colds but I know that Boneset and Buffalo Herb Tea will do the work. When everything fails I am so glad you have some herbs that will bring us back to health.

THE WONDERFUL CHEMISTRY OF PLANT LIFE

There appears to be abundant proof that even the ancient philosophers knew that through the process known as metabolism, plants changed inorganic substances into organic substances. From water, salts, carbon-dioxide plants manufacture carbohydrates, fats, albumens with their all important vitamins. Through their chlorophyll they absorb the kinetic energy of the sun and transform it into potential energy. When man or beast consume these plants this potential energy is again changed into kinetic energy. Now we read of the amazing discovery that growing plant tissues emit ultra-violet light, capable of stimulating cell divisions and growth. This has been demonstrated by three eminent scientists of the Institute of Pathology, Western Pennsylvania Hospital, Pa., Ralph R. Mellon, N. Von Rashevsky and E. Von Rashevsky.

Plant Juices and Human Blood—The noted German scientific author and publisher, W. Weitzel, has published a new book entitled "The Mystery of Plant Blood." In it he illustrates how plant blood and human blood are closely associated and how the Vitamins in the juices of green plants change into the hormones that course in human blood. This scientific masterpiece is a powerful testimony of the value of roots and herbs in building up our health and resistance to disease.

ALKALOIDS NOT AS EFFECTIVE AS HERB TEAS

That the isolated active principle of an herb (alkaloid) is far less effective than the herb itself has been demonstrated by a large number of scientists foremost of which are Prof. Rubner, Hindhide, Horace, Fletcher and especially Prof. Tschirch; probably for the reason that most plants contain more than one substance of therapeutic action, as well as certain substances that alter or soften certain acrid principles of the plants.

In the mad endeavor to aid the medical world to keep their remedies secret or to improve on nature, chemists have isolated certain active principles of herbs (alkaloids) but after 50 years or more it has now been established that they act too harshly.

SECRETS OF ANCIENT SPECIALIST

For thousands of years physicians and scientists studied the art of healing with herbs. Many of these physicians, during the years of their practice, discovered certain herbs far more effective for certain ailments than others. These remedies were jealously guarded, and often handed down from generation to generation. Some of these secrets were lost to the scientific world with the death of the discoverer. Some were rediscovered by other scientists and physicians. Occasionally an herb discovered by the ancients and handed down to scientists in the books of Discorides, Paracelsus, Pliny, Galenus and Hippocrates was used almost exclusively in the treatment of a certain ailment up to modern times—then a chemical was discovered that will produce certain effects in much quicker time and more certain than the herb remedy—and the herb remedy was quickly discarded. After years of drugging with such chemicals, a wide-awake physician discovered that the chemical had some bad after effects—in some cases worse than the original ailment. Among the following are some of these jealously guarded secrets of ancient and modern specialists.

Professor Winternitz, a noted botanist and practitioner of the eighteenth century, treasured the leaves of Bilberry and White Birch as a diuretic in the treatment of Dropsy, retention of the urine and kindred ailments, ascertaining that they were far more effective and less irritating than any other diuretic.

Dr. Froriepp, another German botanist, employed Nettle Tea exclusively in all cases of dysentery.

Dr. Krahn, another noted practitioner and botanist, employed Garden Sage as a specific for night sweats, especially those peculiar to consumptives. Professors Combenale and Lille, prominent scientists, verified the experience of Dr. Krahn.

Dr. Loeffler, German botanist, valued Coughwort leaves highly for catarrhal conditions of mucous membrane of the bronchial tubes and lungs.

The French scientists, Drs. Bodard and Deschamps, declare they have discovered Coughwort leaves as a specific in scrofula and tuberculosis.

Dr. Walser, a noted German physician, recommends the following for Asthma:
3 parts Coughwort
3 parts Plantain
3 parts Sage
1 part Silver Mullein
Place 2 to 4 heaping teaspoonfuls of the above mixture in a cup of boiling hot water, let it cool for 15 minutes, strain and add 2 tablespoonfuls of honey.
Dose—1 to 2 tablespoonfuls every hour.

De Korab, another noted scientist, recommends Elecampane Root in catarrhal asthma, chronic bronchitis and catarrhal affections of the air passages. The tea is made by bringing a cup of water to the boiling point in which is placed 1 to 2 tablespoonfuls of the ground root of Elecampane. When cool, drink 1 to 2 tablespoonfuls every hour.

The following was a highly prized formula of the noted scientist, Dr. von Czarnowski, for inflammation and irritation of the bladder and mucus lining of the urinary passages:
Equal parts Linden Flower
Equal parts Elder Flowers
Equal parts St. Johnswort
Equal parts German Chamomile Flowers
Equal parts Blackberry Leaves
Place 2 to 4 heaping teaspoonfuls of the above mixture in a cup of boiling water, allow to cool, strain and drink one cupful 3 times a day half hour before meals.

Rosemary Wine, as made by the noted German botanist, Paul Dinand, and recommended for dropsy, especially dropsy of the heart.
Directions—Fill a quart fruit jar half full of Rosemary Leaves, pour over this sufficient wine to fill the jar, let it remain for 24 hours, strain.
Dose—2 to 4 tablespoonfuls mornings and evenings. White unsweetened wine is preferable.

Dr. Westen's Blood Purifying Tea:
4 parts Dandelion Root
4 parts Chicory Root
4 parts Witch Grass Root
1 part Fennel Seed
Take 1 or 2 tablespoonfuls of the above mixture, place in a cup of boiling hot water, boil for one minute, let cool, strain.
Dose—2 tablespoonfuls one-half hour after meals.

Dr. Frederick Wolfe, one of the most modern of German reform physicians, reveals two formulas the value of which can only be appreciated by those afflicted with these painful and distressing ailments. He also gives advice on diet that must be carefully followed if results are to be permanent.

For Neuritis, Migraine, Etc.
1 ounce St. Johnswort
1 ounce Primrose Flowers
1 ounce Blessed Thistle
1 ounce Lavender Flowers
1 ounce Sweet Balm Leaves
2 ounces Peppermint Leaves
3 ounces Fragrant Valerian Root

Directions—Mix the above ingredients together; then take one or two heaping teaspoonfuls of the mixture and place it in a cup of boiling hot water; cover with a saucer and when cool, strain and drink 3 cupfuls every day. Either one-half hour before or after meals.

For Gout, Muscular Rheumatism, Etc.
3 ounces Birch Leaves
2 ounces Horsetail Grass
1 ounce Rest Harrow
1 ounce Garden Rue
1 ounce Juniper Berries
1 ounce Yarrow

Directions—Mix the above ingredients together; then take 1 or 2 heaping teaspoonfuls of the mixture and place it in a cup of boiling hot water; place it on back of stove to keep hot for 10 minutes; allow to cool a little; strain and drink while it is still warm 1 cupful one-half hour before or after each meal.

Diet—Avoid meats, fish and sweets and pastries, and alcoholic liquors. Eat fresh green vegetables and fruits, eat only sparingly bread, eggs, cheese. Avoid as much as possible any drinks containing sugar. If you desire sweets, eat honey.

Dr. Ashner of Vienna states that during twenty years of his practice, he has proved that certain plants containing a bitter principle, such as Gentian, American Centaury, Wormwood, Condurango, taken as a tea never failed to relieve Stomach Troubles—often when an operation was considered the only remedy.

Editor's Note—If you desire to use any of the above simple herb teas, you may do so without hesitation, as they are all harmless, but as these ailments are of a serious nature, you are advised to lose no time in consulting only a specialist and dietitian.

HOW TO KEEP YOUNG

Recent experiments have demonstrated that the process known as metabolism, that is the breaking down of waste materials and building up the new cells, is kept in perfect harmony with the consumption of plants and plant juices, such as herb teas, vegetables and fruits. This vegetable matter has a distinct influence on gland activity, and therefore restores and prolongs youth. Vitamines are not the only activating agents of plant life—the organic minerals, cosmic and violet rays and other rays combine in a mysterious way to benefit mankind. As an example in Water Cress and Spinach are found radio-active calcium that has a decided influence on the rhythm of the heart beat.

VITAMIN E—THE SEX VITAMIN

According to Prof. Herbert Evans of the University of California, Vitamin E is the fertility or sex vitamin.

Water cress, growing along brooks and streams, is one of the best sources of Vitamin E.

L. B. Mendel and H. V. Vickery, noted scientists of New Haven, Conn., report to the Carnegie Institution of Washington, as follows:

"We have demonstrated an abundance of Vitamin E in the green leaves of water cress."

Botanists call water cress Nasturtium Officinale. Mendel and Vickery made the tests upon male and female rats. If these animals eat food which has no Vitamin E they show no fertility. In the case of male rats, there is marked decrease in sex health. The females become barren.

Dr. Karl E. Mason of Vanderbilt University worked with Mendel and Vickery. His research also showed that water cress was rich in Vitamin E. He estimates that the dried leaves of water cress contain three times as much Vitamin E as do the dried lettuce leaves.

In their experiments, Mendel and Vickery fed rats food mixtures in which only water cress leaves had any Vitamin E at all. Yet from the day of birth until maturity, these rats grew up as if they had sufficient Vitamin C. They were repeatedly mated, and showed perfect health.

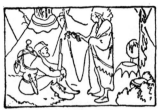

ANEMIA

Anemia is a condition of the blood in which there is a deficiency of red blood corpuscles. It may be present in many diseases and conditions.

Symptoms—Unnatural pallor of the skin (yellowish green), loss of strength, shortness of breath, headache, nervousness, coldness of the extremities, heart palpitation.

Treatment—Fresh air; good, nourishing food rich in minerals, especially iron; keep bowels open. Eat goat cheese daily. Take a good herb tonic tea, and consult a specialist.

The Herb Doctor's choice of botanical Tonics are: Walnut Leaves, Gentian, Angelica Root, Wild Strawberry Leaves, Red Raspberry Leaves, Asparagus, Spinach.

—Tonic Tea.......
Rocky Mountain Grape
Gentian
Marshmallow
Sacred Bark
Turtlebloom
Yellow Root
Fennel Seed
Jamaica Ginger
Anise Seed
Thyme
Juniper Berries
Colic Root
Bearberry Leaves
General Tonic—Improves the appetite.

I want to send in a recipe as Blood Builder and cure for Anemia. Take the leaves of the Black Walnut Trees, which should be picked before the nuts form, and make a tea from them the same as an ordinary tea. Drink a cupful three times a day. Writes Mrs. R. D., East Liverpool, Ohio.

My daughter who lives in Mexico was recently a great sufferer from Anemia, following an attack of malarial fever. A Mexican woman seeing her sad condition told her of a simple remedy which the common folks use there to cure themselves of this condition. She at once tried the remedy and was soon restored to health and strength. She has since told many of this remedy and in every case, almost miraculous results followed in a short time. But in long standing cases, it is necessary to continue the use of the medicine for a considerable time, even sometimes a year. The remedy is, just take the Black Walnut Leaves and make a tea of them, drink it like any other tea. Take lots of it, drink it with your meals, drink it between meals, whenever you want a drink of water. It is not poisonous and will not hurt you. Use a small handful of the dried Walnut Leaves to a pint of boiling water, steep until as strong as you like, but on the whole it is not bad to take. While taking this tea, use plenty of good nourishing food to build up your body also. Writes Miss A. B., Allentown, Pa. (Copied from the "Golden Age.")

Editor's Note—Do not expect results from herbs that are over a year old.

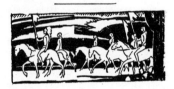

My husband had asthmatic attacks until he couldn't sleep anl he took your Wild Plum Bark Tea and now he is relieved. He can lie down and sleep as quiet as a baby. Writes E. F. B., Clarinda, ?—?.

Black Walnut Leaves are very good for Bloodlessness and Anemia.

I have found Sumach Berries made into a tea very beneficial for Diabetes. Writes Mrs. L. B., Shawnee, Okla.

To tone up the system and circulation:
Gentian Root, Rocky Mountain Grape Root, and German Chamomile, and one teaspoonful of powdered Golden Seal, also 2 tablespoonfuls Cascara Bark, place in a well covered can or fruit jar. Mix thoroughly by shaking, steep one heaping tablespoonful in a pint of boiling water, let stand until cold, strain, and take ⅓ cupful three times a day. Good for anyone who is tired and run down for loss of appetite, etc. Writes Mrs. J. E. S., Arcadia, Indiana.

ANIMALS

For Tape or Round Worms in a dog, don't feed him all day, then give 3 tablespoonfuls of Castor Oil in the morning, whether he wants to drink it or not, and at night give him 3 drams Kamala, next morning give another dose of Castor Oil, then you can feed him again. Repeat this in 10 days if necessary. It cured our dog

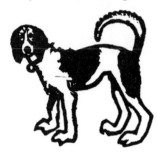

For Running Fits in Dogs—Give a piece of Blood Root about the size of the first joint in the little finger or same amount in powdered form. Give three times a day for three days, then discontinue three days and so on. Then you can also give a tablespoonful of Gun Powder in sweet milk after this. Hope this hint may be of use to someone. Writes H. C. S., Juniata, Pa.

Try a handful of Huckleberry Leaves and make a strong tea, give 1 to 2 teaspoonfuls three times a day and will stop the bowels; so is it good for Dysentery in Calves and All Stock. Writes M. C. M., Bolivar, La.

Hog Cholera—You can add this recipe to your book. I know it should be for herbs, but this is not for man but has been tried for Hog Cholera, and will clean the hogs out. Use about twice a year Jalap, which will clean them out, then give them carbolic acid in sour milk, a tablespoonful to 12 quarts of milk. They will never have any pigs die with cholera. I have used it for years. Writes Mrs. T. H., Seney, Mich.

Editor's Note—It will be necessary to partially powder the Jalap with a nutmeg grinder.

For little puppies with Worms and Distemper, give a teaspoonful of Sulphur and the same amount of lard mixed, every three days for two or three doses. Be sure they do not get wet while using this or they may get stiff joints. Writes Mrs. E. H., Sesser, Ill.

To cure Cholera in chickens put Poke Root and May Apple Root in their water. Writes Mrs. W. F. N., Middletown, Tenn.

Poke Root kept in drinking water will prevent Cholera in chickens. Writes V. M., Esto, Ky.

Remedy for Heaves—Mix 2 ounces of Lobelia with 4 ounces of Oil Cake (6 oz. 25c.) Put this with oats or other light feeding of your horse, 3 times a day. Do not work the animal and sprinkle the hay if it is very dry or dusty. The above remedy cured a horse for us after she was old and thin, and even given up to die; she got well and afterward raised the most beautiful colt we had ever had on our place. Writes Mrs. M. E., Oklahoma City, Okla.

In the spring, when horses are out of condition and fail to shed their winter coat and seem sluggish, don't clip off the hair and give them cold or possibly pneumonia, but get some good clean Red Puccoon or Blood Root as it is usually known and put a teaspoonful in their food a couple of times and they will not only shed their hair nicely but will get in better condition. Writes G. L. M., Odin, Ill.

Editor's Note—I would suggest that you ask for the powdered blood root as it is more easily handled.

I have a recipe for you which applies to horses, but as it is valuable I wish you to print it in your Almanac. In the Spring time when starting the horses in the Spring work, especially colts being used for the first time, apply a wash made from White Oak Bark, for it will toughen the tender skin. Writes W. K., Baltic, Ohio.

For Coughs and Colds in Horses, take Sumach Bark, grind with a food chopper or purchase it ground, and feed a handful in the feed twice a day for a week. Writes E. L., Troy, N. Y.

Worm Cure for Horses—Use Poplar Bark ground, feed a handful twice a day in the food.

For Colic in Horses or Cattle there is no better or quicker relief than a pint of melted lard mixed with two tablespoons of Turpentine. Drench as warm as possible, and if not relieved in one or two hours repeat same. This is a sure cure. My father and mother have saved several cows and horses that were so bad they would have been dead before a veterinary could have arrived. Writes Mrs. A. C. S., Mansfield, Ohio.

Editor's Note—I don't know much about cattle. This seems rather ugly to take.

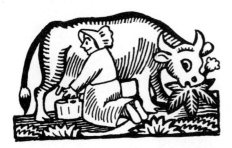

For Cows That Have Caked Bags—
Use the cut Horse Radish Root and feed twice daily a pint or so in the feed, 2 or 3 doses in general, and this should be enough, but if not, give another dose. Writes Mrs. A. K., Caro, Mich.

Sunflower Seed has almost completely cured my neighbor's horse of Heaves. Writes J. McC., Utopia, Ont., Canada.

I know Poke Root boiled until the strength is all out will kill and cure Fistula in Horses, for I have cured several myself in that way. I use a syringe to get it into the tubes. Writes L. L. R., Liberal, Mo.

For Cholera in Turkeys and Chickens give one teaspoonful of powdered Alum followed by water made yellow with Golden Seal or Barberry Root. This has saved me several dollars. Writes Mrs. A. W., Saltville, Va.

Here is a recipe for Hog Cholera. Make a strong tea of Sampson Snake Root and then make this into a dough and give to the hogs. Mrs. T. B., Flowery Branch, Ga.

Make a salve of Bittersweet Roots and it cannot be beat for Cows with Swollen Udders. Two or three applications well rubbed in will do the work. Writes C. B., Mercers Bottom, W. Va.

Here is a recipe if you care to print it. I had chickens who died from running of the bowels, and I did all I could for them. Everyone said there was nothing to any avail, until one day a lady advised that I get the real Olive Oil and put enough of it in their feed so as to bind it together, give every other day. I did so and my chicks are alive yet today. Writes A. M. H., Aurora, Colo.

APPENDICITIS

Treatment—If the case is severe and an abscess has formed, consult a specialist at once. Rest in bed. Give only liquid foods and sparingly, and keep bowels open.

Appendicitis—It is advisable to abstain from food, other than hot lemonade until all pain, inflammation and fever have subsided. Then nothing but orange juice for a few days. Avoid foods which constipate: for example, meats, fried foods, tea and coffee, white bread, white sugar.

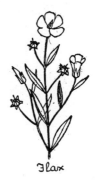

Flax

I am sending you a recipe for appendicitis. Take half teaspoonful Flax Seed three times a week, follow with only two doses the second week. Writes M. E. J., Yale, Okla.

For Appendicitis—I cured a woman the doctors said had to be operated on. She took one ounce of Olive Oil three times a day and rubbed turpentine on to take out the pain. Writes C. H. S., Ludington, Mich.
*Editor's Note—*May be O. K. in some incipient cases.

In either Chronic or Acute Appendicitis, give patient a cup of Olive Oil. This saved my sister when they said she could not live through the night, and we have seen it work wonders in other cases, too. Writes M. B., Washington, W. Va.
*Editor's Note—*We must not forget that there are some cases that cannot be cured except by draining the pus. Try the above if you wish, but consult a specialist.

To keep away attacks of Appendicitis, take plenty of Olive Oil. Writes Mrs. B. B., Norwalk, Ohio.

I would like for you to find a place in one of your books for a cure for Appendicitis. We have told this to several who were ready to go under the knife, and their doctors were astonished when they found them so well, and I can give references about this. This recipe came from a surgeon in the Hoosier State: You take the Timothy Seed, which can mostly be obtained at any feed store; 25c worth will be sufficient to make for the whole family, as the children love it. Take a cup of the seed and pour over a quart of boiling water, boil a minute or so, strain, sweeten, and drink either hot or cold, although hot is best, but if not possible to keep hot you can take it cold. In using this you can even feel the inflammation begin to boil right out of the appendix. Writes Mrs. S. C., Lima, Ohio.

For Appendicitis—Take pan hot water, put in 2 tablespoonfuls Salts and 1 Turpentine. Wring turkish towel or flannel cloth as hot as can be borne, put on side. Keep still and pain will soon be gone. Writes M. E. S., Timblin, Pa.

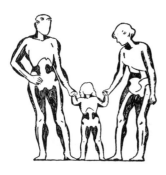

ARTERIOSCLEROSIS OR HARDENING OF THE ARTERIES

This is a serious condition. Consult a specialist. Deep breathing is of wonderful aid in the treatment. Low breathing is one of the chief causes of this ailment.

The Herb Doctor's choice of botanical Tonics are: Mistletoe, Yellow Dock Root, Life Everlasting, Mormon Valley Herbs.

My father-in-law lay waiting, yes, just waiting, to pass on. He could raise his voice only to a whisper. The doctors gave him two days to live. He received two letters, one from a relative in the East and one from a relative in the West. Each said that Garlic would cure Hardening of the Arteries and High Blood Pressure. It so happened that they had a neighbor who had it growing in her garden. They rushed it to him and cooked it and gave him a dish of it. In a remarkably short time he felt better, so they kept right on making that the main part of his diet for a day or two. In six days he was downtown to his blacksmith shop.

It was all so remarkable that the news spread like wild fire—so much so that for a long time he was receiving letters from all over the United States, wanting to know what he could say about it. Writes Mrs. S. J. S., Ottawa, Kan. *Editor's Note*—Thank you for this simple remedy.

Take Black Haw, make a tea, drink about a pint a day, sip all along during the day, and it will surely cure high blood pressure.

Take 1 tablespoonful of Hempseed and crush, place in a quart jar and fill with cold water, drink a small amount at a time until a quart is consumed in a day. This recipe is the one that I used for High Blood Pressure and it will drive the blood down. Writes M. S., Fresno, Ohio.

I am sending in a remedy for High Blood Pressure, and it is the best and surest thing I know of as it cured three persons that had given up. Take Garlic, might be strong, but it does the work. Writes I. R. Y., Le Roy, Kan.

High Blood Pressure—Take Mistletoe and Angelica Root, ground fine, two teaspoonfuls of each, place in a pint of water and bring to the boiling point, allow to cool. Drink two or three cupfuls a day.

    —Mistletoe Comp..
    Mistletoe Twigs
    Sassafras, bark of root
    Marshmallow Root
    Licorice

Very soothing to the kidneys. The only tea we have containing so large a portion of Mistletoe. May be used freely wherever the therapeutic action of Mistletoe is indicated. Mistletoe is the only herb mentioned in the U. S. Dispensatory as a treatment for high blood pressure.

APPETITE, TO IMPROVE

Try Dogwood for the appetite. Place a handful of the root bark in a quart of water. Boil to one pint; let set for an hour, strain, and take one tablespoonful three times a day. Writes Q. V. M., Quitsna, N. C.

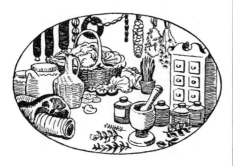

Wahoo Bark, White Oak, Golden Seal, Sarsaparilla, Wild Cherry Bark and Boneset in equal parts with ½ gallon of water, boiled down to one quart and take a tablespoonful three times a day and upon retiring. This is very good for poor complexion, loss of appetite, and it is very good as a health builder. Writes J. H. J., Kansas City, Kan.
Editor's Note—Seems to be a sort of a cure-all. Properties: Mainly astringent and tonic.

My father always prepared the following formula as a Spring Tonic and it Improves the Appetite. Pour boiling water over Wild Cherry Bark, Shell Hickory Bark, Prickly Ash Bark and Mullein and let stand awhile, then help yourself. It surely is fine to give you strength. Writes Mrs. M. H., Ringos Mills, Ky.

I have tried this for myself and I am now trying it for my sister and it works fine. I was so weak, no appetite. I fixed a tea of the following and drank four and five cups a day and one cupful upon retiring at night: 1 part of Wild Cherry, 1 part of Re Alder, and 1 part of Cedar. Pack it tightly in a pitcher and cover with hot water. Writes L. M. L., Jacksonville, N. C.

The Wild Plum Bark was excellent. I feel like a new person and I have gained a wonderful appetite while using the Bark and feel so much improved. Writes Miss M. D. G., Yaphank, N. Y.

As a good tonic for the appetite: Sassafras Tea in the spring and Sulphur and Sorghum Molasses mixed into a pill in the fall. Take a pill each night. This is good for some simple sores that break out in the fall. Writes Mrs. G. N., Farmington, Mo.
Editor's Note—First thing you know, you will have our five million readers pill rollers and then where would I be?

Take 1 oz. of Gentian Root, ½ oz. of Colombo Root and ½ oz. of Scullcap Herb, pour on 2 pints of cold water, simmer gently for twenty minutes, let stand for a little while and strain. Drink a wineglassful one hour before a meal to procure a good appetite and take two hours after a meal in Belching and simple Indigestion Have found this an excellent tonic for relief of the aged and Dyspepsia.

--Hop Bitters......
    Hop Flowers
    Buchu Leaves
    Prickly Ash Bark
    Buffalo Herb
    Rosemary Leaves
    Sassafras
    German Cheese Plant
A fine tonic. The main ingredient is Hop Flowers, the same that gives good beer the refreshing and tonic properties.

This is the only recipe that I have not seen in your herb book. It is for a Spring Tonic. Take 2 tablespoonfuls of Senna and 2 of Sarsaparilla Bark and boil in a quart of water. This is very good for that tired feeling in the Spring. Writes C. C., Kansas City, Mo.

Here is a Good Tonic Remedy—Six teaspoonfuls of Hickory Bark, 3 of Poplar Bark, 8 of Sweet Gum Bark, 8 of Wahoo, 2 of Sassafras and 2 of Fringe Tree. After all are mixed well, use 1 heaping teaspoonful into a cup of water, and take 3 times a day, a large mouthful at a time. Writes E. H. Y., Wilmington, Va.

Tonic—Gentian Root and Colombo 1 ounce each, 5 gills of boiling water, reduce or boil down to 4 gills, strain and take a half wineglassful 3 times during the day.

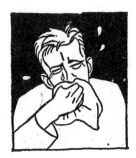

ASTHMA

Asthma is known by occasional paroxysms of difficult breathing, lasting from a few hours to several days, coming on at intervals, to be followed by remissions, during which the patient breathes with comparative ease. The attack returns again, either at regular intervals, or is provoked by exposure to cold, damp air, severe effort or even mental emotions; during the attack, the respiration is labored, wheezing, sighing, loud; accompanied with anxiety and frequent cough. Sometimes the lips and face become bluish, and toward its close, or even during its entire continuance, free expectoration of mucous.

Treatment—It is doubtful if the same botanicals will affect every person in the same degree, therefore we can only list such as have been found useful as Antispasmodics and Carminatives. The Herb Doctor's choice of botanicals are: Wild Plum Bark, Skunk Cabbage, Wild Cherry Bark, Elder Flowers, Elder Berries, Horehound, Mullein, Nettle, Speedwell, Elecampane, Celandine, Grindelia;
There are also a large number of common household remedies such as: Eating raw onions, red cabbage, raw linseed oil.

***

Asthma—It is considered that the diet has been very faulty before such attacks can develop; too great a fondness for carbohydrate foods, starches and sugars. Discontinue the use of all carbohydrate foods for a while—white bread, pastry, potatoes, all cereals and refined white sugar. Eat freely of citrus fruits and green leafy vegetable salads.

—Juniper Berry Comp.....
Juniper Berries
Sassafras Bark
Gentian
Wild Clover Tops
Bluets
Horehound Leaves
Fennel Seed
Wormwood Leaves
Rosemary Leaves
German Cheese Plant
This tea was popular in the late Eighteenth Century and is still having a good sale. It is a mild diaphoretic and tonic. It will find many uses.

***

Asthma—"A syrup made from the bark of Wild Plum is a sure cure for asthma. It has cured six cases in this town alone. The syrup is made by steeping a handful of the bark of Wild Plum into a quart of water. Boil down to 1 pint and add sugar to make a syrup. Dose, 3 or 4 tablespoonfuls during the day." Writes C. D. S.

***

Asthma—Here is a helpful recipe. Cocklebur tea is a cure for asthma; two handfuls steeped in a quart of water and a cupful taken three or four times a day. Also the Wild Plum Bark you mentioned in your book is a sure cure. Writes Mrs. J. T. D., Cedar Rapids, Iowa.

***

Asthma—I wish to contribute this recipe for your almanac. For asthma—Take one ounce of Spikenard, Elecampane, Comfrey, Horehound, and one-half drachm Lobelia. Pulverize, and steep in one pint of honey. Dose: One tablespoonful every half hour until relieved. Writes Carl B., Walnutport, Pa.

***

For Asthma—Take one quart of Sunflower Seeds, put in a half gallon of water, boil down to one quart of water, strain, add one pint of honey and boil down to a syrup. One teaspoonful three times a day is the dose. Writes A. P., Bremen, Ala.

***

For Asthma—Make a pillow of Life Everlasting, sleep on it for asthma, for my aunt did this for her little son and it cured him.

***

A lady at Yellow Springs, Ohio, tells me that she cured herself of Asthma by using for her common drink a tea made of Chestnut Leaves. The tea may be sweetened and its use should be continued for two or three months. Writes F. L. S., Auburn, Me.

I am writing you to tell you how much good the Plum Bark has done my brother and myself. I have had asthma for fifteen years and my brother has had it for ten years and we have tried everything without much success until we took this plum bark and now the attacks are only light. Writes Miss E. K., Newport, Ohio.

For asthma attacks:
1 tablespoonful grated Indian Turnip
1 handful Hickory Bark
1 handful Maiden Hair
1 cupful strained Honey.
Cook Hickory Bark first in one quart of water, then add the roots and simmer a while longer, strain through cloth and add the honey. Dose: One teaspoonful for a child and 1 tablespoonful for adults, three or four times daily. Writes H. D., Plain City, Ohio.

I know a good household remedy that I have been using three years and find it just fine. Fig Leaves for Asthmatic attacks. I gather them as soon as they begin to dry and put them away and as I feel the attack coming on I smoke them and they give instant relief. Writes Mrs. M. M., Arlington, Tenn.

I received the two boxes of Wild Plum Bark for my father-in-law. After taking the first box, he has found great relief. I hope it will do as much good for others as it has for him. Before he started to take the tea he was unable to sleep in his bed for weeks, having to sleep in his chair. Writes E. H., Southbridge, Mass.

I received a dollar's worth of Plum Bark a year ago and it did me more good than anything I ever used before. I got asthma every year for the last forty-three years and a year ago I had no attacks of it worth mentioning. Writes N. S. M., Springtown, Pa.
My grandfather who was troubled with Asthma slept on a pillow stuffed with Field Balsam. He said this helped him more than anything he could find to use. Writes Mrs. R. E. W., Little Falls, W. Va.

Mullein Leaves, dried and crumbled up, smoked as you would tobacco in a cigarette or pipe, is also an excellent relief in cases of Asthmatic attacks. Writes G. S. H., Scottsville, Ky.

Wild Plum Bark was very helpful to my ten-year-old son when he had asthmatic attacks and hay fever this fall. Writes Mrs. D. O., Marion, Ohio.

Coughwort has done me more good than anything I ever used for a cough and I have been bothered with asthmatic attacks and a cough for twelve years and have taken only one 25c package. Now I can sleep all night. Writes R. J., Marianna, Fla.

I tried the recipe given in your old edition of the "Herbalist" calling for Mullein Leaves, Horehound, Lungwort, Sage and Sweet Root in equal parts for Asthmatic attacks, and it helped just wonderful. Writes Miss A. B., Baltimore, Md.

Will you please send me one package each of Wild Cherry Bark, and Wild Plum Bark, at 25 cents each? Honestly and sincerely they have really relieved me of asthma, but I still take them for good measure.—Mrs. J. E. DeM., Cheyenne, Wyo.

For Asthmatic attacks: Take the flowers and leaves of Life Everlasting. Make a pillow of it and sleep with it under your head at night. Writes Mrs. S. H., Kountze, Texas.

For Asthmatic attacks, add a handful of Wild Cherry Bark to one quart of water, boil, strain and add one cupful of best honey and take one tablespoonful four times a day. One spoonful on arising and one, one hour after each meal. Writes M. F. B., Milo, Iowa.

My wife had the Asthma and my brother had a little red book called "The Herbalist" and in this book I read about Wild Plum Bark Syrup. I made some and gave it to her and since then she has not had an attack. That was three years ago. I have the book yet and I consider it very valuable. Writes C. M., Wellsville, N. Y.
Father has used Mullein Leaves as a smoke for Asthma for years, and it has helped him more than any medicine, for which we spent lots of money. Writes Mrs. C. D. C., Salem, Ohio.

I am sending for two more 25c boxes of Wild Plum Bark. I sent for one trial box as I have bronchial asthma and I am glad to say I received immediate relief. Writes Mrs. N. C. J., Bellefontaine, Ohio.
Asthma attacks: One teacupful of Lobelia Leaves, steeped for a half hour in a pint of boiling water. The dose is one tablespoonful every fifteen to thirty minutes until free spitting of mucus is produced. Writes M. L. K., Fayetteville, N. C.

For Asthma—Take: one-half of a 25c size package of Horehound, Comfrey, Spikenard, and Elecampane Root. Soak in one gallon of water and boil down to one quart, strain, add one pint of honey and boil until thick like syrup. Take a teaspoonful 3 or 4 times a day when needed. Writes Mr. J. S., Mason City, Iowa.

Feather pillows are very bad for Asthma patients. Replace them with Hops placed in the pillow and note the great help: Writes Mrs. C. M., Jeannette, Pa.

Asthma—Here is a remedy for Bronchitis, Asthma, which should be continued for a long time. Two drams Marshmallow Root, 2 drams Licorice, ½ ounce Linseed, ½ ounce Iceland Moss, 2 drams Golden Seal, 2 drams Life Root, 2 drams Pleurisy Root. Simmer slowly in quart of water, stirring all well. Strain when hot, add 2 ounces of sugar. Take a wineglassful 4 times a day, and should be kept in cool place too. Writes G. G., Providence, R. I.

Asthma Cure—This has cured many cases of long standing if faithful in its use until cured. Grate ¾ teaspoonful of Skunk Cabbage Root and ¼ teaspoonful of loaf sugar, even measure. Grate only as needed. One teaspoonful of above before each meal. Place dry on tongue, wash down with little water. Take this until cured, and in very severe cases it takes 6 months. Writes Mrs. W. R., Massillon, Ohio.

For Asthma—The Wild Plum Bark sure is fine for asthma as I have tried it and my 12-year-old boy too. Writes Mrs. W., Haskell, Ark.

I wish to inform the public through you that I have been using Wild Plum Bark:
For the last couple of days I have had a severe Sore Throat; last night my throat seemed to be swollen. Before retiring I took about three swallows of Wild Plum Bark, which I had prepared, and awoke this morning with no Sore Throat. It has left me entirely. I cannot praise this remedy enough. Writes E. G. S., Tampa, Fla.

I have been pleased so much with Plum Bark for asthma until I hardly know just what to say, but I will say that was a God-send to me, and I can't thank you enough. Writes Mrs. J. D., Bessemer, Ala.

Just a few lines to let you know that the Wild Plum Bark surely has done me good. Before I received the bark I had a spell of asthma every night so bad until at times I thought I would never get my breath, but since taking the Wild Plum Bark I haven't had even one spell. I wouldn't be without Wild Plum Bark. Writes L. L., Albertville, Ala.

Your Wild Plum Bark is surely good for Asthma. I've bought quite a few of your herbs for my father and it has helped him wonderfully. A few months ago he was very bad but now he is feeling fine. Writes Mrs. E. W. S., Ruso, N. D.

I have tried Wild Plum Bark syrup for Asthma, and it has done more good than any other medicine used. I had a bad attack for about four or five weeks. One day a neighbor got your Almanac and showed it to me. I purchased a 25c package of Wild Plum Bark from you, which I made into a syrup, and I haven't had a spell of Asthma for 15 months. Writes E. Mc. D., Long Island, Kan.

Editor's Note—If folks would only read every one of these little recipes they could save themselves many doctor bills and much suffering.

Asthma—My husband had Asthma for over 40 years and we just spent all we made trying different doctors and hospitals without much or any good. Since we have got your Almanac and tried Wild Plum Bark. Now, sir, everyone that sees him working around the place asks, "My, what have you been taking?" and when he tells them they say it sure must be wonderful. It is sure a pity we did not know this 40 years ago. Writes A. E. M., New Florence, Mo.

I had the Asthma so badly and I got the Wild Plum Bark and made a syrup of it, like it says in the book. That was last fall I started taking this, and I haven't had a touch of it since. Writes Mrs. J. H. L., Nowata, Okla.

Wild Plum Bark is excellent for Asthma. A friend of mine was cured with Wild Plum Bark after suffering for 35 years. Writes Mrs. W. C. D., Bluefield, Va.

I have spent a lot of money for medicine for Asthma in the last three years, and with no results, but I received your Almanac and read about Wild Plum Bark and I purchased some and sleep now from the first night on. Writes A. N. N., Fallon, Nev.

I just want to tell you the good Wild Plum Bark has done for me. I have suffered for 15 years with Asthma, and this Spring I was down for 12 weeks that I couldn't walk across the floor, and three doctors gave me up, when one of my neighbors, a Mrs. J. G.—, ordered me a box of Wild Plum Bark and it put me on my feet in a week. I certainly can never say enough for it. Writes M. A., Winchester, Va.

Just a few lines to praise the Wild Plum Bark, for my son has had Asthma since the age of six months and he is now 17 years old and we have spent a fortune to get medicine for him. It would not be bad if it helped him, but it was always the same story, and we even spent a year in Colorado for relief. As he got older the spells would get worse, but now the second cup of this Wild Plum Bark helped him out, and it is now haying time and he never had an attack where other times he used to have very bad spells during that time, so I am sending for more. Writes Mrs. A. L., North Adams, Mass.

I am using the Wild Plum Bark Tea, and one teaspoonful of whole Mustard Seed before bedtime and upon arising for Asthma and Bronchitis. It sure has been helping me wonderfully and I wish you would pass the news along. I have given this a long trial and can testify to the wonderful help received. Writes C. E. K., Detroit, Mich.

*Editor's Note—*I don't doubt this a bit.

Wild Plum Bark. Have used this over a year, and I am greatly improved, but still keep it on hand to use occasionally. Wild Plum Bark sure has done wonders for me. Writes Mrs. T. A., English, Ind.

Lately I handed a young man an Almanac, and advised him to use Wild Plum Bark for Asthma. Now he reports that it has worked wonders and he never feels the least sign of it unless he eats too much. Writes Mrs. F. E., Battle Creek, Mich.

A cough syrup made of Wild Plum Bark and sugar just can't be beat for Asthma. Writes Mrs. F. C., Oak Hill, Ohio.

Asthma—The Wild Plum Bark I purchased from you cured my boy of Asthma. I say cured, because he does not get it any more. Writes Mrs. J. G., Colver, Pa.

Wild Plum Bark has certainly helped my little daughter. She had Asthma so bad I had tried everything that I could think of or heard of, but since she has been taking the syrup from the bark of the Wild Plum, I can say she hasn't had an asthma spell this winter. I am sure thankful for this remedy. Writes Mrs. R. W., Crawfordsville, Iowa.

The writer advised a Mrs. B., of Cincinnati, Ohio, to send and get Wild Plum Bark for the treatment of Asthma for her son, who is badly afflicted. His attacks came on twice a week, thinking every one would be his last. No matter what they did, under the treatment of doctors, specialists, the spells came on just the same. Have been using the Wild Plum now 6 weeks and not a spell from the first dose. The boy has gained 5 pounds and his complexion has changed to a rosy color. Writes F. P. L., Williamsburg, Ohio.

*Editor's Note—*Wild Plum Bark and, in fact, all of our herb teas are so harmless one wonders why everybody does not use them.

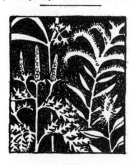

The Wild Plum Bark is excellent for Asthma. The lady for whom I ordered the trial package on June 29th, did not realize she had Asthma after taking the first cupful of the tea. In fact, she even forgot to make the tea on one or two occasions during the trial treatment. Writes A. A. W., East Akron, Ohio.

I have been using your Wild Plum Bark for Asthma for some time and it has done wonders for me. I have suffered nine years. Writes O. S. R., Goldsboro, N. C.

I have been a great sufferer of Bronchial Asthma. I have taken about every kind of medicine and inhaled smokes of all kinds. I have about $200.00 worth of serum in my arms, and so on. I have been in bed by the month and been like this for 12 years. A friend sent me one of your books and it had Wild Plum Bark marked in it, so I sent and got one package for only 25c and if it was no good I would not be out very much. I prepared it, and began to take it, and I was not able to sleep nights either, and had to smoke some asthma herb 5 or 6 times a night and many times during the day, while I coughed myself nearly to death. I had not taken the Wild Plum Bark 3 days when I did not have to get up nights and I do not have to smoke now at all. I have just begun on my second package and have not been so well in 14 years. I shall continue to take more of it if I need it, but I do not think I shall need much more. Writes Mrs. G. E. T., Arlington, Vt.

Editor's Note—Many others could save many dollars if they would but come back to nature.

BABY

Treating the Baby—The less medicine you give the baby the better for it. Don't run to the medicine chest every time baby cries. Keep it clean, dry and warm and nature will do the rest. In cases of Colic or Constipation use medicines below. Writes Mrs. J. M., of Milwaukee, mother of eight healthy children.

For Constipation—For children over one year give one-half spoonful castor oil. If child is much troubled with constipation give one-half teaspoonful pure olive oil every evening before retiring, for a month or more, until every sign of the disease has vanished.

For Colic—If the child is restless and continually crying it is most likely suffering from colic. Give one-half teaspoonful Fennel Tea made as follows, every half hour if necessary.

2 teaspoonsful Pure Fennel Seed.
2 teaspoonsful White Sugar.
2 ounces boiling water.

Do not allow the water to boil after the seed has been added. If the child has spasms, apply warm flannels to the abdomen. Be careful not to scorch child.

When troubled with Colic it is well to hold the child in an upright position and to tap gently on the back. This allows the gas to escape.

Catnip Tea is useful for Colic in Babies. Writes Mrs. C. S., Pleasant Ridge, Pa.

Peppermint Tea is good for babies when they are cross or have a Cold. It is also good for adults when the tea is made strong. Writes D. McD., Flora, Ill.

Here is a good recipe for babies. When one is cross, take Sang Root. Make a tea and sweeten to taste. Give it to the child every one or two hours. I have tried it and found it to be very good. Writes Mrs. W. H. G., Forest City, N. C.

Here is a recipe for Baby's Bowels that I have tried, and several of my friends have, with good results. Take a piece of Sweet Flag Root about ½ inch long, chip up fine ½ teaspoonful of Catnip, ⅓ teaspoonful of ground Allspice and boil in 1 teacupful of water for 5 minutes. When cold, give a teaspoonful every hour until relieved. Peppermint Tea is also good for Baby's Sick Stomach. Writes Mrs. R. E. B., Edinton, N. C.

Editor's Note—I would prefer to leave out the ground Allspice for a very young baby.

Catnip Tea is fine to give babies for the Colic. It is also good for Nervous people. Writes Mrs. W. F. N., Middleton, Tenn.

For new-born babies whose kidneys have failed to act, make a tea of a handful of Watermelon Seeds and a half pint of water. Feed the infant a spoonful frequently until results are obtained. Writes Mrs. U. M. H., Marion, Ind.

A remedy which I have always used for Babies' Colic. Make a tea of the Catnip Leaves, add sugar to taste, and give to baby in the nursing bottle or by teaspoon. Writes Mrs. L. P., Galloway, Ohio.

Catnip—A tablespoonful steeped in a pint of hot water is good to give little babies for Colic; if they will not drink it, it can be sweetened, or the mother should drink a large cupful before meals, that is, a nursing mother. Writes

Ginseng Tea will cure infants from Colic. Writes G. W. B., Cassard, Va.

Just a weak tea of Catnip is good for babies with Colic. Writes A. B., New Vienna, Ohio.

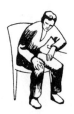

BACKACHE

The Old-Fashioned Plaster—Judging from the great number of inquiries we get for Back Plasters and Chest Plasters, it appears that these will again become as popular as they were 40 years ago. Like Roots and Herbs, they have been succeeded by more powerful drugs, but gradually people are coming back to these good old standbys—and their values in certain ailments are being rediscovered. When you get tired drugging yourself try one of these plasters —they are great and harmless.

Back Plaster—Helpful in Lumbago, Tired and Lame Back, etc.

Belladonna Plasters—The good old-fashioned kind, used for the same purpose as the above.

Chest Plaster—Useful in Coughs, Colds, Asthma, Whooping Cough, etc.

Here is a recipe that may be useful to someone. I knew a man that hurt his back in lifting weights and the work he was doing at this time was of a very bad nature for one that had anything the matter with his back, and so he only grew worse every day. He tried all kinds of remedies, doctors, and specialists and spent his money all ways to try to get a remedy that would do him good. Finally he tried a tea of the plant that I know well, that comes from England, Pellitory of the Wall. A little climbing plant that will cling to a wall like the Boston Ivy. He used this tea, putting a handful of the dried herb in a jug and poured over a quart of boiling water, and when cold he drank a teacupful 2 or 3 times a day. In about 6 weeks or 2 months he was completely cured, and it never returned, although he continued this heavy lifting at work. Writes A. W. H., Calgary, Alta., Canada.

A tried and true remedy for Backache: Take a large handful of Horsemint, steep in a pint of water, drink a cupful at bedtime. Writes Mrs. W. B. S., Winslow, Ark.

For Backache—Take Devils Shoestring Root, as much as you can hold between the thumb and forefinger, and boil it into a tea. Drink this and inside of 36 hours it should do the work, for I have tried it and know it is good. Writes R. A. C., Seminary, Miss.

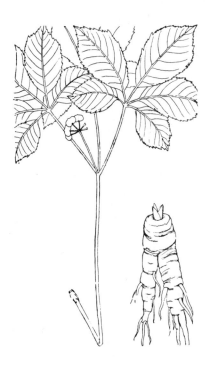

GINSENG
(Panax Quinquefolium.)

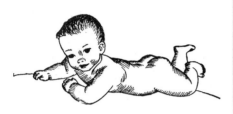

BEDWETTING OR INCONTINENCE OF THE URINE

(Also see Bladder Trouble.)

Often occurs in persons of advanced age and in childhood. It consists of frequent desire to pass water, and often an inability to retain it beyond a short period. It may arise from irritability of the organs, due to renal calculi (gravel stones) or to an acid condition of the urine and through a puncture with a catheter; the latter cases cannot be cured or relieved with medicine.

Treatment—Drink soothing Demulcent drinks with slight Astringent properties.

The Herb Doctor's choice of botanicals are: St. Johnswort, Water Plantain, Buchu, Kava Kava, Sumach Bark and Berries.

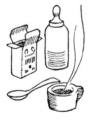

Bed Wetting Remedy—This is a scientific combination of absolutely harmless herbs that will quickly strengthen and purify the kidneys and bladder. It is invaluable for the cure of bed wetting, catarrh of the bladder, gravel and all urinary troubles.

To a quart of boiling water add a box of St. Johnswort, 4 tablespoonsful Water Plantain and 2 tablespoonsful Bearberry Leaves, boil down to one pint. When cold strain; add 1 or 2 cupsful of honey. Dose—Children, 1 teaspoonful on awakening in the morning and on retiring at night. Adults, 3 teaspoonfuls.

Here are my favorite recipes: **For** Bedwetting: Use a half teaspoonful of Pumpkin Seeds, dried, and if you want you can grind them in a food chopper. Pour one-half cupful boiling water over the half teaspoonful and let stand for 30 minutes. Then sweeten with honey or sugar. Take it before meals. In severe cases take it three times a day for three days, then once thereafter. This amount given is for small children, 4 years old or so, but the amount given can be judged according to the age of the child. Writes Mrs. W. B., Green Bay, Wis.

Have you ever heard of Pipsissewa? It is fine for Bedwetting and should be given a trial. Writes O. V. M., Duncannon, Pa.

For Bedwetting—Let the patient drink a tea of Sumach Berries, steeped in boiling water. These berries are sour but a sure cure. Writes H. B. A., Walled Lake, Mich.

—Venetian Herb Tea for
    Children ......
Bearberry Leaves
Cheese Plant
Corn Silk
Sassafras, bark of root
St. Johnswort
Horsetail Grass

Mild Diuretic and Astringent. Harmless to children. One of the main ingredients of this formula is St. Johnswort—considered an old household treatment for bedwetting.

Bed Wetting—Make a tea of Wintergreen Leaves. Use instead of water when thirsty. Writes Mrs. F. I. McI., Indiana, Pa.

—Venetian Herb Tea for
    the aged.......
Bearberry Leaves
St. Johnswort
Catnip Leaves and Flowers
Horsetail Grass
Cheese Plant
Angelica Root

Incontinence of Urine—High protein foods, meats, fish, poultry, eggs, old cheese should be avoided, also all condiments such as salt, pepper, mustard and vinegar, which are irritants to the kidneys. Fruits and fresh vegetables, with a few flaked nuts or cottage cheese will be the most suitable foods. Drink soothing demulcent drinks with slight astringent properties.

In the year of 1904 my mother had bladder trouble. She suffered pain. A woman doctor told her it was irritation of the neck of the bladder and for her to get Horsemint, the kind with the purplish bloom, gathering it while it was in bloom and drying it. Put a handful in a granite pan and pour boiling water over it. Let set until cool and drink two or three cupfuls a day, drinking a large mouthful or two at a time. She did this for two months every day and she has never been bothered with the terrible pains since. Writes Mrs. E. G., Pride, Texas.

Editor's Note—There are numerous variations of bladder troubles where Horsemint is of doubtful value, but it is harmless.

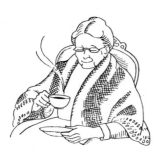

Flad Seed is good for Bladder. Use one level tablespoonful to a quart of water, steep and drink it cold one wineglassful every five hours.

Cleavers Herb is good for the Kidneys. One ounce to a pint of water, boil for a few minutes and drink a wineglassful every five hours. Writes Mrs. A. S., Pittsburg, Kan.

Now, I will tell you what Slippery Elm Bark did for me: Two weeks ago I was suffering from Bladder irritation. I happened to read in the Almanac about Slippery Elm Bark, so ordered some. When it came I drank a cupful of the tea at night and the next morning I was feeling some better, and in a few days my troubles were gone. Writes Mrs. D. V., Atlanta, Ga.

Editor's Note—Slippery Elm is a most soothing demulcent and emollient, but that's all.

I suffered from Bladder irritation and took Elder Flower Tea and it relieved me. Writes Mrs. V. L. H., Columbus, Ohio.

I sent for some Juniper Berries for my son for his kidney and bladder trouble. He had tried all kinds of medicines without doing him any good. The Juniper Berries helped him very much and I am now sending for another order of them. Writes Mrs. M. H. Burlington, Iowa.

I tried Pumpkin Seed Tea and after two weeks it passed something ½ in. x ¼ in., cone shaped and covered with small crystals and verp sharp points. The tea increased the flow of Urine and reduced the inflammation. Writes G. M. S., Mainville, Pa.

Yarrow is good for Bladder. Take a handful of the leaves and boil in one quart water, down to one pint, let cool and drink in place of water. It acted well for me. Writes J. F. M. J., Sylvatus, Va.

There is relief for Bladder irritation and this is it: Mix Peach Tree Leaves, Cornsilk and Marshmallow Root and use 1 teaspoonful to a cup of boiling water and let stand until cool. Drink this every day. I have used this recipe myself. Writes Mrs. H. M. C., Chariton, Iowa.

For bladder irritation: This has been known to relieve it. A tea made of the mixture of Flax Seed, Mayapple Root, and Horehound Leaves. Boil all together and drink the tea. This has helped many bladder irritations. Writes Mrs. S. A., Camp Point, Ill.

I am writing you regarding my case of bladder irritation for which I took your herb teas and for which the result seems to be perfect satisfaction and would certainly recommend the Wild Alum Root and Jezebel Root to anyone ailing with chronic systitis. Try it and be convinced. I drank the teas nearly eighteen months and for nearly three months now I have been in good health as far as the bladder is concerned. Writes L. H., Brooklyn, Iowa.

I am sending a recipe for Bladder irritation. Take one small package of Senna Leaves, one small can of Cream of Tartar, pour one quart of soft water over the Senna Leaves and simmer to one pint, strain and cool, add Cream of Tartar and a little sugar. Take a tablespoonful after meals and before going to bed. Writes Mrs. J. J. W., Oakhurst, Okla.

A tea made of Pumpkin Seed is very good to stimulate the Kidneys Writes S. C. M., Nortonville, Ky.

Here is a remedy for difficult urine. Take the leaves of the Gravel Weed and make a tea of it and drink it and it will give relief. Writes J. T. W., Monticello, Ark.

I am enclosing a sample of a little plant that grows in the hills and is used by the Indians for the Kidneys. They take a handful of this plant, the leaves, and make a tea and drink a half teacupful three or four times a day for the kidneys or where one has to get up frequently at night to urinate. This is a very good remedy. Writes L. S., Peoria, Okla.

Editor's Note—The sample was genuine Mouse Ear leaves.

I could not sleep nights and was up several times with kidney action, and when I did sleep, I had very bad dreams and I did not have an appetite, so I sent for the herbs for the aged and middle-aged, which are Butternut Bark, Marshmallow Root and Rocky Mountain Grape Root. I am 65 years old and by the time I took the tea for a week, I slept fine, didn't have to get up at night and I have a good appetite. Also I seldom have wild dreams. I think I will be all right by the time all these herbs are gone. Writes S. B., Luzerne, Iowa.

Have been telling people what wonderful results I have had by using your herbs. I had a temporary kidney difficulty which was cleared up by the following herbs: Yarrow, Burdock Root, Horsetail, Juniper Berries. I had also been taken with indigestion from time to time and this is also gone. No doubt, one of those herbs also did the work. Writes Miss E. R., Mauston, Wis.

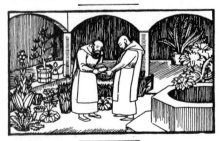

I have used the tea of fresh Prince's Pine and it is a great drink for encouraging the kidneys. Writes F. J. W., Stirling City, Calif.

As a stimulant diuretic, fifteen teaspoonfuls Juniper Berries, fifteen teaspoonfuls Watermelon seed, two teaspoonfuls Dandelion root, cut fine, three teaspoonfuls Hops and two teaspoonfuls Flaxseed. Put all together in three pints of water, boil down to one quart, strain. The dose is a waterglassful four times a day. Writes Mrs. A. L. S., South Bend, Ind.

For Stones in the Kidneys and Bladder—Take equal parts of any three or more of the following:

Horsetail Grass	Knotweed
Shepherds Purse	Agrimony
Rose Hips	Broom Tops
Bearberry Leaves	

Directions—Place 1 or 2 heaping teaspoonfuls of the herb mixture into a cup of boiling hot water, let it stand until cool, strain and drink 1 or 2 cupfuls a day—a large mouthful at a time.

In Retention of the Urine — Take equal parts of any four or five of the following:

Horsetail Grass	Shepherds Purse
Birch Leaves	Sage Leaves
Juniper Berries	Broom Tops
Am. Centaury	Yarrow

Directions—Place 1 or 2 heaping teaspoonfuls of the herb mixture into a cup of boiling hot water, let it stand until cool, strain and drink 1 or 2 cupfuls a day—a large mouthful at a time.

I have used your Black Walnut Leaves for Anemia with results and also Marshmallow Leaves for Bladder trouble for my little 2-year-old boy when two doctors couldn't help him and this tea gave grand results.—Mrs. L. R. S., New Philadelphia, Ohio.

Trailing Arbutus is a soothing diuretic for easing bladder irritation. Use one ounce to one pint of boiling water. Steep to make an infusion. The dose is one-fourth teaspoonful every three hours. Writes Mrs. N. T., Chetek, Wisconsin.

Princess Pine is a wonderful tea for stopping bedwetting. Writes Mrs. W. B. B., Many, La.

Take Sampson Snake Root, make a tea and drink it through the day, a large swallow at a time, also at bed time. This is a very good remedy for Flux. Writes G. T. H., Trenton, Tenn.

For bedwetting make a strong tea of Wintergreen Leaves and drink one cupful in the early part of the day. Continue until the trouble ceases. Writes Mrs. J. P., Hartford, Wis.

A tea made of Trailing Arbutus is really very valuable for soothing bladder irritation. Writes Mrs. D. C. D., Bluefield, W. Va.

For bladder take equal parts of Smartweed, Corn Silk, Peach Tree Leaves and make a tea. I used to get up as often as six times a night, but I don't any more. Writes W. T. C., Strong City, Kan.

One of our household remedies. Take the herb of Horsemint and make a tea and drink a cupful twice a day. It is very good for irritation of the Bladder. Writes M. E. C., Kansas City, Mo.

I used your Saw Palmetto Berries, Gentian Lutea, Star Root, mixed. It stopped irritation of the bladder. It is a very good tonic. I used your Viro Tonic, too, and know it is a great medicine for those who have nervous trouble. Writes E. A., Gatzke, Minn.

Last year I had irritation of the bladder and suffered with burning and straining. I read where Couch Grass was so good and bought some of this herb. Just a few doses of it and I was greatly relieved. Writes Mrs. E. L., Marlboro, New York.

Buchu leaves steeped are good to ease bladder irritation. Writes R. E. Y., Neon, Kentucky.

Relief for bed-wetting. My little grand-daughter wet the bed until she was seven years of age. Her mother tried most every kind of patent medicine without results. A friend advised Corn Silks, just a small handful of the Silks in a cup of boiling water, let cool and strain, and drink morning and at bed-time. One cup of this Corn-silk Tea relieved this child. Writes Mrs. R. M., Aberdeen, S. D.

Editor's Note—Every farmer should get acquainted with these simple household remedies.

For irritation of the bladder get a package of Water Pepper. Put one-half of it into a pint of water and steep like tea. Drink half of this tea while it is hot and in one hour drink the other half and your irritation will often be better. Writes Mrs. L. W., Cedar Rapids, Ia.

Buchu leaves is one of the best known remedies to soothe the irritation of the urinary organs. Best results are obtained from the infusion made from an ounce of the leaves in two pints of boiling water. Two or three soup-spoonfuls, four or five times daily. Writes M. L. K., Fayetteville, N. Car.

Trailing Arbutus is a soothing diuretic for easing bladder irritation. Use one ounce to one pint of boiling water. Steep to make an infusion. The dose is one-fourth teaspoonful every three hours. Writes Mrs. N. T., Chetek, Wisconsin.

I don't think your Prince's Pine can be beat for bedwetting. I have never known it to fail when given a fair trial.

I have used your Black Walnut Leaves for Anemia with results and also Marshmallow Leaves for Bladder trouble for my little 2-year-old boy when two doctors couldn't help him and this tea gave grand results.—Mrs. L. R. S., New Philadelphia, Ohio.

Trailing Arbutus is a soothing diuretic for easing bladder irritation. Use one ounce to one pint of boiling water. Steep to make an infusion. The dose is one-fourth teaspoonful every three hours. Writes Mrs. N. T., Chetek, Wisconsin.

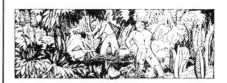

I sent for some Juniper Berries for my son for his kidney and bladder trouble. He had tried all kinds of medicines without doing him any good. The Juniper Berries helped him very much and I am now sending for another order of them. Writes Mrs. M. H., Burlington, Iowa.

I tried Pumpkin Seed Tea and after two weeks it passed something ½ in. x ¼ in., cone shaped and covered with small crystals and verp sharp points. The tea increased the flow of Urine and reduced the inflammation. Writes G. M. S., Mainville, Pa.

BLADDER TROUBLE

(Also see Kidney Troubles.)

Inflammation of the Bladder—The symptoms are pain in the region of the bladder with severe burning and irritation, difficulty or inability of passing water, and almost constant desire to urinate.

Treatment—Take 1 or 2 Annistan Tablets if necessary, to relieve the pain. Hot water bag applied to the region of pain is often beneficial. Take a soothing and cooling Demulcent botanic tea, and consult a specialist.

The Herb Doctor's choice of botanical Demulcents are: Cubeb Berries, Marshmallow Root, Cheese Plant, Dog Grass, Corn Silk.

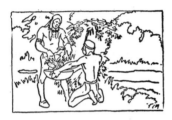

—U. U. Tea......
Palmetto Berries
Bearberry Leaves
Licorice
Cubeb Berries
Juniper Berries
Althea Root
Sweet Fern
Pipsissewa
Fennel Seed
Bluets

The experienced herbal physician will recognize this as a very valuable formula. It is a mild diuretic and tonic with emolient and soothing properties to the urinary passages.

—Wild Swamp Root Compound
....
Swamp Lily Root
Marshmallow Root
Bearberry Leaves
Cheese Plant
Sassafras, bark of root
Buchu Leaves
Horsetail Grass
Bluets
Corn Silk

Mild, soothing Demulcent and Diuretic, very pleasant to taste and of many uses.

Inflammation of the Bladder—Take a handful of dry Hops. Pour a quart of boiling water over them. Allow the tea to cool, and drink a glassful three times a day. You can sweeten to taste. Writes Mrs. G. B. S., Preston, Neb.

Editor's Note—I believe Marshmallow Root is still better.

Horse Radish Root is fine for Weak Back, Bladder and Kidney Troubles. Writes Mrs. P. H., Chase City, Va.

In the year of 1925 I suffered nervous breakdown caused from a 30-year hard strain. I had painful scalding urine; God himself knows what I suffered. I had pills from drug stores, also medicine from the doctor, none helped. My case continued. In one of your Almanacs it states that this painful, scalding urine is caused by over-worked, inflamed glands of the bladder. I sent to you for 1 package of Bearberry, 1 package of Goose Grass. I made a tea of this that helped me. What joy now! I use the tea off and on; my health is improved since using your herbs. Writes Mrs. F. F., Tama, Iowa.

BITES

There was a girl bitten by a mad dog and nearly a year elapsed before the poison became active. When the fits came on, it required two stout men to overpower her. A stranger finally advised a treatment for her of Poke Root powdered. When he saw a Fit was coming on, he gave the first dose and it was lighter than those preceding it. He continued the treatment and cured the girl. The dose of the Poke Root Powdered was what you could lay on the round point of a table knife. Writes L. J. F., Chillicothe, Ohio.

Editor's Note—Here is a remedy that is not to be sneezed at, if you know what I mean.

Rattlesnake Bite—Henry Steward, a farmer of Springfield, Neb., in a letter to the "Great Divide," published in Denver, Colo., says that he was bitten by a big Rattlesnake last August and that Wet Salt counteracted the poison —this is well worth knowing. He said, "I was about 60 rods from the house and my finger was swollen to about once its natural size and my arm felt like there were a thousand bumblebees stinging it. We wrapped it up with Wet Salt and put some in the bites. My finger was stiff for two months. After I put salt on it, the hurting stopped and in 20 minutes I went back to work." Writes E. E., Jacksonville, Ill.

Place wet mud where you have been stung by bee or wasp and it will take out the pain. Writes Mrs. H. E. T.

Remedy for Snake Bite is to use Saltpeter, just wet with a little water and apply to the bite. Writes Mr. W. J. O., Forest Hill, La.

My grandfather was an Herb Doctor. He says: Lobelia is a very valuable herb in case of Snake Bites. Writes Mrs. J. R. L., Vinemont, Ala.

I will send you a remedy for Snake Bite. Bind common Soda on the bite and pour on Cider Vinegar. It will draw the poison. Writes W. F. L., Garnett, Kan.

Carry Rattle Snake Master in your pocket and a snake won't bite you. Writes D. K., Pochahontas, Tenn.

Editor's Note—Well, I'll be ——.

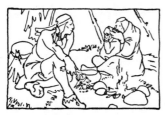

Whoever is bitten by a snake or mad dog and immediately takes Sweet Oil and washes the wound with it and then puts a rag three or four times doubled up and well soaked with the oil on the wound every three or four hours and drinks a couple of spoonfuls of the oil every four hours for a few days will surely find out what peculiar virtues the Sweet Oil possesses in poisons. Writes F. E. K., Bunker Hill, Kan.

Editor's Note—But in the meantime call a doctor. You cannot take a chance on a mad dog or snake bite.

Snake Bites—Take a handful of Wild Touch-Me-Not, and make into a poultice, then apply on bite. Then also make a tea by steeping a handful into a pint of boiling water, and drink as hot as you can. Writes J. T. F., Alexander City, Ala.

Wasp or Bee Stings—Take Epsom Salts, heap up on place where you have been stung, then put a bandage around to hold salts at proper place. Use water to dampen this, and it is excellent for stings. Keep dampened until relieved. Writes Mrs. B. E. C., Friendsville, Tenn.

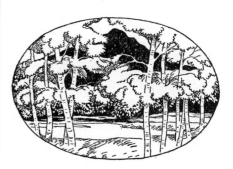

A recipe that is good for Snake Bites, and almost any kind of swelling. Make a poultice of Wild Violets. I have tried this as well as many others, and it has cured. Make into stiff poultice and bandage to the surface. Writes Theo. R. B., Lacour, La.

Here is a recipe for Santa Fe Stings, which I did not see in your Almanac. Take a quart of sweet milk and 2 handfuls of Cockleburrs, green if possible, make into poultice, and place in granite vessel. Pour milk over them, stir well to extract the virtues, then it is ready to apply. Put this lotion on 6 times the first day, and 4 times the rest until cured. This is tried and true. Writes R. F. F., Choctaw, Okla.

Hydrophobia and Snake Bites—Preventive and Cure—Take the bark of the White Ash, commonly called Black Ash, peel off the bark, boil it to a strong decoction and of this drink freely, one gill three times a day for 8 or 10 days.

Two boys and a sheep were bitten by a mad dog. While this remedy was being prepared, the sheep began to be so afflicted with hydrophobia it was unable to stand. It was drenched with a pint of the Ash Root ooze. A few hours after drench had been given, the animal got up and began grazing with the flock. The two boys were given the remedy and no effects of the poison were ever discovered. Writes J. S. B., Pittsburgh, Pa.

I am sending you a recipe for Snake Bite. Take one onion, a teaspoonful of salt, one of Turpentine, cut the onion up very fine, mix with salt and turpentine, and apply to the wound. Writes W. D., Meadow View, Va.

Bee Stings—Rub Onion on the sting. This will stop it instantly. I have tried it numbers of times and it works. Writes G. B., Palisade, Colo.

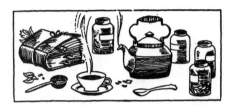

BLOOD PURIFIERS

The botanicals listed are mostly of a mild alterative nature. Here again proper diet, fresh air and sunlight build up resistance to disease, and medicine and drugs, except for local application, are quite useless.

The skin is an index to health. It is like a barometer, indicating the state of our body and certain organs. It demands scrupulous cleanliness. The pores should be kept open. There is no better tonic for the whole system than bathing in cold water followed by a vigorous rubbing.

It is common practise to treat eruptions of the skin by means of external applications, but eruptions rarely form upon the surface of the skin unless there is something wrong with the system. Therefore, there is the necessity of treating all such eruptions with internal remedies in addition to the external applications.

Blood Purifier—Use a tablespoonful of Saffron Flowers to a cupful of boiling water, let steep a few minutes, strain, use an earthen bowl when steeping. Sweeten to taste, and give a few teaspoonfuls several times during the day. Writes E. L., Fairmount, Minn.

Here is what is known as the Famous Blood Remedy:
1 pound Sarsaparilla
2 ounces Quassia Chips
2 ounces Senna Leaves
2 ounces Licorice Root
3 ounces Yellow Dock

Boil all the mixture in a gallon of water, over slow fire for six hours. Strain, and lastly add one-half teaspoonful Oil Wintergreen and two pounds of sugar. Dose—One dessert spoonful before meals. Used in Dropsy, Rheumatism, or any form of Blood Disease. Must be kept cool. Writes A. D. D., Sedalia, Mo.

For a spring tonic and blood purifier and cleaner, make a tea of Sassafras, and if you desire you can break in a little Red Elder. Drink like coffee or tea. Writes O. C. C., Marietta, Ga.

Mormon Valley Herbs Compound— This is a scientific compound of Indian and modern botanicals. It is a scientific blend of herb simples that we offer with the greatest confidence for its powerful astringent and mild tonic properties.

The main ingredients of this remarkable preparation is a plant known and highly prized among one tribe of Indians as ''The herb of the Sun'' and Skookum Plant by another tribe. In Utah, it is called Mormon Plant. It grows in the valleys of Utah and as far south as Mexico. It is one of the main ingredients of several widely advertised remedies and tonics.

This preparation has proved of such value that we can sincerely recommend it. When a certain preparation is widely advertised, it is usually over-rated; however, this particular formula surely is worthy of attention for ailments in which these agents are indicated. It has the further advantage of being absolutely harmless.

Besides the M rmon Plant, this formula has other ingredients of proven quality, making it one of the very best preparations we have. It may be used externally as a cleanser for old and running sores as well as internally.

—Mormon Valley Herb
    Compound......
    Mormon Valley Plant
    Black Cohosh
    Licorice
    Gentian
    Fennel Seed
    Bluets
    Wild Cherry Bark

A powerful Astringent with tonic properties, a tea of hundreds of uses. May be used internally or externally as a wash for sores and ulcers. A book could be written on the varied usefulness of this remarkable compound. Look up the various ingredients in any good book on medicinal botany.

I would like to contribute what I know to' be a fine Blood Remedy. Steep equal parts of Burdock, Wild Cherry Bark, and Red Sassafras in boiling water and drink a swallow three or four times a day. Writes W. B., Rupert, W. Va.

Here is a herb recipe which is a blood purifier. Single handful of each. Pleurisy Root, Queens Delight, Sarsaparilla, bring to boil in a quart of water. Dose, a wineglassful 3 times a day. Writes T. H. Jewett, Texas.

A medicine that father always used in cases of Bad Blood, has been tested and never failed: Bitter Sweet Root, Elder Bark, Cypress Leaves, and Sarsaparilla, a pint of each, put all together in 2 gallons of water, boil down to 1 gallon, strain, add a preservative and it is ready. Writes R. D. J., Wann, Okla.

Editor's Note—Alcohol is the best preservative. Seven pounds of Granulated Cane Sugar to each gallon of liquid will make a thick syrup that will keep if kept moderately cool.

Blood Purifier—A good blood purifier:
2 ounces Sarsaparilla
2 ounces Yellow Dock
2 ounces Bitter Dock
2 ounces Stillinga
Take a teaspoonful one-half hour before each meal, increase to a tablespoonful. If too strong add water. Writes Mrs. G. W. S., West Monterey, Pa.

Blood and Pimples—For blood or pimples, or breaking out of any kind: Strawberry Leaves, gathered fresh and boiled, strained through a flannel cloth to gather the hairs on leaves and drink a glass of tea three times a day, after meals. Writes Mrs. G. B., Bellevue, Idaho.

For Blood Poisoning—Pulverize Slippery Elm Bark and Sassafras Bark. Mix in equal parts. This is to be put into a pan with enough water to be absorbed. Put into a gauze bag and apply to the affected area. It is the finest remedy I know of for blood poisoning from spiders, insects, snake bites and injuries. Writes Dr. F. W. C., Newark, N. J.

Here is a home remedy which is fine for the blood:
3 teaspoonsful Cream of Tartar
3 teaspoonsful Sugar
3 teaspoonsful Sulphur
Mix these and take 1 teaspoonful for adults at bedtime for nine nights. Children according to age. Writes K. H., Carmine, Tex.

I am sending two remedies which have been used in our family for years: Take 2 big handfuls of Rattleweed, put in a stone jar and cover with a quart of boiling water and let cool. Drink a big swallow 3 times a day. This is a good Blood Purifier.

A tea made from the bark of Sassafras and drunk instead of water is good for Thinning the Blood.

Blood Purifier—Drink a tea made from Red Willow Bark. Writes I. H., Jackson, Mich.

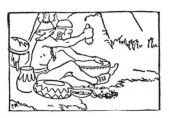

Blood Purifier—Four parts Sassafras Bark, 3 Sweet Weed, 2 Hops, Anise Seed and Am. Sarsaparilla and 1 of Buckthorn Bark. Mix well, put 2 tablespoonfuls in a quart of boiling water, let stand until cool; drink a wineglassful 4 times daily. Dr. L. E., New Lexington, Ohio.

Blood Purifier—Find a Red Sycamore tree, chop off about two gallons of chips. Put in boiler with 2 gallons of water and boil down to 1 gallon. Sweeten with any syrup or sugar, to improve taste. Drink 3 times daily, 1 cupful before meals. A blood purifier that will destroy germs in the blood, causing old stubborn sores to heal quickly. Writes A. E., Rockford, Ind.

Sassafras Tea in the Spring makes the sluggish blood thin. L. A. G., Michigan City, Ind.

Tea from Wild Grape Root is good blood purifier. Writes Mrs. J. S., Arcadia, Ind.

—Yellow Dock Clover
    Compound .....
Yellow Dock Root
Red Clover Flowers
Stillingia Root
Poke Root
Prickly Ash Bark
Rocky Mt. Grape Root
Elder Flowers
Marshmallow Root
German Cheese Plant
Tinn. Senna Leaves
Sassafras, bark of root
Am. Sarsaparilla Root

A Mild Alterative. A scientific blend of 12 different botanicals in which Yellow Dock predominates. A very fine tea. All patent so-called ''Blood Purifiers'' are composed of one or more of these various botanicals. Yellow Dock is one of the botanicals richest in organic iron.

I am sending you an herb and fruit remedy for the blood, a purifier, that I have been using for many years with good results. A pound of figs, 2 lbs. prunes, 1 lb. of raisins, 1 stalk celery, ¼ lb. water cress, 1 oz. of Wintergreen Herb, 1 oz. of Birch Bark, boiled in 1 gallon of water for 2 hours over a slow fire, then when cold add the juice of 6 lemons and a pint of honey. Dose, a wineglassful 3 times a day. Writes E. H. D. N. D., Davenport, Iowa.
Editor's Note—Looks reasonable.

Quack Grass Roots and Violet Roots have been used as a Blood Purifier in my mother's family for over one hundred years. Mrs. O. C., Cadillac, Mich.

Blood Tonic—Take the Spicewood Bush, break up the limbs in short pieces, about 3 inches long. Put about 3 handfuls in a boiler. Pour on about 1 gallon of boiling water and let set about 1 hour on back of the stove. Sweeten and drink about 3 or 4 cups daily for about 1 week. This makes a light pink tea. Writes A. E., Rockford, Ind.

I am using Mormon Valley Herbs and they are good for the Blood. They helped me out in great shape. I had the cramps in hands and feet so bad I could not work and now they are gone, and I am only on my second box. Writes F. J. M., Juliaetta, Idaho.

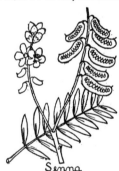

Senna

—Clover Blue Flag
   Compound ....
Red Clover Flowers
Blue Flag Root
Juniper Berries
Rocky Mountain Grape
Tinn. Senna Leaves
Alex. Senna Leaves
German Cheese Plant
Blue Gentian
Lesser Periwinkle Leaves
Mild Alterative and only slightly laxative. A fine tea.

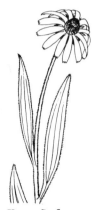

Kansas Sunflower

—Kansas Sunflower
   Compound.....
Kansas Sunflower
Prickly Ash Bark
Poke Root
Bluets
Rocky Mt. Grape Root
Marshmallow

Mild Alterative. Most of the highly touted and advertised blood tonics and blood purifiers are composed mainly of one or more of these simple ingredients.

Bleeders' Disease—There is always a deficiency of calcium or lime in the diet when there is a tendency to hemorrhage. The foods which are richest in calcium are nettles, water cress, dill cabbage, lettuce, dandelions, spinach, Swiss chard, chives, radishes, cottage cheese, turnips, whey, milk, lemons, onions, and leeks. Squeeze out the fresh juices of any of the above and drink suitable quantities whenever desirable in addition to regular meals.

BOILS

Boils are too common to require a description.

Treatment—Cover the boil with a piece of gauze.   After pus or matter has formed the boil should be opened with a needle that has been passed through a flame and carefully wiped. The pus can be very gently pressed out and a fresh dressing of Feronia Ointment applied.

The Herb Doctor's choice of mild botanical Alteratives and Tonics are: Inner bark of Birch, Yellow Dock, Seven Barks, Queen's Delight, Prickly Ash Bark, Strawberry Leaves, Red Raspberry Leaves, Blue Flag, Rocky Mountain Grape Root, Elder Berries, Elder Flowers, Chickweed, Tetterwort and Violet Leaves.

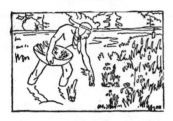

Boils—I have used this myself, and I know it is good for boils and sores:

1 cupful Yellow Poplar Bark
1 cupful Sumach Berries
½ cupful Senna Leaves

Put all in ½ gallon cold water. Let stand 5 or 6 hours, and strain. Take a half cup of the tea 3 times a day for 8 or 10 days. Writes T. L. F., Paris, Miss.

Abscesses or Gumboils—Make small poultices of equal parts of ground mustard and flour and mix into a paste with Glycerine. Put in small sterilized bag or cloth and apply over the diseased part within the mouth, and on the outside you can administer cold applications, but never hot or it will draw the abscess or boil to the outside of the cheek and leave an unsightly scar. Change the poultice every 15 to 20 minutes, and then when it breaks use a good mouth wash. Writes Mrs. A. A., Charleroi, Pa.

Boils—One should avoid high protein foods, meat, fish, poultry, etc., and feed largely on fresh fruits, fresh green vegetables and a moderate supply of nuts or cottage cheese.

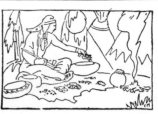

Boils—I am sending a recipe for Carbuncles: Take Wahoo Bark and put in water and when it gets slimy, put bark and all in a cloth and bind it to them, and you will not even feel it draw it out, and it will burst them. Writes Mrs. J. W. Chattahoochee, Ga.

Here is a remedy that has been used in our family for years for Boils and Nail Wounds or any Inflammation. Take Catnip, boil in water until the water turns green, leave the leaves in, then thicken with corn meal or wheat bran, cook into a poultice and apply as hot as a person can stand and it will draw and give relief where most anything else fails. Writes Mrs. R. S.,

Boils—First swab with warm water to soften the skin, then apply Eucamint thickly over the boils, covering them with a soft white cloth. Repeat application every two hours. Do not rub.

Boils and Pimples—Take a whole nutmeg and grate until you have a third of a teaspoonful, add a little sugar (possibly the same amount, or to taste), pour on ½ cup of boiling water, and keep covered until cool enough to drink. Take this three mornings in succession, omit three mornings. Do this, until you have taken it nine times. Writes Mrs. M. D. R., Edmonds, Wash.

Boils and Pimples—I am an old trapper and have received the following formula from an old Indian. It has cured me of boils. I used to be afflicted with these boils every year. At times I would have from 1 to 14 at a time. Take the inner bark of Birch, about a teacupful of the bark to a quart of water. Boil a few minutes and drink in place of water. Writes J. F. M., Sharboquo, Ont., Canada.

For Boils, Felons, or Abscesses—Get a large handful of Ironwood and boil in 1½ pints of water down to 1 pint, let cool, strain and thicken the ooze with meal. It is the best I know. Writes E. T., Peel, Ark.

I am sending you a remedy that cured me of Boils. I had six or seven of them at one time, and doctors failed to do me any good. Take equal parts of:

Wild Cherry Bark
Burdock Root
Poplar Bark
Sassafras Bark

Boil all together until strength is taken from it, then strain, add sugar to the juice and boil to make a thick syrup. Take a tablespoonful three times a day or more if it does not move the bowels too freely. I have not had a boil since taking this remedy and that was ten years ago. Writes Mrs. M. R. P., Jefferson, Ohio.

Fuller's Earth is good for Boils. Make a salve of Leaf Lard and Fuller's Earth and mix well. When the boils open dust the Earth dry on it to heal. Very good also for animals. A $2,000 horse was saved by this. The hoof was rotting and Fuller's Earth Salve helped him. Writes Mrs. S. C., Maywood, Calif.

For a Felon and Boils take a piece of Gum Camphor the size of a large hickory nut and dissolve in a good ounce of Turpentine and bind a cloth on the Felon or Boil and keep the cloth wet all the time with Turpentine and Camphor. Writes Mrs. H. M., Nebraska, Pa.

When a young man, my father had Boils continually. He got several handfuls of Burdock Roots and boiled down to a syrup and took four tablespoonfuls a day. The boils soon disappeared and he never had another. Writes B. E. W., Evansville, Ark.

Take Plantain Leaves and boil for about half a minute, put the leaves on a boil, cover with cloth at night. This will draw out the inflammation from the boil. Writes T. J. B., Lublin, Wis.

A good poultice for Boils and Carbuncles: Mix equal parts of Slippery Elm and Liquid Honey to a consistency of cream, and apply with cotton wool. Writes W. E. R., Melbourne, Australia.

Since your Burdock Root helped my husband relieve his system of boils so easily and quickly, we both feel that we have made a discovery—herbs certainly are the best kind of medicine and we intend to try some more! Writes Mrs. J. L. J., Sulphur Springs, Tampa, Fla.

Take Yarrow Leaves and boil them with Wheat Bran and make poultices for boils. It sure will bring them to a head. Writes C. C., Almira, Va.

I was bothered with boils until several years ago when an old man told me this recipe. Take equal parts of Wild Cherry bark, Burdock Root, Poplar bark and Sassafras bark, boil in water until you have the strength of the roots; strain and add sugar to make a thick syrup. The dose is one tablespoonful three times a day or more if it doesn't make the bowels move too much. I have not had a boil since trying this and this same recipe has helped others. Writes H. J., Coulterville, Ill.

Make a tea of White Oak bark and thicken with meal for boils. Writes D. E. M., Garnett, Kan.

As a poultice for application to boils use ground flaxseed. Put about a tablespoonful in a dish, wet with a little hot water to make a paste and apply to the sore over night. This is very good. Writes Mrs. N. L. A., Sheldon, Wisconsin.

Take a small handful of the roots of Indian Physic and put in a cup, pour boiling water on them in the morning and let it stand. Drink before retiring at night. I drank some 30 years ago and I have not had a Boil since.

Editor's Note—Old Tamarack says the inner bark of Sweet Birch is even better.

For Boils and Sores—Boil Sassafras Root and make a tea about the color of coffee or as strong as you like. Sweeten and drink 2 cupfuls a day for about a week. Children like it too. Writes A. C. W., Meigs, Ga.

Garden Sage and Cornmeal made into a poultice is good for Boils.

Golden Seal made into a tea is good for the Flux. One tablespoonful every two hours until relieved.

Alder Bark Tea is a good laxative for infants. Scrape the bark down, give warm and sweetened. Writes Mrs. M. E., Monticello, Ky.

Editor's Note—Please don't—Prune juice is so much better tasting.

Use Mullein as a wash or a poultice after a boil has discharged. Writes N. N. G., Ludlow, Wash.

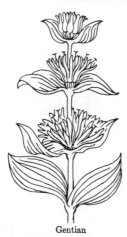

Gentian

Anyone afflicted with Boils can get relief by making a tea of Gentian Root, and drinking a cupful morning and evening. Try this two or three times a year; a week's treatment and you will not be bothered with boils or infections, as it is a great blood purifier, too. Writes A. W. B., Indianapolis, Ind.

The center stems of Plantain that have the seed on are good to cure Boils and Bad Blood. Make a strong tea and drink. Writes Mrs. J. W., Green Forest, Ark.

Editor's Note—Cannot do any harm—if not effective.

I know that Burdock Tea will stop Boils, almost at once. Make a medium strong tea and take a cupful a day. To any one that has tried other things, medicines, etc., without success, just try this one. Writes Mrs. A. T. Y., Sheridan, Ore.

For Blood Poison, Boils and All Kinds of Swellings—Take the bark of Slippery Elm and make a poultice. Apply to the affected parts and it will give relief. Writes R. G., Timbo, Ark.

Here Is a True Remedy for Boils— Take the bark of Tag Alder and make a tea of same. Drink 2 cups a day. This cured my father of boils when other remedies failed. Writes M. H., Hillsboro, N. C.

Peach Tree Leaves poultice is good for Felons, Boils, or other risings. Writes Mrs. E. C. G., Inka, Ill.

For Boils—Take Sycamore Bark and make a tea. Drink instead of water. This is a sure cure. Writes Mr. K. M., Arcanum, Ohio.

For Boils—Take Powdered Slippery Elm Bark and mix with lard. Make this to a paste. Cover the boil. When this becomes dry apply a new one until the boil is completely drawn out. Writes Mrs. O. L. S., Greensburg, Ind.

A friend of mine used Burdock Root to cure a Boil and he said it helped him. He boiled the root and soaked the cloth in it and put on the affected part. Writes C. B., Waverly, Iowa.

For Boils—Cut the Burdock Roots and fill a quart can, then pour on boiling water. Take ½ glass 3 or 4 times a day. It will purify the blood and check the recurrence of boils. Writes M. C., East Columbus, Ohio.

Abscess—Take ground fine Leptrandra Roots, boil down and make poultice. It can't be beat. Apply hot as can be borne to the skin. Writes N. H. E., Alum Rock, Pa.

Boils—I am sending you a recipe for boils, which I have used myself, and know several others that have used it also, and it cured them as well as myself. Take Elder Bark, pour boiling water over it, let steep on back of stove for hour, and drink the cupful during the day. Writes Mrs. J. P. C., Adel, Iowa.

For Boils—Take a piece of rosin, and one-third as much lard, melt together. Put this plaster on boils and it will take out the core. Writes Mrs. D. E. J., Smethport, Pa.

I can give you a remedy for Boils that cured my husband after suffering for several years. Take a teaspoonful of Cream of Tartar and Sulphur, and mix, and use a teaspoonful of the mixture, and eat dry. Writes Mrs. T. D., Moulton, Iowa.

Am sending you a recipe for Boils, Pimples. Take a handful of Balm of Gilead Buds, and half a pint of hog's lard, 1 teaspoonful Sulphur, also 1 of Spirits of Turpentine, fry them all together and apply upon going to bed. Writes M. B., Gilmore, Ky.

Boils—A sure cure for Boils or Carbuncles: Take the Bark of Sycamore and boil in half gallon of water for 2 hours; drink as a tea. Writes A. C., Metz, Ind.

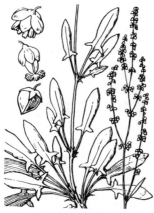

Sheep Sorrel

Salve for Boils, Etc.—Take a small handful of Sheep Sorrel, steep in a half cupful of fresh lard, then strain and cool. It makes a fine salve for boils, cancers or abscesses. Writes Mrs. J. H. M., Toledo, Ore.

Editor's Note—I am sure this will not affect a real cancer.

I myself have used this with good effect, for a boil on my wrist that became very painful and large without suppurating. Bandaging with a saturate solution of Epsom Salts in vinegar, reduced the swelling and relieved the inflammation, and the boil did not suppurate. The poison therefore must have been reabsorbed by the blood and let out of the system in a more orderly route. The bandage must be kept moist, otherwise it becomes dry and crusty. Writes P. W. G., Adamsville, R. I.

For Carbuncles and Boils—Equal parts of Mutton Tallow or Vegetable Oil Soap, shaved fine, Castor Oil, Camphor Gum, and Beeswax. Melt all together to form a salve that draws and heals. Apply by spreading on clean white cloth. Poppy Seed can be added to this mixture, too.

I had an awful Boil on the calf of my leg and it was awful stubborn, and everything I did was no good. My husband went to the woods, gathered some Slippery Elm Bark, which we dried and soaked in warm water, putting it on a cloth and applied it and within two days the boil was gone. Writes Mrs. D. K.

For Boils—Take 3 whole Nutmegs, chew good, a little bite every hour until the three are used up. This helped my husband who had boils for three years. Writes Mrs. G. W., Ann Arbor, Mich.

Take Peach Tree Leaves, break or chop up fine, boil in water, thicken with flour, and a few drops of Turpentine, make a poultice, and put on the boil when warm. Writes D. D., Humphrey, Ky.

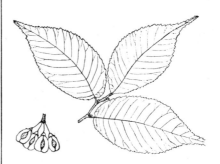

SLIPPERY ELM

For Boils—Take just enough Slippery Elm to cover a boil and pour enough boiling water over it to make a paste. Then put on a cloth and place it on the boil. This will draw it to a head. Writes Mrs. K. R. M., Chelan, Wash.

For Boils—Take 3 whole Nutmegs, chew good, a little bite every hour until the three are used up. This helped my husband who had boils for three years. Writes Mrs. G. W., Ann Arbor, Mich.

Eczema—Eczema and other skin diseases are evidence that the regular eliminatory channels have not been clearing out toxins as fast as they accumulate, and too much of high protein foods. A fruit, nut and fresh vegetable diet is recommended, especially green vegetable salads.

BRIGHT'S DISEASE

The symptoms sometimes are so obscure as to escape attention until an incurable condition is presented. Usually there is pain in the back, too frequent, thick, muddy, or clear frothy urine; general weakness; drowsiness and debility, or continual headache, dizziness and rheumatic pains in the back of limbs, all pointing to defective action of the kidneys. If this disease has become well established or chronic it is considered incurable, but if the symptoms are recognized early it will respond to treatment.

Treatment—Consult a doctor. Herb Doctor's choice of botanical Demulcents and Diuretics are: Horsetail Grass, Marshmallow Root, Cheese Plant, Bearberry Leaves, Sassafras, Globe Flower Bark or Root, Huckleberry Leaves Bugle Weed.

Editor's Note—Diabetes and Bright's Disease are very serious ailments that require very careful and individual treatment. It is of the greatest importance to consult a specialist and especially a dietitian as soon as possible.

Bright's Disease—Take two ounces of Thimble Weed, Button Snake Root and Sweet Bugle. Mix thoroughly and steep a tablespoonful into a cupful of boiling water. Drink this at least three times during the day and I am sure a great improvement will be apparent. Writes Mrs. G. R., Oak Harbor, Ohio.

Bright's Disease—Follow same treatment as Diabetes. In place of water drink a tea made by steeping one teaspoonful German Cheese Plant in a cup of boiling water for half hour, add one-half teaspoonful Rochelle Salts. Drink at least three cupfuls a day. Take sweat baths.

For Bright's Disease or Bladder Trouble—Take one ounce each of Couch Grass, Blue Cohosh, and Juniper Berries and Buchu Leaves and mix them well. Take one pinch of the mixture and pour half a pint of boiling water. Steep and drink during the day. This is a doctor's prescription. Writes Mrs. C. N. B., Randsburg, Calif.

Here is a recipe that I hope may aid some suffering soul. Take a teaspoonful of Ginger and pour boiling water on it, and cover, let it steep and strain later.

I had a brother that had Bright's Disease and Dropsy. I got Queen of the Meadow Roots and made a strong tea of it and it cured him after three doctors said he would be in his grave. Writes O. W. L., French Creek, W. Va.

Editor's Note—We have not yet discovered all of the remarkable properties of this root. It should be used more.

Fresh air, quietude of mind and outdoor exercise are beneficial. Chilling must be avoided. Tea, coffee, alcoholic drinks, cheese and fats must be prohibited. Frequent warm baths are useful and perspiration can be induced by infusion of Asclepias tuberosa. Marshmallow root and peach leaves are soothing and promote the flow of urine. All irritating and highly stimulating agents must be avoided.

For Bright's Disease—Mix together one box each of Jamaica Sarsaparilla and Corn Silk and a half box of Cleavers and four teaspoonfuls of Spearmint. Steep a teaspoonful of the mixture in a cup of boiling water until cool. Drink one or two cupfuls during the day. Writes A. P.

My son has Bright's Disease, so the doctors say, and their medicine didn't seem to help him. A friend told me of your herbs and I sent for a dollar package of your Bugleweed Compound.

He has gained five pounds since taking it. Writes Mrs. H. W., Muskegon, Mich.

Bright's Disease—All high protein foods should be avoided—meats, fish, poultry, eggs, cheese, dried peas and beans, lentils. All condiments, especially salt, pepper, mustard, vinegar should be abstained from. Patient should be put on an absolutely salt-free diet. Fresh fruits and fresh green vegetables are always to be recommended.

BRONCHIAL TROUBLES

(Also see Lung Troubles.)

In affections of the pulmonary organs, diet, sunlight, and proper nursing can do more than medicine. Local remedies are often useful. The botanical demulcents, diaphoretics and refrigerants and expectorants listed here can merely aid Nature and do not constitute a panacea.

Bronchitis—Is an inflammation of the mucous membrane lining the air passages of the throat and chest, shown by hoarseness, cough, fever and soreness in the chest.

The Herb Doctor's choice of mild expectorants are: Mullein, Coughwort, Horehound, Sundew, Yarrow, Linden Flowers, Honey, Marshmallow, Figwort and Flax Seed.

Cough Syrup—Take equal parts of Wild Cherry Bark, Mullein Leaves, Horehound, and boil all together to make tea and strain, then add Sugar or Honey to make the syrup. Writes Mrs. J. S. B., Whitwell, Tenn.

Bronchial Troubles—Here is a recipe that I have not found in your book. It has cured my wife of bronchial troubles that she has had for years, in the winter time she could hardly sleep at night for coughing. An old Negro woman gave the remedy and it has cured her and others. Take two large handfuls of Mullein Leaves, steep in one quart of water down to a pint, and add a cup of honey. Writes F. A. M., Marked Tree, Ark.

To a pint of Flax Seed tea, add the juice of two lemons, add 3 tablespoonsful sugar. Take a teaspoonful every half hour until relieved. This is very good for Bronchitis. Writes Mrs. E. C. S., Billings, Okla.

Here is a remedy for Bronchitis or Bronchial or in fact other Coughs, my mother used and it helped me when I was very sick with Bronchitis: Take a cupful of Flax Seed, boil in a quart of water, add 3 lemons and add either ½ cup of honey or a box of Rock Candy, and it will surely loosen the cough. Take by tablespoon as often as you like. The Flax Seed, of course, is strained out when boiled, and then the juice of the lemons added. Writes Mrs. W. S. B., Browns Valley, Minn.

Red Clover Blossoms are good for Bronchitis, all kinds of colds, is a good blood purifier and is excellent for asthma, flu or grippe.

1 cup dried Red Clover Blossoms
2 level tablespoons Ground Flaxseed
1 pint boiling water

Mix these ingredients and steep for an hour, strain, add sugar and the juice of a lemon. Be careful not to boil this mixture for that will kill its healing quality. Drink hot, and best when taken at bed time. Writes Mrs. H. D., Aitkin, Minn.

I had an Inflammation of the Bronchial Tube very bad and the phlegm nearly choked me to death. A young man who knows these herbs came to my house and said to me: "If I only knew where there was some Mullein, I could help." I didn't know where to get it, and he left, but he came back and this is what he did: Heated the Mullein Leaves in warm vinegar, then put on my neck and chest and later made me drink a cup or two of Peppermint Tea and it helped me very much. Writes Mrs. F. N., Mascoutah, Ill.

Editor's Note—A knowledge of the medicinal value of herbs will save you many dollars and much suffering.

Here is a good recipe to try out and it sure is the best that ever was for consumption or bronchitis:

2 parts Hickory Bark
2 parts Wild Cherry Bark
1 part Indian Turnip
1 part Wahoo Bark
1 part Calamus Root
¼ part Garlic

This is a positive cure for consumption. Take a teaspoonful of all and let steep for 30 minutes and sweeten with honey and glycerine, a teaspoonful of each. My forefathers have cured over 500 cases with this and it is only one of over 200 recipes I have for you, as I have spent most of my time in the study of medicines.

Editor's Note—Thank you for your kind letter and recipe. Will gladly publish such of your recipes as we can find space for. When taking any treatment for consumption it is of prime importance to get plenty of fresh air and sunlight and good wholesome food. The above recipe is quite harmless but cannot be efficient by itself.

For Catarrhal Colds and Bronchial Affections, inhale the fumes of singed Mullein Leaves, scatter the leaves on a hot skillet and breathe in the smoke that will rise. Writes L. G. P., Cains, Pa.

BRUISES AND SPRAINS

Take Red Oak Bark, boil in water, then remove the bark, thicken with Wheat Bran or Corn Meal and apply to the Bruise. My son was accidentally shot, the bullet going through his big toe. An old soldier told me this remedy was used during the Civil War for gun wounds, so I applied it and the swelling soon disappeared and the wound healed up immediately. Writes J. H. B., Van Alstyne, Tex.

For a Bruise—Add a pint of Boiling Water to a handful of Peach Tree Leaves and simmer until the leaves are tender. Apply the hot leaves and bandage and soak the bandage with juice from the leaves. Submitted by Mrs. F. R., Milton, Ind.

A good remedy for Sprains is to get White Oak Bark, put in a quart of water, a large handful, then boil down to a pint and bathe the sprain with it often. Writes E. P., Ft. Dodge, Iowa.

For Bruises, take Chamomile, steep, then strain and use hot as can be borne with compresses, cover with a dry cloth to retain heat. Have used this with success especially with children, having their legs bare in the summer, etc. Writes C. E. W., Cleveland, O.

A splendid recipe for Strains, Sprains and Bruises. Take Red Oak Bark and Mullein. Use two-thirds as much Mullein as Red Oak. Put in a vessel, cover good with water, and boil and simmer until the ooze is strong, strain, add a little Salt and a little pure Apple Vinegar to it, then thicken with Wheat Bran or Corn Meal. Apply as a poultice and renew every 6 hours for about three or four times and you will be surprised to see how much better you are. Writes C. F. W., Gainesville, Ga.

Take Sumach Bark and Wheat Bran, make into a poultice and apply hot for Stone Bruise. Writes Mrs. D. E. B., Sevierville, Tenn.

Liniment—This is good for all kinds of aches. I have used it for years and given it to a great many. One cup turpentine, 1 cup vinegar, 1 egg. Mix all together and shake well. Writes L. O., Seattle, Wash.

Our boy got his foot mashed by a big heavy horse jumping on him, striking his foot with a heavy shod foot. The pains were severe and caused a chill, followed by fever and delirium. We placed the foot in a poultice of Inner Bark of Slippery Elm. This drew the soreness and fever, also the swelling out. Then the place broke and the flesh was dressed with a salve made from thick Sweet Cream and Peppermint Leaves which were fried slowly. We made the salve fresh daily. Writes Mrs. L. L. M., Willow Springs, Mo.

Editor's Note—This poultice is good—

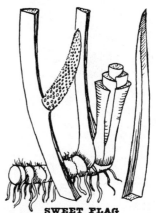

SWEET FLAG
(Acorus Calamus—Arum Family)

A farmer while at work about a threshing machine fell and sprained and bruised his elbow so bad that two doctors told him that they could do nothing for him, but take the arm off. But the man would not consent. A neighboring farmer told him to have made a poultice of Calamus Root, and renew it twice a day. This was done and in a few weeks the arm was well and the man was able to go about his work. Writes Dr. A. W., Davenport, Ia.

Editor's Note—Be sure to ask for powdered root if desired for a poultice.

For Sprains—Steep for 5 minutes or so a generous supply of Smart Weed, bathe the part with the warm tea and, if convenient, bind the weed on the sprained part. This has been found very good for man or beast. Writes A. B., Lincoln, Kan.

BURNS

The best remedy I have ever known tried for Burns. Get Bear Grass Root, boil and make a strong tea of about a good handful of the root. Cook down low, strain the tea, put about a half cupful of Hog's Lard in it, cook water out of this. Writes Mrs. M. E. T., Gordon. Ga.

For Burns—Two ounces Linseed Oil, 2 ounces Sassafras Oil, 1 ounce Coal Oil. This is fine for burns. It will exclude the air and stop the pain, thus healing the burn. Writes Mrs. N. D., Glasgow, Missouri.

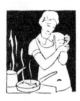

I am sending a recipe for Burns. Take Chestnut Leaves, boil them into a strong tea. Wash the burn in the tea. If the burn should get dry and crusty, soften with some kind of salve or oil first, and then use this tea. Writes A. H., Linden, W. Va.

Here is my Recipe for Burns—½ pint Pure Linseed Oil and 2 ounces powdered Sulphur. Mix well and apply at once. When my baby was a year old he fell and stuck his hand into the mouth of a heating stove full of fresh live coals and burned it so it looked parched and wrinkled. I had to go out to get the medicine and it was at least 30 minutes after he was burned before I got it fixed and put on. It was burned so deep that it made a bad sore, but this fixed it up and never even left a scar. Writes Mrs. J. C. R., Asher, Okla.

To draw out fire when one is burned, take the White of an Egg, and scrape a little Alum or use Powdered Alum, beat the two together, put on the burn, and you probably will not need only two applications. It will do the work and is cooling. Writes Mrs. E. A., Willmathsville, Mo.

Burns—White Lily Root made into a salve will cure a burn without a scar. Writes Mrs. A. V., Louisville, Ky.

Gum Plant Tea—Is cooling for all kinds of Burns. We find it better than anything else. It is also fine for Asthma taken internally in small doses. Writes S. H., Vallejo, Calif.

For Burns—Get Witch Hazel Bark and add 2 quarts of water, boil down very low, take out the bark, add fresh Hog Lard, let come to fry, strain, and apply. It sure will relieve. Writes M. I., Augusta, Miss.

Cold water is the great remedy for Burns, because it excludes the air and is immediately taken up by the burned blood and the dead skin that has been burned, putting them under the solvent process of water, and so the water itself is taken up and passed into the dry, burned, cooked, roasted places where the blood has been congested or cooked, and all these particles are soaked up or liquefied in a very short time, so they may be taken up, removed or thrown off by the vital force, for water is the natural solvent of the body. All the time the person is in the water, or that the water is being applied to any cases of burn it is of the utmost importance that the person should have pure air to breathe, and liberal quantities of water should be drunk as well. Writes Mrs. E. D., Dowagiac, Mich.

As burns are more or less serious, one should always have on hand a good reliable remedy, something that can be applied instantly. I am sending you the best remedy I know of. Take equal parts of Rosin, Mutton Tallow or Pure Lard, melt together and put in a container, glass or earthenware, that may be closed up tight. If Poppy Buds or Flowers can be procured fry these first, strain, then add the Rosin, etc. This eases the burn and it will never blister, if used at once. Writes Mrs. E. M., Willow Springs, Mo.

Here Is a Wonderful Remedy for Burns—Two tablespoonfuls of powdered Camphor mixed with 2 tablespoonfuls of pure Hog's Lard, apply at once and if the air has not got to the burn will not blister and won't hurt you after 5 minutes. Writes Mrs. T. B., St. Helena, Calif.

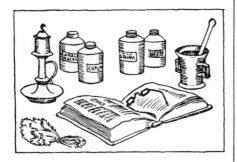

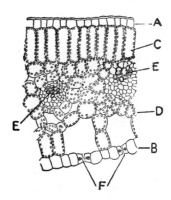

For Burns—Make Burn Salve, ½ pint Pure Olive Oil, 2 ounces Spermaceti, and 2 ounces of White Wax, heat until all is melted, mix well, when cool it is ready for use. This recipe is very good and will heal any burn. Writes Alfred G., Cabot, Pa.

Apply raw Linseed Oil thoroughly and liberally covering the Burn, repeat until cured and it will not leave a scar. Writes Mrs. R. K., Sentinel, Okla.

An old standby for Burns is Witch Hazel, also moistened Baking Soda. Writes R. B., New York City, N. Y.

Take the bark of Red Oak and boil down until you have an ooze, and this is very good if used to sores and burns. Writes Mrs. E. McA., Quinlan, Okla.

My Recipe for Burns—Use Linseed Oil on Burns of any kind. Have used it for years, and there will be no blister. Writes Mrs. M. B., Manchester, Tenn.

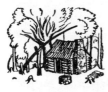

BUNIONS

I am sending a recipe which has proved to be a sure cure for Bunions: Take a 2-inch square of yeast bread, 2 tablespoonfuls of shredded Catnip and a tablespoonful of Sweet Milk and boil together until thick. Make into a poultice and put on the bunion night and morning until four poultices have been used. Writes Miss L. S., Tremont, La.

PLANT LABORATORY

Twenty years ago I told my readers that the chemical laboratory of a single blade or grass would make our finest man-built laboratory look like a pig pen; clumsy, crude and incapable of producing what a single blade of grass is manufacturing day after day.

The illustration above shows the intricate, yet orderly network of cells of a leaf enlarged 400 times. It represents a cross section of a leaf one four-hundredths of an inch in thickness; not any thicker than an egg shell. A shows the top skin (epidermis), B the lower skin, C, D, E and F the inside cells of the leaf.

The tissue between the upper and lower skin (epidermis) is called Mesophyll (or middle leaf). Meso means midst—and phyll means leaf. In this ilustration the tissue is in the shape of palisades, (Fig. C) is rather firm, but the mesophyll underneath these palisades is soft. In this soft mesophyll (D) the cells have open spaces between them. F, the little stomates (or mouths) on the lower skin open directly into these larger cells. Air passes through these mouths (or stomates) of the skin into the cells where the gases needed are absorbed by the mesophyll. Through the leaf the plant absorbs the sunlight which yields the energy whereby its work is done. From the sunlight green plants derive their energy which is stored in the food they make. E in the above illustration shows the vascular bundle or veins which penetrate every particle of the leaf and through which the water and other substances are carried from the roots, through the stems to the leaves of the plant and it is here where inorganic substances are transformed into organic substances; here is stored the force which sustains all life.

—Bavarian Herb Tea,
Elder Flowers
Rocky Mt. Grape Root
Juniper Berries
Anise Seed
Black Mallow Flowers
Fennel Seed
German Cheese Plant
Mullein
Coughwort
Turtlebloom Leaves
Marshmallow Root

The history of this tea dates back to the days of the benevolent old Pastor Kneipp of Bavaria. We have improved the original formula by addition of a few botanicals of Indian origin. It is still sold in foreign countries under the name of ''Catarrh Tea.'' Judge of the formula by the ingredients.

Unfailing Catarrh Remedy—Equal parts of Gum Arabic, Gum Myrrh and Blood Root, all in powdered form, mix and use as a snuff.

Editor's Note—I am afraid the Blood Root will irritate too much.

Here is a Good Recipe for Catarrh—I know of a case where the doctors didn't do any good and this man used the juice of Lemon mixed with Honey. This should be snuffed up the nose 4 times a day. Writes P. A. S., Mt. Angel, Ore.

Editor's Note—I would advise to dilute this with warm water at first and gradually cutting down on the water until it can be snuffed up without irritation. Looks like a good and sensible treatment.

I got this recipe from an Indian 74 years old and he claims it a positive Catarrh remedy. Use the dried cut Peppermint Leaves to snuff into the nostrils. Writes Chief D. F., and submitted by Capt. M. J., Chicago, Ill.

For Catarrh of the Head—Use the dried Peach Tree Leaves as a smoke. Writes G. A. B., Mt. Creek, Ala.

Editor's Note—Here you are, you Michiganders: Peachtree leaves seem to be good for lots of things. I am using them for my hair.

For Catarrh of the Head—Take equal parts of Cubeb Berries and Wild Cherry Bark, and smoke a pipeful each night for 12 months. Retire as soon as through smoking. It is stimulating and has cured serious cases in my home.

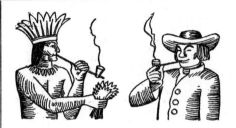

CATARRH

Is a chronic inflammation of the mucous membrane lining the nasal cavities. Its principal symptoms are, profuse discharge of thick mucous, nose is stopped up, difficulty in breathing. There is sometimes pain across the forehead.

Catarrh — Almost every person is troubled with catarrhal inflammation of some kind which is slowly but surely devitiating the blood and poisoning the system. The majority of the laity are of the opinion that the prime symptom of catarrh is a clogged condition of the nostrils, and as long as breathing through the nose is not difficult they are free of the disease. This is a serious mistake.

Foul breath is a sure indication of catarrh. The seat of catarrh is the larynx and pharynx and inner channels of the nose and throat. To treat chronic catarrh successfully it is indispensable to apply a healing agent to the diseased membrane and to take a blood purifying and tonic remedy; also to keep the mouth and teeth clean by the use of antiseptic mouth washes and tooth powder.

As a local soothing agent, one or more of the following may be used: (1) Nasal Powder for snuffing up into the nostrils, (2) Nasal Smoke.

Bronchitis—In all bronchial troubles there is evidence that the sufferer has been eating too freely of carbohydrate foods, starches and sugars. Omit from the diet, bread, pastry, cereals, sugar, milk, coffee and tea, fried foods, potatoes and all starchy foods until the system is thoroughly cleared up. Fresh fruits, especially the citrus ones, and fresh vegetables are very acceptable.

Catarrh—Crush 1 ounce of Flax Seed and a half ounce of Licorice Root in 1 pint of boiling water for 2 hours, filter, and add 1 ounce of Lemon Juice. This is a good drink in cases of Catarrh. Dose—3 to 5 tablespoonfuls daily. Writes D. J. C., Corfu, N. Y.

Mullein Leaves smoked by persons having Catarrh is supposed to cure it. Writes V. M., Esto, Ky.

Catarrh Specific—Two parts Powdered Golden Seal, 2 parts Gum Camphor, and 1 part Powdered Blood Root. Mix well and use as a snuff twice daily. Writes M. F. B., Milo, Iowa.

Cubeb Berries for Catarrh—A new remedy for Catarrh is crushed Cubeb Berries smoked in a pipe emitting the smoke through the nostrils, and after a few trials, this will be easy to do. If the nose is stopped up so that it is almost impossible to breathe, one pipeful will make the head clear. For Sore Throat, Asthma and Bronchitis, swallowing the smoke effects immediate relief. It is the best remedy in the world for offensive breath and will make the most foul breath pure and sweet. Sufferers from that horrid disease, ulcerated Catarrh will find this remedy unequalled and a month's use will cure the most obstinate case. A single trial will convince anyone. Eating the uncrushed berries is also good for Sore Throat and all Bronchial complaints. After smoking do not expose yourself to cold air for 15 minutes. Writes O. R. S., Portland, Ind.

Cubebs—If the nostrils are stopped so as to prevent easy breathing take crushed Cubeb Berries and smoke them in a new clay pipe, forcing the smoke through the head and nostrils. The head will be as clear as a bell in 5 minutes so that one can breathe naturally all night. Use this remedy only before retiring or when you can remain indoors as it is said to open the pores to the extent of placing the system in great danger if exposed to the air very soon after using. Cubeb smoke disinfects and heals and will cure Catarrh if used every night regularly. Writes O. R. S., Portland, Indiana.

For Catarrh—Use the dried Sumach Leaves and smoke them in a clay pipe twice a day, and we are sure you will find them good. Writes E. L., Troy, N. Y.

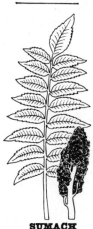

SUMACH

Dried Mullein Leaves made into a cigarette and smoked, inhaling the smoke will cure Catarrh. Writes Mrs. J. D. Mc., Lake Charles, La.

Take Yellow Dock Root, Burdock, Dandelion, Red Clover Flowers, 4 ounces of each to 2 gallons of water, add a good handful of Hops, boil slowly for 1 hour, strain and cool, then add a cake of Yeast; when fermented strain, set in a cool place, and take a small wine glassful 3 times a day, and this should be very valuable for Catarrh. You can also get the dried Mullein and smoke it 3 times a day. Writes Mrs. M. W., Latham, Ohio.

This recipe was given me by a friend whose father-in-law was one of the old doctors years ago, and he said it was a fine Spring Tonic when one was run-down and tired out. My mother found it to be as he said:

1 ounce Burdock
1 ounce Yellow Dock
1 ounce Sarsaparilla
1 ounce Dandelion

Dose: One-half teaspoonful 3 times a day. Writes Mrs. G. H., Mapleton, Minn.

Make a strong tea of Wild Cherry Bark. Then take a tablespoonful of the tea in half a glass of water 4 times a day. This is a very good Tonic. Writes Mrs. C. F., Oak Hill, Ohio.

CHILLS AND FEVERS

In these ailments as in most others, Nature does the curing. Medicines, whether of organic or inorganic origin, can merely aid in the process by building up resistance. The botanicals listed are mostly diaphoretic in their action if used as hot infusions; if used cold they act as mild tonics and aromatics.

Sage Tea given freely, slightly sweetened will break up a severe Cold and Fever. This was given to a child with a severe cold and fever and it surely helped. Writes Mrs. J. H., Knoxville, Ia.

Five Finger Grass used in tea is useful for Fevers in young or old. Writes Mrs. C. S., Pleasant Ridge, Pa.

Tea made of the herb called Balm is good for inward Fevers. Writes S. B. W., Lancaster, Ky.

For Chills—Take a small handful of leaves or stems of Pennyroyal. Make a tea, drink a cupful or two a day for a week or so. May be sweetened if desired. I used this on myself over 50 years. Writes A. W. of Woodmen, Colo.

Fevers—Steep 1 ounce of Fever Weed to 1 pint of water and drink freely when cold. This will relieve Fever.

For Chills and Ague—Take Powdered Alum, put in white muslin sack a teaspoonful, and wear around the neck, so it will hang on the breast; also one on the back. Wear for 30 days and you will never have any chills. Writes J. H. S., Davis, Ill.

Editor's Note—If this is not a mind cure— then it must be something else.

Tag Alder is good to cool fever, and so is Salt in water and bathe with it. Writes Mrs. A. V., Witts Springs, Ark.

Here is a recipe that I did not see in your list. Take the leaves of Sweet Basil, a teaspoonful, steep in a cup of boiling water for 10 minutes, and sweeten. Drink 3 times a day and will cure any kind of Fever, for I know of a case doctors gave up and this cured her. Writes Mrs. R. McQ., Kokomo, Miss.

As a pioneer, my mother tested many valuable recipes and I remember well that Boneset Tea is very good for Chills. Writes Mrs. E. O. B., Carthage, Mo.

Editor's Note—I agree with you.

Willow Bark is very good for Ague and Fever. Writes L. W., Coldwater, Miss.

—Florida Tea.......
  Sweet Flag Root
  Jamaica Ginger Root
  Juniper Berries
  Clove Buds
  Cubeb Berries
  Sassafras Bark of Root
  Senna Alexandria Leaves
  Oregon Grape Root
  Cassia Bark

This is an excellent diaphoretic if taken hot. Useful in Fevers, Ague, and to break up a cold.

—Jesuits Fever Bark
  Compound......
  Jesuits Fever Bark
  Jamaica Ginger
  Clove Buds
  Cascara
  Licorice Root

A useful substitute for Quinine. **Try** it for Colds, etc.

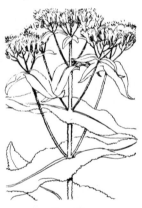

Boneset

Chills—I will send you my mother's recipe for Chills. Take Boneset and make tea and drink it as hot as possible, and it sure will break the Chills, and it is harmless. Writes Mrs. O. W. H., Russelville, Ala.

For Chills and Fever—Take Smart Weed, make a tea, drink cold, and note how useful it is. Writes Mrs. W. W., Fremont, Neb.

For Fever—Take a teaspoonful of Cream of Tartar to one cup of water. It never fails to break a Fever. Writes Mrs. A. J. C., Vining, Minn.

Black Snake Root is fine in most cases of Fever. Writes S. H., Vallejo, Calif.

Fever Flowers—In Central America and Mexico there grows a plant commonly known among the Americans and foreigners as Fever Flowers, but which the natives call "Jamaica." The flower petals of this plant yield a most delightful thirst satisfying and cooling drink, very similar to lemonade. The name Fever Flower was undoubtedly given to this plant on account of its cooling effect in Fevers. Recently a physician, who lived many years in these tropical countries visited with me and presented me with a quantity of these flower petals. My experiments, very limited up to this time, prove the value of this plant in allaying fevers. I am of the opinion that these flower petals are rich in Vitamins A and B and certain minerals—and in another decade will be heralded by the medical profession as a wonderful new discovery.

The directions for using these flower petals are as follows: Place 3 to 5 petals in a glass of slightly sweetened water, allow it to stand an hour—and you will have a golden orange, cooling drink. It occurs to me that these flower petals could also be used in flavoring pies and custards.

Tea or Sweet Balm Leaves is the best fever medicine that I know of. Just put the leaves in a cup and pour boiling water over them and drink for Fever. Writes H. L. T., Benton, Ky.

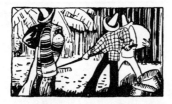

Editor's Note—Sweet Balm Leaves and all other medicinal plants and leaves lose their virtue after they are a year old.

When I was a young girl, I took down with Fever and as we were some 5 or 6 miles from a doctor and had just moved in a strange neighborhood, mother wrote her brother who was a doctor. He wrote to give me as much Boneset Tea, sufficient to make me vomit, and then to give me 2 or 3 cups a day, a few swallows at a time, with just enough Cayenne Pepper to make it a little hot. Said it would break any case of Fever and no doctor bill to pay, and it sure did the work. Writes Mrs. E. W., Summerfield, Fla.

Over a handful of the dried Peach Tree Leaves, pour a pint of boiling water, let steep 15 minutes, and sweeten if desired. This tea cured my husband of Chills and Fever to which he was subject for many years. This tea has also helped others to whom I have offered it. Writes C. R. R., Toledo, Ohio.

For Chills and Colds—Use a tablespoonful of clean Flax Seed, pour over boiling water, let stand 30 minutes in warm place on stove, then add a tablespoonful of Honey and some Peppermint, then strain all. Take this in the morning and before going to bed for 3 or 4 days. It is also important to keep the bowels in good condition. Writes Mrs. W. B., Green Bay, Wis.

Chills and Fever—Take the leaves of Mullein, boil to make a strong tea. Sweeten and drink two cups a day, for three days. Writes Mrs. C. E. O., Longton, Kan.

Fevers—Take the buds out of the tops of Ragweed, make a tea and drink about two cups a day. Will break Fevers. Writes Mrs. P. G., Detroit, Mich.

Editor's Note—Yes and so will Boneset leaves and flowers.

Chill Tonic—One pound powdered Gentian, 4 ounces powdered Rhubarb and Aloes, 2 of powdered Ginger, 2 of Baking Soda, 2 of powdered Cinnamon, and a pound of Brown Sugar. Dose: 1 teaspoonful in a glass of water, 3 times a day. This has been successfully used in the south. Writes J. D. M., Pennsboro, W. Va.

For Fevers give Indian Sage and Senna Tea. Take the same amount of each and fill a common cup half full of the herbs, fill with hot water. Let stand half hour. Give 2 tablespoons every 2 hours until you have given 3 or 4 doses. Writes T. L. F., Water Valley, Miss.

I have tried Life Everlasting for Colds and Fever and know it is very good. Writes Mrs. W. L. H., Cottondale, Ala.

Fever—I have a good cure for Fever. Take a teaspoonful of Elder Blossoms to a cup of hot water, and drink as hot as you can, go to bed, and sweat. I have cured my children of flu when it was so bad, using this in the Fevers. Writes Mary P., Academy, S. D.

Editor's Note—Yes, this is very good.

We have tried this recipe for Fever and Colds and find it very useful for children: Make a strong tea of Elder Flowers and Pennyroyal, and give cold in the day time and hot upon retiring. This is also useful to run down a Fever. Writes E. R. M., Lewis, Ind.

Dried Wild Sage made into a tea is also one of the best remedies I have ever used for Fever, and it's very, very good for babies during the teething period. Writes Mrs. P. C., Ennis, Texas.

For Fever—Take a big handful of Mullein Leaves and boil into a strong tea, sweeten and give. This helped my little girl when nothing else did. Writes Mrs. W. R., Dillen, Ark.

Here is a little Recipe which no doubt will interest many—Just take the Camphor Gum, hang around the neck in a little bag between the shoulders, and it will surely break up Chills. Writes W. R. N., Paducah, Ky.

Fevers of all kinds, also Influenza— ''I am sending in a recipe of an herb remedy which I have known to cure Fevers of all kinds, and it is a sure shot for the Influenza, because it cured me and my family. I was in bed for four weeks and the doctors could not do me any good and my mother made me some tea out of Peach Tree Leaves. Take 2 teaspoonsful of the leaves and place in a cup of boiling water. Let cool. Then strain and sweeten with Honey or Sugar.'' Writes I. S., Marlin, Texas.

Fevers—One of the best remedies for Fevers of any kind is Blue Cohosh. Writes Mrs. D. R. G., Leon, W. Va.

Fevers—Steep 1 ounce of Fever Weed to 1 pint of water and drink freely when cold. This will relieve Fever. Writes Mrs. R. V., Angelica, N. Y.

Make a strong tea of Elder Flowers, Leaves, or Bark. Dose: ½ teacupful of the tea, ½ teacupful of fresh sweet milk, add 1 teaspoonful of Sugar. Two or three doses every hour will stop the Fever after a Chill or Ague. Writes R. C. R. A., M.D., Haynes, Ala.

Add to a quart of water, three handfuls of Witch Hazel, White Oak Bark, and Apple Tree Bark. Boil down to a pint and strain. Add half a pound of lard, and simmer till the water disappears. This is very good for piles. Writes Mrs. J. C. E., Jovele, Utah.

CHOLERA

When I was in Illinois I took Cholera Morbus and nothing would stay on my stomach. I started for town and when reaching my boarding house, the lady of the house asked me what was wrong. After telling her, she said I can relieve you. She took a teaspoonful of Wood Ashes (Charcoal) and put it in a teacup of water, stirred it up and let it settle. Then gave it to me 1 teaspoonful at a time. In a half hour I was relieved. We have a neighbor whose son took down with Indigestion too and in a few days nothing would stay on his stomach. The doctor did all he could, but the boy kept getting worse. When I arrived the doctor had gone and they told me he could do nothing, so I told them about the water and wood ashes. They seemed to think no one but a doctor could do any good, by finally convincing them that it would do no harm, we gave the boy some. First he began to feel sicker and wanted to vomit, but we kept on until he was easy, and relieved. The first or second teaspoonful may come up, but wait a while and still give and it will prove good. Writes H. L., Severy, Kans.

Use Wormwood Tea for Cholera Morbus and Cramps, and it will be very useful, for I have found it so. Writes J. M. W., New Plymouth, Ohio.

Burdock also cured a baby of Cholera Infantum after the M.D.'s said nothing could save it from dying, and this is a true fact. Writes J. L. L., East Gastonia, N. C.

Cholera Morbus—Take 2 ounces of the leaves of Benne, put them in ½ pint of cold water, and let soak an hour, give 2 tablespoonfuls hourly until relief is experienced. Writes Mrs. M. H. McG., Los Angeles, Calif.

Euca Leaves Compound—This is a combination of leaves from California that have given such good results as a foot bath, in those conditions in which hot applications to the feet are indicated or have been found helpful, that we have been persuaded to add it to our list. Steep a handful of the leaves in a half gallon of hot water, stir awhile and when it cools down, use as foot bath before retiring.

COLDS

For Cold or Stopped Up Head—Put 1 teaspoonful of Camphor in a cup of boiling hot water, inhale this steam, and you will find it surely does help. Writes Mrs. M. C. P., Shelbyville,

To Break Up a Cold—Drink Ginger Tea upon going to bed. It will cause a good sweat and make one sleep well. To break up a hard cold, 1 teaspoonful of Ginger in a glass of cold water, no sugar or milk, drink and go to bed at once. Writes Mrs. L. S., Cocolalla, Idaho.

Cough Syrup—Put 1 quart of Horehound to 1 quart of water, and boil it down to 1 pint, add 2 or 3 sticks of Licorice, essence of lemon. Take a tablespoonful three times a day, or as often as cough may be troublesome. Writes O. R. S., Portland, Ind.

I want to pass along my tried and true remedies, so I am sending this Cough Syrup recipe:
1 pound Dates
1 pound Figs
1 ounce Sage
4 quarts Rain Water
Boil down to 1 quart, strain, add 10c worth of Rock Candy, and take as often as needed. Writes Mrs. A. J. B., Mansfield, Ohio.

For Colds on Chest for Children—Take a flannel shirt and grease with lard, the breast part and between shoulders, then take 3 Nutmegs, grate fine and sprinkle on the shirt and let them wear it for three days, then renew and wear three more days. This I know is true for I used it, and my father broke pneumonia on one of my sisters with it. Writes Mrs. J. J., Etty, Ky.

Editor's Note—I know that if this treatment is taken the child must be kept warm and indoors. The slightest exposure would aggravate the ailment.

Fever Weed is the best thing to break up a cold. I have tried it upon going to bed, drinking a cupful of the hot tea. Writes F. A., Ritner, Ky.

Coughs—Take a double handful of Wild Cherry Bark to 1 quart of water, boil to a strong tea, strain, add equal part of honey, and boil down to thin syrup. Take 1 teaspoonful three times a day. Writes Mrs. A. G., Dawson, Ala.

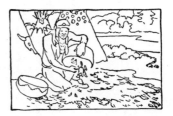

I am a part Indian and I sure do believe in herbs, and all my people do, too. Here is a home remedy for Colds. Use equal parts of Mullein, Horehound, Sycamore, and Wild Cherry. Make a tea, drink it hot. It can be taken cold, but hot is best. Writes R. B. S., Noblesville, Tenn.

For Coughs—1 tablespoonful Honey, yolk of egg, 1 teaspoonful Olive Oil (which can be gradually increased to a tablespoonful). Mix well and taken morning and evening should cure coughs, cigarette coughs and even T. B. Beat this together well, and take all in one dose. Writes Mrs. A. N., Petoskey, Mich.

All winter I hardly had a bad cold. As soon as I felt one coming on I took a cup of hot sage tea and in no time the cold was gone. Writes M. K., Marshfield, Wis.

In cases of common chest colds, phlegm can be raised and the patient greatly relieved by giving glycerine in teaspoon doses every fifteen minutes until relieved. It surely helped me when I had a cold. Also one drop of household ammonia in a teaspoonful of lard and beaten to a froth and used to rub on the chest will relieve simple colds. Writes Mrs. C. I., East Peoria, Ill.

For Common Cough and Cold Relief—Take a tablespoonful of flaxseed and boil for several minutes and strain. Add lemon juice, sugar and butter and boil again for a few minutes. This is harmless and relieves coughs due to colds. Wrties E. L., Brentwood, Mo.

For relief of coughs and colds, take hot tea at bedtime made from Coltsfoot. Writes Mrs. S. B. H., Charlotte, N. Car.

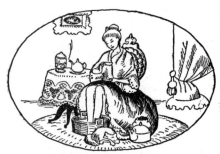

WHEN COLDS THREATEN

A hot tea of St. Johnswort will produce profuse perspiration and stops cough. Writes J. W., Parrish, N. C.

Melt a little lard, put a small quantity of Turpentine in it or Eucalyptus Oil in the lard, then while warm rub well over neck, lungs, back and around nose and ears, cover chest and back with flannels. This is very good for colds in babies. Also give the baby a laxative. Writes Mrs. H. E. T.

To Break Up a Cold—Take 4 lemons and roast in oven until the juice comes through the skin, remove all the juice from them, and strain. Take 3 tablespoonfuls of Horehound and steep in water, then strain and add enough sugar to make a thin syrup. When cold add the lemon juice, and bottle. Writes Mrs. G. L., Pontiac, Mich.

Colds—Get some Feverfew, make a tea and drink hot at night. It is good for colds and flu, which I have tried with good results. Writes C. E., Sardis, Miss.

Catarrh or Cold in Head—For catarrh or cold in the head, smoke dried Mullein Leaves, as you would Tobacco, only forcing the smoke through the nose. Also, with the mouthful of smoke, close lips tight, hold nose with thumb and finger and force the smoke into the upper parts of the nose and ears. Writes Mrs. A. W., Portsmouth, Ohio.

Coughs—Make a strong tea of Wild Rose Roots, add sugar or Honey to make a good syrup. Take as any other cough remedy. Writes Mrs. G. W., Greenfield, Mo.

Spikenard (Life of Man)—Take 1 ounce of the root to 1 quart of water and extract so that you will have 1 pint of liquid. Take 1 quart of good molasses and make a thick syrup, add both together, while hot, so that there will be a little over 1 quart when done. Set away to cool. Dose—a teaspoonful as often as needed. This makes one of the best cough syrups known to this part of the country. Strictly a home remedy. Writes L. M. A., Bangor, Me.

Flax Seed for Colds is very good. Use 1 teaspoon in a cup of boiling water and drink, preferably at night. Writes Mrs. W. M., Manitowoc, Wis.

For Coughs—Equal parts of Horehound, Elecampane Root, Comfrey Root, Spikenard and Wild Cherry. Boil in 1 gallon of water, down to 1 quart. Strain and add 1 pound Honey. Take a tablespoonful when cough is troublesome. Writes Mrs. A. W., Portsmouth, Ohio.

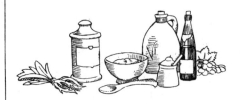

MUMPS

Is known by the sensitive swelling of a gland in front of and below the ear, on one or both sides. It is attended with fever and pain when chewing. It usually passes off in three or four days, but is sometimes dangerous if the patient is chilled. Complications may arise that may be more or less serious.

Treatment—Put patient to bed.

The Herb Doctor's choice of botanicals are: Sweet Balm, Chamomile Flowers, Elder Flowers. Use chiefly with the addition of Lemon Juice as refrigerant teas; if taken hot they act as diaphoretics.

Catnip Tea will take away the pain in Mumps, if some is taken hot. Whenever they start to pain, use it hot. Have used this with my children and it's wonderful. Writes Mrs. J. P. B., Chelsea, Okla.

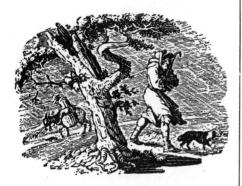

COUGHS

For Coughs—Take Wild Cherry Bark, boil down and strain, then mix with honey. Writes C. B. C., Martin, Tenn.

For a Cough—Take a large handful of Life Everlasting, Chestnut Leaves, Wahoo, just a small amount of White Snake Root and Mullein Flowers. Boil in ½ gallon of water until all the strength is out, then strain, sweeten, and boil into a syrup. Writes E. M., Okey, Ohio.

A strong tea of the Boneset will break up a bad Cold quickly. Just make and sweeten to taste. Writes Mrs. L. P., Galloway, Ohio.

An old Pottawatomie remedy, used as a Cough Syrup: Four handfuls Sycamore Chops, 2 Prickly Ash Bark, 2 Wahoo, 1 Wild Cherry, 1 Horehound, 1 Sweet Flag. Put all together in a gallon of water, boil down and strain, add Sugar and 1 teaspoonful of Ginger. When you have a quart, stop boiling and allow to cool. Take a tablespoon 3 times a day. Writes M. C. B., Pawhuska, Okla.

I made a cough syrup of Mullein Leaves at 25c per box and Sugar as given in your "Almanac," and it helped my boy's cough, and within two days he coughed very little. Writes Mrs. F. B., So. Connellsville, Pa.

Editor's Note—If mixed in equal parts with Coughwort Leaves it is still better.

I must say a word in favor of Coltsfoot. It is the best remedy I have ever taken for colds. It is surely a great relief to know that there is a tea that one can take, and not ruin their stomach with drugs. Writes F. McC., Cressina, Pa.

For Colds in the Head—Smoke Golden Rod Tops and Life Everlasting mixed, 2 or 3 times a day and also before going to bed. Writes Mrs. H. C., Jacksonville, Ala.

A cold in the head or Coryza begins with an attack of sneezing and feeling of stuffiness in the head, accompanied by inability to breathe through the nose. In a few hours there is a profuse watery discharge from the nose, which becomes inflamed and painful. There is frontal headache, with a loss of sense of smell and taste; slight fever. All these symptoms may become more severe if the cold persists for a length of time, temporarily affecting the hearing and irritating the throat from the constant mouth breathing. In a week or so the nasal discharge becomes purulent, and the upper lip may become badly swollen. The duration of a common cold is usually from one day to three weeks.

When a cold is coming on we recommend that the system be made alkaline as quickly as possible. To do this we recommend to take eight neutralizing tablets every two hours for three doses, a glass of warm water to be taken along with the tablets. This makes the system alkaline, as can be tested by touching litmus paper with secretions from the nose and urine.

Best Cough Remedy—
    1 oz. Thoroughwort
    1 oz. Slippery Elm
    1 oz. Stick Licorice
    1 oz. Flax Seed
Simmer together in 1 quart of water until strength is extracted. Strain carefully, add 1 pint of best molasses and ½ pound of loaf sugar, simmer them all together and when cool bottle tightly. A few doses of 1 tablespoonful at a time will alleviate the most distressing cough of the lungs, soothes and allays irritation, and if continued subdues any tendency to consumption; breaks up entirely whooping cough and no better remedy can be found for croup, asthma, bronchitis and all affections of lungs and throat.

Pine Needles boiled in a little water, strained and enough sugar added to make a syrup is fine for Colds. I tried it for the children and they like it so much better than what can be bought, and it does so much better for them. Writes Mrs. C. C., Winston-Salem, N. C.

For Colds—Slice 1 Lemon, rind and all in small bowl, with ½ teaspoonful of Ginger Root, pour on 1½ cups boiling water, and sweeten with Honey. Drink as hot as possible upon retiring. Writes Mrs. R. T., Mason City, Iowa.

To break up a Cold just drink Boneset Tea. Writes M. B., Concord, Tenn.

Scald a large handful of dried Elder Blossoms with 2 cups of boiling water, let stand about an hour, strain and drink hot. Sugar may be added if desired. It is best taken just before going to bed, and it is very good for Colds. Writes Mrs. M. L., Newport, Pa.

Here is a fine Remedy for Colds—Burn a little Pine Tar on the stove every morning. The fumes will surely relieve a Cold and prevent one, too. Writes Mrs. B. M., Kaw, Okla.

Tonsillitis and Quinsy—No food whatever. Warm lemonade or water when thirsty, until fever has subsided and pain has gone. Then orange juice for two days. Afterwards a vegetarian diet, no meats or meat broths. Feeding will surely retard recovery.

Laryngitis—Sufferer has probably been rather too fond of starchy and sugary foods, taken more carbohydrates than the oxygen breathed can oxidize. Eat more fruits and salads. Avoid tobacco and constipation.

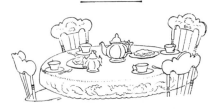

Take the juice of 1 Lemon, 2 tablespoonfuls of Honey and 1 of Butter, warm and mix together. Sip a little at a time for Coughs. Writes N. S., Schenectady, N. Y.

Take a tablespoonful of Garden Sage, and simmer in a teacup of water for 1 hour, or boil for a few minutes, then sweeten and strain through a cloth. Give to the children every few hours for Colds and Coughs. I have never known it to fail in cases of common Coughs or Colds. Writes Mrs. D. L., Alabama City, Ala.

For Coughs and Colds in Children—First soak feet in Mustard and hot water and upon retiring give Catnip or Ginger Tea as hot as can be taken, go to ged and cover up well. It will produce a sweat which will loosen the obstinate cold. Writes M. K., Boston, Mass.

Editor's Note—Whenever an herb tea is taken as a diaphoretic, i. e. to produce a sweat, great care must be taken that the child is kept covered and warm.

This simple remedy was given me by an old Indian Doctor. For Colds: Take hot Ginger Tea and squeeze into it the juice of 1 Lemon. Drink as hot as you can take just before going to bed. Writes B. H., Era, Texas.

For Coughs and Colds—Take Wild Cherry Bark, about 4 ounces to a quart of water, boil down to a dark red and strain, then add a cup of Sugar and boil to a thick syrup. Take 1 big swallow 5 or 6 times daily, and it will loosen up the cough. I tried this myself, and it done great work. Writes W. F., Summerland, Miss.

For Coughs and Colds—Take 1 quart of Boneset to a gallon of water, put vessel on stove and let come to a boil. Strain and add 3 lbs. of Sugar, 1 Lemon and 1 Orange. Put into a crock and let ferment for 1 month, strain, bottle for use. It improves with age. The above makes one of the best wines I ever tasted and will cure a severe cold when other remedies fail. It should be in every home. Writes J. M. I., Bellwood, Pa.

Two tablespoonfuls of Castor Oil and 1 of Ginger in a large size tumbler of Dark Syrup. One teaspoonful every hour is fine for Colds, Hoarseness, etc. Writes O. C. C., Marietta, Ga.

Cough Syrup—This remedy has been in our family for years and we have it on hand at all times. Use 1 ounce of Chestnut Leaves, steeped in a pint of boiling water, let stand until cool, then strain and add a pound of loaf Sugar, heat and stir till dissolved then add one drop Anise Oil. Writes M. A. S., Royal Oak, Mich.

For Coughs—Take plenty of Chestnut Leaves, boil in iron kettle, from a gallon down to a half gallon, strain, put in about 2 pounds of Brown Sugar and boil down to a quart. Take a teaspoonful 3 times a day. This cured me when doctors said it would turn to T. B. Writes Mrs. E. A. W., Good Springs, Tenn.

I tried the recipe calling for Sumach Berries for Cough as given in your Almanac and it sure is fine. I paid 75c for a bottle of almost the same thing at the drug store. Of course, these come dried, but it is no trouble to prepare. Writes Mrs. G. C. H., Birthright, Texas.

This cold recipe has been in the family for years. One handful of Blackberry leaves, two or three of Peppermint leaves and one of Horehound. Put in a pan with about one quart of water and let simmer until about two cupfuls or a little less remains; then strain and add two tablespoonfuls of honey. Shake well before taking, about three times per day. Writes S. C. H., Cincinnati, Ohio.

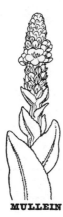

MULLEIN

Coughs, Colds, Etc.—This herbal preparation is unexcelled for coughs, colds, etc.:

1 tablespoonful Mullein Leaves
1 tablespoonful Horehound
1 tablespoonful Elecampane
1 teacupful cane sugar

Place the above in a quart of water, and boil down to 1 pint. It is then ready for use. Dose—Tablespoonful when needed. This sure is a wonderful remedy. Writes W. D. T., Rose Hill, Ill.

Consumptive Cough—"1 teaspoonful of Wild Cherry Bark. Add sufficient boiling water to make a tea. Let simmer. Never boil as boiling takes the virtues out of the tea. Use this as a beverage in place of coffee, tea, etc., at meal times and otherwise. An excellent remedy for all coughs and colds." Writes Miss L. G., Ann Arbor, Mich.

Cough Remedy—Take an ounce of Indian Turnip and steep in a pint of water. This should be taken three times during the day. An excellent remedy for coughs. Writes Mrs. B. R., Brooksville, Ky.

Balm of Gilead Buds steeped in sugar to make a syrup will cure a Cough of long standing. Writes G. D. B., Endeavor, Wis.

Here is a recipe for Coughs: Take 2 handfuls of Boneset Leaves and 2 handfuls of Carpenter's Square herb (more commonly called Figwort) and 3 tablespoonfuls of Horehound and about a gallon and one-half of water. Boil for an hour, strain and add 1 pound of sugar. Boil this down to a thin syrup and take every 3 hours until relieved. Writes Mr. G. H., Bourneville, Ohio.

As every Herbalist knows Horsemint or Desert Mint is an invaluable remedy for Colds, Flu, etc., but what some do not know is that the matured tops or seeds are even better than the leaves. I discovered this when I wished to gather some and cold had killed the leaves. They should be crushed before using. Writes L. M., Bogalusa, La.

Some years ago I had a strangling Cough. I nearly choked and my eyes would almost bulge out of my head, when coughing. I had some dried Elder Flowers and I purchased some Rock Candy, made a tea of the Elder Flowers and boiled the Rock Candy in it. I drank a few swallows every time I thought of it and the next day I was cured of my cough. Writes Mrs. L. M., Elkhart, Ind.

The following Cough Syrup recipe is excellent for children and can be given as often as needed. Dose: Half teaspoonful, according to the age, up to one year, after they are a year or more, use the full teaspoonful:

1 ounce Horehound
1 ounce Elecampane
1 ounce Comfrey

Boil the ingredients in 3 quarts of water until 2 quarts remain, strain, add 1 pint of sugar and boil until you have a quart. Writes Mrs. L. D., Merom, Ind.

Here is my Recipe for Coughs—Take ½ pint of Pine Tar, 1 pound of Granulated Sugar. Put this into a quart of water and boil 1 hour slowly. Let cool and strain and take ½ teaspoonful every 3 or 4 hours. Writes Mrs. J. R. C., Rockingham, N. C.

Two tablespoonfuls of Ginger Root and three of Brown Sugar. Mix all together and take by one-eighth teaspoonful doses every time you have a Coughing Spell. Writes J. P. K., Summerville, Pa.

Recipe for Coughs—Take Wild Cherry Bark and Flax Seed, boil together, then strain and add Sugar to make the syrup. The dose is a tablespoonful 3 times a day. Writes Miss T. B., Chase City, Va.

Coughs and Colds—Use an ounce of Oil of Tar, also a ½ ounce Oil Origanium, for it is very beneficial for Coughs and Colds. Use 3 drops of the mixture on Sugar. Writes Mrs. R. R., Casnovia, Mich.

Coughwort surely done me a world of good and, thanks to your book, I am now able to get up and work a little, but before nothing did any good. Writes M. McC., Norwalk Ohio.

Sea Wrack or Bladder Wrack is offered for over-fatness, but I have found it one of the best articles for a Flu Cough. One box of it to a pint of water, strain and mixed with Honey, take 2 teaspoonfuls at a time when needed for the cough. It surely is a good remedy. Writes Mrs. L. E., Eastside, Ore.
Editor's Note—Probably on account of its Iodine content.

Here is a Recipe for a good Cough Syrup—Take Sumach Berries, boil down from a quart to a pint, add sufficient Sugar to make a thick syrup. It is fine. It cured my nephew of a measle Cough, when doctor's medicines failed. Writes R. H., Wallingsford, Ky.

Take a square of Camphor Gum, and light it, leaving to burn slightly, then inhale the fumes, and repeat this for 10 minutes and it will break up colds. Writes Mrs. H. D., Galena, Ill.
Editor's Note—When camphor is burned it throws off a black soot that it very annoying. A better plan is to place the camphor on a hot plate or in boiling hot water.

Here is my home remedy. Take the Sumach Berries and steep or boil down into a syrup by using Sugar or Honey and take a spoonful when needed to stop Coughs, and it should do this in a short time. Writes Mrs. H. H., Wheeling, Mo.

For Colds—One drop of Iodine in a glass of water, once every hour for 3 hours, is very good. Writes Mrs. N. S.,

Here is a Cough recipe for your columns. Take bark of Wild Cherry, a small handful, same amount of Mullein Leaves, and Horehound, boil all in quart of water down to 1 pint. Strain and bottle, and take as often as necessary. Writes A. C. L., Murrycross, Ala.

Here is a good tea to use as a remedy for Colds, Fevers; steep a teaspoonful of Sweet Elder Flowers and Wild Ginger Root, equal parts in a cup of boiling water for 20 minutes, and drink all at once hot. Then go to bed and cover up warm. Writes A. O. R., Staples, Minn.

A real good Cough Syrup—Put 2 ounces of Flax Seed in a quart of water, boil 5 to 10 minutes. Put a handful of Hops in a quart of water, boil until all the strength is out. Then, strain the Flax Seed and Hops put together, then add ½ pint of good Horehound Tea to suit taste and juice of 2 small or 1 large Lemon, and Rock Candy, boil this mixture down to 1 quart, add enough Sugar to make a syrup, and honey could be added to the mixture also. Take 1 tablespoonful every 2 hours. Writes Mrs. B. M., Richmond, Va.

I am sending you a cold remedy which has been used in my family for forty years and always with good results. In one-half gallon of water put a box of Mullein, Old Field Balsam, Peppermint, Pennyroyal and a quarter box of Wild Cherry Bark. Boil down to a strong tea. Dose is a teacupful three or four times a day. Writes Mr. B. F. S., Marietta, Ohio.

For relief of coughs and colds, take hot tea at bedtime made from Coltsfoot. Writes Mrs. S. B. H., Charlotte, N. Car.

For Coughs and Colds—Take 1 or 2 Lemons, bake in the oven till tender, squeeze juice in a pint of Honey, stir thoroughly. Dose: One or 2 teaspoonfuls, I have used it for bad Colds and Coughs, and it is soothing to the throat.

Coughs—We have proved this remedy for coughs many times in rearing our family:

    1 box Seneca Snake Root
    1 box Horehound
    1 box Coltsfoot
    1 box Licorice

Put Licorice in water to soak until dissolved. Steep the herbs separate in 1 pint of water. When well steeped, strain together and boil down to 1 pint, add 1 pint New Orleans Molasses. It is ready for use. Dose—1 tablespoonful four times a day, or when the coughing spell comes on. Writes Mrs. A. E. B., Tujunga, Calif.

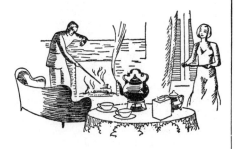

Coughs, Colds — Take Elecampane Root and make a strong tea, sweeten to taste. The amount of the root to be used is judged from the strength you wish to make the tea. The dose is a tablespoonful when needed. Writes W. D. T., Rose Hill, Ill.

Coughs—Take a double handful of Pine Needles to a quart of water, boil for 15 minutes, strain and add 1½ cups of sugar, boil to a thin syrup. This is excellent for coughs; take 2 teaspoonfuls night and morning. Writes F. S., Mena, Ark.

Coughs—Equal parts of Horehound, Elecampane Root, Comfrey Root, Spikenard and Wild Cherry. Boil in 1 gallon of water, down to 1 quart. Strain and add 1 pound Honey. Take a tablespoonful when cough is troublesome. Writes Mrs. A. W., Portsmouth, Ohio.

Spice Bitters—Use Golden Seal, Poplar Bark, Bayberry and Sassafras, Unicorn, Cloves, Capsicum, 4 ounces of each and 4 pounds of Sugar. Put to 1 ounce of this powder, 1 quart of Sweet Wine, let it stand a week or two before using it. Dose: One wineglassful 2 or 3 times a day. Writes Mrs. M. H. McG., Los Angeles, Calif.

This remedy was given by a woman through a magazine that all subscribers pass along every true and tested remedy for poor suffering humanity. It is a sure cure for Coughs, Lung Troubles, etc. It cured me of a hard persistent Cough. Take 2 ounces each Rue, Sarsaparilla, Horehound, Sage, Elecampane, and Indian Turnip. Mix well and divide it in half and make only half of it up at a time for it will likely sour if the whole amount is made up at once. Put into a granite kettle with 6 quarts of water, and boil down until when strained there will be a quart, add 1 pound of Sugar to this liquid and simmer until it looks about as thick as Cough Syrup. Dose: One tablespoonful before each meal. It may be necessary to begin with less and gradually increase to required amount. It is also a good tonic. An excellent plan is to smoke dried Horehound Leaves at the time of using this remedy too. Writes M. M., Stilwell, Okla.

Here is a cure for Croup, Colds and Hoarseness I wouldn't be without: Dissolve a cake of Camphor Gum in Kerosene and apply to throat, and it will give almost instant relief for Croup. Do not cover or it will blister the throat. Writes Mrs. W. R., Pershing, Iowa.

Editor's Note — Warning: For Membranous Croup give raw Pineapple juice and call a specialist without delay.

Coughs, Colds, Etc.—Maiden Hair Fern. A delicate species of fern. Leaves is the part used, and it is a tonic, expectorant, refrigerant, astringent. Excellent, cooling drink for fevers, coughs, colds, hoarseness, asthma, pleurisy, erysipelas. Used freely in decoction or syrup. Writes C. P. J. Bedford, Va.

Colds—For tight colds in the chest and lungs, take equal parts of each of the following herbs: Lungwort, Balm of Gilead Buds, Sweet Gum Bark, Wallwort, Water Plantain and Butterfly Weed. Mix these together, then take teaspoonful of the mixture and place in a teacup, filling the cup with boiling water, steep 30 minutes and drink the whole cupful as hot as possible upon retiring at night. Writes Mrs. S. E., Cincinnati, Ohio.

I am sending you a recipe my mother and I used for Colds and Coughs. Take a quart sauce pan half full of Cherry Bark, add water to fill the pan, and boil until it is a real dark color, strain and add enough Sugar to sweeten a little. Boil again until it becomes a syrup. Let cool and add ½ teaspoonful of Glycerine and ½ teaspoonful of Camphor and take a teaspoonful every half hour. I never use any other cough syrup for my children. Writes Mrs. A. S., So. Dennis, N. J.

Best Cough Syrup—
1 ounce Thoroughwort
1 ounce Slippery Elm
1 ounce Stick Licorice
1 ounce Flax Seed
Simmer all together in 1 quart of water until strength is extracted. Then strain and add 1 pint of Molasses and ½ lb. of Sugar. When cold bottle tightly. Dose: 1 teaspoonful as needed. Writes Mrs. J. J. S.

For Coughs—Here is an excellent remedy. Take Tamarack Bark about 2 handfuls and steep in water enough to make 1 quart, also about a pint basin of Hops, then boil in water enough to make another quart, add 1 cup dark Molasses, 2 cups of Sugar, simmer down to 1 quart. Have given this medicine to several people and they all say it is fine. One lady used it that was troubled with Bronchitis and she said it was the best remedy she had found. Writes Mrs. W. E. H., Bentley, Mich.

Here is a Recipe for Cough Syrup— Take double handful of the Holly Leaves, also a large handful of Mullein, and a large handful of Wild Cherry Bark, pour over this half gallon of cold water. Place over the fire and boil down to 1 quart, then strain, add 1 cupful of Granulated Sugar and boil again until you have a pint, cool, and bottle. Dose for adults is 1 tablespoonful every 4 hours, while for children, 1 teaspoonful every 4 hours. I have tried this myself many times and have never yet known it to fail in curing a Cough. Writes Mrs. J. H., Barthell, Ky.

For Coughs due to Colds—Put a medium size handful of Wild Cherry Bark, a medium size handful of Horehound and a medium size handful of Pennyroyal Leaves in 1 quart of water, boil for 15 minutes, strain, put 1 pound of Sugar in the liquid and boil down to 1 pint or until it becomes a syrup. Take a teaspoonful at a time when needed. Writes D. M., Mapleville, Md.

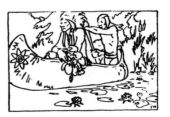

Another Cough Remedy you may say, but a good one.
Use Horehound Leaves, Hops, Wild Cherry Bark, Chestnut Leaves, in equal parts, and a pound of dark Brown Sugar to 1 quart of water, boil to thick syrup. The dose is a teaspoonful as often as needed. Writes Mrs. L. D., Peculiar, Mo.

I am sending you a good Cough Medicine. I have used it myself and have given it to others that had a bad cough after Pneumonia and it cured their cough. Boil 1 ounce or 4 tablespoonfuls of Flax Seed in a quart of water for ½ an hour, strain and add to the liquid the juice of 2 Lemons and ½ pound of Rock Candy. If there is a soreness and general weakness from the cough add ½ an ounce of Powdered Gum Arabic. Writes Miss B. T., Richmond, Ind.

I wish to tell you what we find about Garlic. We eat it by the spoonful for Colds. Those who do not like the taste, I recommend that they take a mealy, baked potato, open it so it is fluffy and put the Garlic in it and douse with either butter or gravy. You can then swallow it without chewing and do not notice it at all. It will stop a cold in the head and throat in a few days and prevent one for some time after. We eat it in the winter for that purpose. Writes C. L. B., North Fork, Calif.

Make a tea of Sycamore Bark and Chips; boil until dark red and sweeten and drink for Colds. Writes Mrs. H. T. B., Potosi, Mo.

Editor's Note—If you want results from herbs, you must positively get them fresh.

Here is Mother's Recipe for Coughs— Take the Shaggy Hickory Bark, boil in water until the juice is dark brown, strain, put in Sugar to make a syrup, and take a teaspoonful every few hours. Writes Mrs. G. E. S., LaFayette, Ga.

When you have a cold get dry Mullein leaves and smoke them. Roll them into a cigarette. Writes C. H. W., Bennell, Fla.

I am sending you a cold remedy which has been used in my family for forty years and always with good results. In one-half gallon of water put a box of Mullein, Old Field Balsam, Peppermint, Pennyroyal and a quarter box of Wild Cherry Bark. Boil down to a strong tea. Dose is a teacupful three or four times a day. Writes Mr. B. F. S., Marietta, Ohio.

Here is a Cough Syrup that cured my uncle when it was said to be in the first stages of Consumption. Take 1 package of Boneset, and a pound of Sugar, boil to a syrup. Take a mouthful as often as desired. Writes Mrs. W. W., Fremont, Neb.

An excellent Cough Syrup can be made from equal parts Mullein and Horehound steeped in sufficient water to make a strong tea. Strain, add a cupful of Sugar to each cupful of tea, and cook until it is a thick syrup, take as often as needed, and it is harmless. Writes Mrs. M. C., Clover Lick, W. Va.

I want to say that Wallwort is great for Colds. Writes F. F. P., Wilton Junction, Iowa.

Editor's Note—Yep. Make it into a tea and drink plenty of it. A teaspoonful to a cup of boiling water.

Take equal parts of Hickory Bark, Mullein Leaves and Seven Barks, put in 3 quarts of water, boil for 2 hours, strain and put Sugar in, then boil down to a pint of Syrup; very good for Chronic Coughs. Writes F. W., Elmer, Mo.

Am sending you a formula for a good Cough Remedy.
2 ounces Horehound
2 ounces Mullein
2 ounces Flax Seed
Put in 1 quart of water and boil down to a pint, add Honey to taste. Take tablespoonful at a dose as needed. Writes F. G., Columbus, Ohio.

Cough Syrup—Take equal parts of Wild Cherry Bark, Mullein Leaves, Horehound, and boil all together to make tea and strain, then add Sugar or Honey to make the syrup. Writes Mrs. J. S. B., Whitwell, Tenn.

Prescription for Coughs, Congestion, Inflammation of the Lungs, etc.—Which has been used successfully and handed down through 3 or 4 generations, and even cured Tuberculosis, when doctors in large cities said there was no help for them at all and that patient could not live. Take a good handful of the dried Elecampane Root, put in granite ware vessel, and put on enough water to make a quart of tea when steeped. Let steep slowly for 3 or 4 hours, but do not let it boil. Strain, and to a quart of tea add a cup of strained Honey, 1 teaspoonful Cayenne Pepper. The dose is 1 tablespoonful 4 or 5 times a day, and one upon going to bed. If you bottle this article as you should, then shake it well before you use it. Writes W. E. F., Ontario, Center, N. Y.

Mother rubbed the children's chest with Goose Grease for Colds, and I know it is good. Have also heard that a drop of the Goose Fat dropped in the eye affected with Cataract will cure it, if used every day until cured. Writes Mrs. J. H., Portland, Ore.

My folks would get the Indian Turnip, dry it, and in the winter they would grate it, mix with Honey and give for Coughs and Colds. I am sure if others would use it, even if they purchase it, it would be of service. Writes Mrs. M. E., Paxton, Ill.

Take the Elder Flowers, place in a vessel and pour boiling water on them. This gives off steam and when inhaled is excellent for tight Cold on chest. Writes W. H. M., Brookville, Kan.

I am sending you a recipe that I have tried, and many of my friends have tried also, and find it a real cure for Coughs of all kinds, including Whooping Cough. Take equal parts of Red Clover Flowers, and Sunflower Seeds. If the Sunflower Seeds are whole, chop them up and then make into a strong tea; later make into thick syrup and give a teaspoonful every hour. Writes Mrs. C. G., Ellington, Mo.

For Cold or Stopped Up Head—Put 1 teaspoonful of Camphor in a cup of boiling hot water, inhale this steam, and you will find it surely does help. Writes Mrs. M. C. P., Shelbyville, Tenn.

Here Is Another Recipe for Colds—Just make a tea of Witch Hazel and sweeten and drink at bed time. This surely is good for bad colds. Writes Mrs. E. C., Slagle, La.

Indian Cough Syrup—Elecampane and Indian Turnip, 1 ounce each and a pint of Honey. Steep the Elecampane and Indian Turnip in ½ pint of hot water for ½ hour, then add the Honey after it has been strained, and the dose is 1 tablespoonful as often as cough or tickling requires it, and take at least 3 or 4 times a day. Writes A. D., Lebanon, Ore.

There are many Cough Remedies and I want to contribute mine. Cough Syrup. One box Life Everlasting, 1 box Boneset, to a half gallon of water, boil down to 1 quart, then strain, and add 1 cup Sugar, boil down to 1 pint. Writes M. H., New Ross, Ind.

Take a cloth, flannel one if to be had, and grease thoroughly, then sprinkle thick with Nutmeg, and place on the throat and chest, and in a short time will relieve Colds or Croup. Writes Mrs. W. P., Cloverdale, Ind.

Editor's Note—But not membranous croup. Call a doctor.

A Cough Remedy very serviceable for Bronchitis—One package Elecampane, 1 package Spikenard, Horehound, Comfrey and Wild Cherry and a ½ lb. of Rock Candy. Put roots in 1½ gallons water, boil down to a pint, strain, add the Rock Candy. A half pint of Honey can be added instead of the Rock Candy. The dose is a tablespoonful every 3 hours, and children according to their age. Writes Mrs. E. W., Dayton, Ohio.

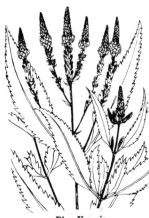

Blue Vervain

Blue Vervain (Verbena Hastata) is the best medical herb that grows out of the earth. I have frequently used it for Colds, and Suppressed Menstruation without a single failure. Writes J. R. R., Hot Springs, Ark.

Horseradish Root is not only a food but made into a tea and then add Sugar to make a thin syrup is fine for sore throat, and cold in the chest. Drink a tablespoonful 3 times a day or oftener. Writes S. H., Vallejo, Calif.

Recipe for Cough Medicine—Take a quart of Hops and place in quart of water, boil down to a pint, strain, add a pint of Vinegar and some Sugar, and boil down to a pint. Take a teaspoonful as a dose, and as the cough gets lighter, let up. This is my mother's old and tried remedy. Writes J. S., Oregon, Ill.

I am giving you a recipe for a Cold. Take a handful of dried Mint Leaves (Spearmint) put in a kettle and pour on enough hot water to make about 2 pints of tea. Cover and let steep for about 15 minutes. Drink this warm before retiring. A little Sugar may be added to sweeten if you desire. It does not matter how much you use of this but 2 cupfuls is plenty. If it doesn't help the first night, try it again. We have used it for a long time, and find it excellent. Writes K. G., Clayton, Wis.

An Old Time Cough Remedy—Use 1 ounce of Horehound and Mullein Leaves to 2 pints of boiling water, let steep 20 minutes, then add a pound of Brown Sugar, 2 ounces of Syrup of Tar, and 4 ounces of Honey. The dose is a teaspoonful every 2 hours until relieved. Writes J. D. M., Pennsboro, W. Va.

A Recipe for Coughs—Take a tablespoonful of Iceland Moss, put in cup and pour boiling water over it and let stand for about 10 minutes. Drink as often through the day as needed. This has been tried repeatedly and if taken regularly will cure the worst cough. Writes Mrs. M. McB., McMinnville, Ore.

For Colds—Take a handful of Dittany to a pint of water, boil 2 or 3 minutes until strength is out of the leaves. Take half for the dose and go to bed and cover up well. May sweeten if you desire, and of course in giving to children, give less according to their age. Writes J. W. W., West, Va.

Take Sycamore Chips, something like a quart of them, cover with water and boil, cook for 4 hours, then strain, add enough Sugar to make the syrup and take 3 or 4 times a day, or even oftener if needed, as it is harmless but is a very good Cough Remedy. Writes Mrs. E. R., Lamar, Ark.

For a Cold in the Chest or Cough— Make a strong tea of Horehound Leaves, mix with equal amount of cooking molasses and boil until very thick and makes a hard candy, which children as well as grown-ups like. Writes M. P., Cleveland, Ohio.

Severe Coughs and Bronchial Troubles —Take an ounce of the following: Horehound, Irish Moss, Flax Seed, Boneset and Licorice, and place in a pan, with a gallon of cold water. Put this on the back of the stove and let it simmer slowly until reduced to one-half gallon. Strain and bottle. Dose— 1 wineglassful 3 times a day. Add sugar if desired. This is one of the best home remedies for such purposes. Writes A. B., Canton, Ohio.

Tea made from Basswood Tree Blossoms is good for breaking up colds, if taken hot before retiring. It has a mild, pleasant taste similar to honey. Writes C. B., Browerville, Minn.

For a Bad Cold—Steep a tea from Smartweed. Drink hot before you go to bed and several cupfuls during the day. I helped many with this where other remedies failed. Writes Mrs. E. K. D., Willowemoc, N. Y.

Make two bags around 3 inches in diameter to go around the entire throat. Make a poultice of equal parts of Flax Seed, Corn Meal and Onions. Fill the bag and apply as hot as can be borne and change about every 20 minutes until the Cold loosens. In my child's case, which was severe, it took about 6 hours. Writes Mrs. F. L. C., Omar, N. Y.

For Coughs and Colds—Take equal parts of Wild Cherry Bark, Life Everlasting and Mullein. Simmer down to a strong tea, add sugar, or honey, and boil until it becomes a thick syrup. Take several teaspoonfuls a day. It is harmless and very good. Writes Mrs. W. P. B., Nauvoo, Ill.
Editor's Note—About 1 package of each to a quart of water—boiled down to a pint.

Use equal parts Hops, Tamarack Bark, and cooking molasses, and a cup of brown sugar. Boil to a syrup and take three or four times daily as a Cough Syrup. Writes Mrs. U., Rhodes, Mich.

For Colds—Make a tea of equal parts of Mountain or American Dittany and Sumach Berries. Drink while hot. Writes Mrs. G. G. D., Coldwater, Mo.

Use a quart of Horehound in a quart of water. Bring to the boiling point, then strain and when cool add 2 cups of brown sugar and make into a syrup. When cold, add the juice of 3 lemons. For Colds, take a teaspoonful as desired. Writes M. L. P., Traverse City, Mich.

Here Is a Good Remedy for a Cold— Eat a little Garlic twice a day or more, for two or three weeks, and you will have no more trouble with your cold. Writes K. A. K., Lancaster, Minn.
Editor's Note—And stay away from the fair sex while taking this treatment. I am telling you something now.

Cough Syrup—Use Cherry Bark, Hickory Bark, Mullein Leaves, Horehound, and Life Everlasting, a large handful of each, boil in 3 quarts of water until a strong tea is made; strain and sweeten, and boil down with sugar to a syrup. We like this better than any other cough syrup. Writes Mrs. W. R., Dillen, Ark.

During the World War when the Flu raged, I became so run down that when the Flu finally got me it left one lung bad.
I doctored with a specialist, but was only getting worse gradually, and, living in a city, I couldn't be out as much as I should. At last I told the doctor I could not afford his treatment any longer, as I was not getting any better. He told me that if I could be where I could live out of doors and rough it, and have fresh fruits, greens, vegetables and eggs and milk that I would start to gain. I left and came back to my old home town and hired a tent and slept out for two years.
I took Mullein Leaves and steeped it a long time, then strained it and added 2 lemons sliced thin, half a cup of whole Flax Seed and half a pound of Honey in the Comb. I let it all simmer slowly until it got down like syrup, then strained again and bottled it. I have taken this medicine a great deal, and it stopped the Cough and I began to gain in strength. Writes H. M. M., Manchester Depot, Vt.

For small children that have a Cold and phlegm in their throat and can't cough it up, give them Lobelia Tea to make them vomit. This will clear the throat of the phlegm. Lobelia is also good for Whooping Cough. Writes M. S. S., Gove, Kan.
Editor's Note—Lobelia Tea is made by steeping a teaspoonful of the herb in a cup of boiling hot water. Let it stand until cool. Dose, 1 to 2 tablespoonfuls for children.

Cough Remedy—To a handful of Horehound add a pint of water, boil until essence is boiled out of the herb. Then sweeten with enough sugar to make a thick syrup. Take a spoonful of this syrup often. Writes Mrs. U. H., Marion, Ind.

Coughs and Colds—Here is a formula for a Cough and Cold remedy that is unexcelled. I have used this for several years without a failure. Far superior to advertised cough remedies.

1 ounce Elecampane
1 ounce Wild Cherry Bark
1 ounce White Pine
1 ounce Mullein
1 ounce Horehound

Place all these herbs in a quart of water and boil down to 1 pint, add sugar to make a syrup. The dose is, for adults, 1 tablespoonful three times a day or as often as the cough is troublesome; for children, 1 teaspoonful as often as needed.

Here Is a Tried and True Recipe for a Bad Cough—I cured my son of one of over a year's standing. Please print this in your good Almanac for the good of humanity. Take the rough or shaggy bark off of Hickory Trees, boil until strength is all out and add sugar after straining the juice. Boil to a thin syrup and take a tablespoonful three or four times daily. It will soon break up a stubborn bad Cough. Writes Mrs. M. D., Bonnie, W. Va.

Editor's Note—I would add an equal part of Coltsfoot Leaves—they are wonderful.

For Coughs—Take Sage, Willow, Horehound, in equal parts, with boiling water, steep until cool, or the strength is extracted, strain, add syrup or honey, and it is excellent for coughs. Writes O. C. C., Marietta, Ga.

There are many Cough remedies but I will send you mine. A 25c box of Horehound, and half box of Lobelia (25c size), cover with a quart of boiling water and simmer down to a pint, strain and add a pint of white sugar and boil to a thin syrup. This is all we ever use for cough syrup and think it is fine. Writes Mrs. E. J., Neillsville, Wis.

For Coughs and Colds—Enclosed you will find a recipe for coughs and colds. Use 1 quart of Mullein and 2 quarts of water, boil down to 1 quart, strain, add a pound of sugar, and use three times daily. This has cured coughs where doctors have failed. Writes H. O. F., York, Pa.

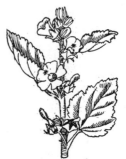

Marshmallow

Cold Remedy—Used in the family for 100 years: Butterfly Weed Root Tea. Used for colds, croup, pneumonia and other lung troubles. Of the dried roots use about 1 teaspoonful to 1 cupful of boiling water, let steep for 15 minutes and drink at bed time for cold. But for one confined to bed, 1 cupful three times a day until relieved. Very valuable. Rub with the following: Melt a small bottle of vaseline, empty, refill with turpentine, empty and refill with kerosene, making three ingredients in equal parts. Mix all three and rub the patient, as well as give the Butterfly Weed Root tea. Will save pneumonia patient after doctor has given up. Writes Mrs. E. B., Macon, Ga.

For Coughs—Equal parts of Horehound, Elecampane Root, Comfrey Root, Spikenard and Wild Cherry. Boil in 1 gallon of water, down to 1 quart. Strain and add 1 pound Honey. Take a tablespoonful when cough is troublesome. Writes Mrs. A. W., Portsmouth, Ohio.

Sacred Bark and Dandelion have nearly cured my sister of the worst cough I ever knew any one to have. She was threatened with Asthma, also, but I believe she will soon be entirely well of it. Writes Miss M. H. J., Monticello, Ark.

Editor's Note—Coughwort leaves or Mullein are still better.

Cough Syrup—Elecampane Root and Indian Turnip, 1 ounce of each and a pint of honey, steep thoroughly and strain. Dose—a teaspoonful or tablespoonful three or four times a day. Writes N. M. H., Andrews, Ind.

Chew Calamus Roots for a Cough—Cherry Bark boiled in molasses until you have a syrup is excellent for coughs too.

Colds—Take a large handful of White Pine Needles, place in about a pint of hot water, let simmer a few minutes. Drink of this tea at night, just before retiring. It is a good remedy for colds. Writes J. W. C., Callaway, Va.

Colds—Here is a very old but a good effective recipe. Take a half teaspoonful of Ginger, 1½ teaspoonfuls of sugar, mix thoroughly in a cup of luke-warm water, and it will break up a most persistent cold if taken at bed time. This is perfectly harmless and brings good results. Writes L. L. M., Bridgton, Me.

Editor's Note—Add Juniper Berries and Elder Flowers and you improve this wonderfully.

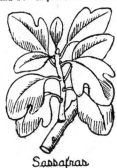

Sassafras

For Cough—Take the blossoms of Basswood and blossoms of Elder Berry, dried, and take a pinch of each, put in vessel that holds about a quart of water, boil it a little while, then strain, and use liquid in place of water. Writes M. S., Thorp, Wis.

Colds—When a baby has a bad cold and it is pretty tight, make a nutmeg poultice by greasing a rag and sprinkle thickly with grated Nutmeg. Then sew all around so as to keep from sifting out, put one on the chest and another on the back. I have raised five children and never used anything else. Writes Mrs. J. P. S., New Bethlehem, Pa.

Colds—I am sending you a recipe that I do not believe has been mentioned, and which is Sassafras used for breaking up colds. Take a handful of Sassafras to a quart of water, and boil it to about a pint, and drink a cupful hot before going to bed. Continue until you are relieved from the cold. I have tried it many times and it proved successful. Writes C. R., Indiana, Pa.

Editor's Note—This is good but could be improved with Elder flowers and Juniper berries.

Dry Cough—Take powdered Gum Arabic, half ounce; Licorice, half ounce; dissolve the gum first in warm water, squeeze in the juice of a lemon, then add squills made into syrup, about 1 teaspoonful, and cork all in a bottle. Shake well before using and take 1 teaspoonful when the Cough is troublesome.

Coughs and Colds—Here is a good tea for Colds and Coughs, which is an old family recipe of ours given by a German doctor:

1 ounce Iceland Moss
3 teaspoons Sweet Wood or Licorice
3 teaspoons Marshmallow
4 heaping teaspoons Brown Sugar
1 Lemon sliced

Boil all for 5 minutes, drink warm at bed time and cool during the day. Writes Mrs. B. M. S., Allentown, Pa.

Colds—When the children have a cold we slice an onion, heap with sugar, let stand a while, then the children can eat all they want. Writes Mrs. J. B. G., Drummond, Wis.

Cough Syrup—This syrup has helped to rid others and myself of severe coughs. Take 2 ounces of Boneset, 1 ounce Sweet Fern, and 2 ounces of Mullein, sugar enough to make a thin syrup, and take 1 teaspoonful four times a day, before or after meals, and at bedtime. Writes Mrs. L. A. S., Eagle River, Wis.

Here is a recipe for colds, coughs and hoarseness. The following is soothing, and healing to most ordinary coughs and colds. One pint of boiling water, two ounces whole flaxseed and the juice of two lemons and sugar. Writes Mrs. A. B., Harper, Wash.

Bull Nettle Cough Syrup—Take a large handful of the dried roots of Bull Nettle, put in a quart of water, boil down to a pint and strain. Add enough sugar and boil to a syrup. Take a tablespoonful every hour until relieved. Dose—for children, 1 teaspoonful every hour. Writes Miss T. R., Henryville, Tenn.

A tea made from the leaves of Yerba Santa is very good for colds and cough. I have a neighbor who uses it exclusively and she claims that if taken at the very beginning of a cold, the cold will be stopped. Writes Mrs. G. T., Tujunga, Calif.

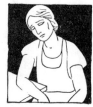

CONSTIPATION

Constipation is usually caused by overlooking matters of hygiene, such as want of sufficient exercise, drinking too little water, too concentrated a diet, irregularities in the time of eating and of going to the toilet; also eating foods that do not contain the necessary amount of roughage, such as bran and coarse vegetables.

The symptoms of constipation are sluggishness, drowsiness, dizziness, no appetite, bad taste in the mouth, bad breath, a full feeling on the abdomen, which is hard upon pressure, and is sometimes distended; there may also be headache and muddy or sallow complexion.

Psylla or Psyllium (Plantago Psyllium)—This product owes its properties to the extraordinary richness in a peculiar mucilaginous substance which the small seeds give out when immersed in water and when eaten gives both bulk and lubrication to food eaten, swelling the same to many times the original size and stimulates the intestines, and when regularly used with our Laxative Tea, Psyllium will secure frequent well-formed stools sometimes as many as three a day.

In taking Psyllium— best results will be obtained in placing 1 heaping tablespoon of the seed in a half cupful of the hot tea, stir well until thoroughly mixed. Do this upon retiring at night.

Psylla Seeds—A drugless laxative, relieves constipation, and an internal lubricant superior to mineral oil. Effective bowel regulator.

Mandrake—One of the best regulators for liver and bowels; a safe and sure physic, often mixed with Senna Leaves. Valuable in jaundice, bilious and intermittent fever, or wherever a powerful cathartic is required.

It has been proven by medical authorities that undigested food had been known to remain in the intestines from two weeks to three months, and even a year. This foul matter forms a coating in the intestines and stomach and even deposits what is commonly known as tartar as on the back of the teeth. The delicate passages through which the bile, juices, etc., pass from the liver and other organs are choked up.

Absorption and secretion are suspended, or partly so.

The stomach and intestines are unable to digest the food properly.

The liver is clogged and overloaded with bile.

The kidneys are filled with decayed tissue and dead corpuscles.

And the blood, which should be filtered and purified, becomes contaminated and poisoned and is pumped through the heart to every conceivable portion of the body from the brain to the toes.

It is not hard to see that such blood, instead of building and repairing the tissues of the body, can only poison the entire system.

It is of prime importance, therefore, that the bowels are put in good condition before attempting to cure any disease of any kind. The formula below is a scientific combination of natural herbs which will prove a revelation to those afflicted with habitual constipation.

For constipation, put 5 or 6 Senna Pods in a glass of cold water at night, drink first thing in the morning, fill glass again, drink at night—throw away and start over again, regulating the number of pods. Writes E. L. M., Oxford, Mass.

Peach Leaves are laxative, and have a sedative influence over the nervous system. They have been used for worms with success. For irritability of the bladder in sick stomach, and in whooping cough, make a tea of one-half of an ounce of the dried leaves in a pint of boiling water. Dose—Take a tablespoonful 3 times daily. My parents used these for several years and found to be a success. Writes E. C. V., Selma, Calif.

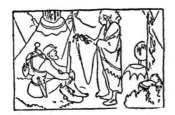

Yarrow boiled and thickened with meal and applied to the stomach will cause movement from the bowels. Writes Mrs. J. H., Tunis, N. C.

Editor's Note—I do not understand just how it can be done.

I can't praise Sacred Bark Tea too much as a remedy for Constipation. I am recommending it to all my friends and neighbors who suffer in that manner. It is especially useful in pregnancy where a gentle but effective laxative is needed almost daily. The pleasant taste, together with its non-griping results is something to be appreciated. Writes Mrs. J. L., Scobey, Mont.

Editor's Note—What do you mean "pleasant taste"? It is as bitter as gall—but good.

For Constipation in children or anyone use Catnip Tea, sweetened, hot, upon retiring and it will make the bowels regular. Children love it. I even give it to children when they feel cross in the day time. Writes Mrs. W. B. Jr., West De Pere, Wis.

Purge—A strong purge is made from the root of Blue Flag, even taken in small quantities, especially when fresh. The inner bark of common Elder is a strong purge, too. Write W. J. P., Whitestone, L. I., N. Y.

Senna Leaves in a tea is a good purgative. Writes Miss E. N., Cowell, Ark.

Red Clover Blossoms made into a strong tea and used to drink the same as table tea will empty the bowels as freely as a dose of salts. Writes A. E. B., Plato, Mo.

Editor's Note—And is far more harmless.

Here Is My Recipe for Constipation— 1 teaspoonful of whole Flax Seed to be eaten raw upon retiring. Writes Mrs. T. M. K., Fairbault, Minn.

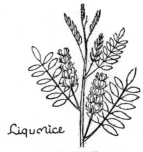

Liquorice

A Laxative Compound—3 parts Sweet Wood and Licorice Root, 2 Colic Root and Senna Leaves and 1 Buckthorn Bark. Mix well as you do all these formulas, put 3 tablespoonfuls into a quart of boiling water, let stand over night, then take a wineglassful morning and evening. If it moves the bowels too freely, then use only half the dose. Writes Dr. L. E., New Lexington, Ohio.

The inside bark of the Slippery Elm soaked in warm water is good for colitis. Writes W. W. C., Bassfield, Miss.

Noticed that you desire recipes, and I am sending you this recipe for Constipation. Take 1 or 2 teaspoonfuls of Flax Seed Meal, stir this into your breakfast food while it is yet warm, eat same as usual, continue this day after day, and you will soon find the stool to become more regular. This remedy is absolutely harmless, but you will find it very beneficial if kept up for some time. You may regulate the dose to suit yourself. Writes P. H. P., Robbinsdale, Minn.

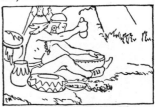

For Congested Bowels—Warm half pint or very near that amount of the best Olive Oil. Put in a fountain syringe and inject into bowel. It is best to raise the person a little so the oil will stay in the bowel, but if the pack is low down it won't stay. This is a sure remedy and will do the work. It takes a few hours for the oil to soften the stools, but if it stays in the bowel it will. I relieved many a person with this. Writes L. W., Cold Springs, Mo.

Here Is a Constipation Remedy—
Take 4 ounces of Senna Leaves, 1 pound of raisins and grind together in a meat grinder and then shape into small balls the size of a large marble. Eat one every other night, and drink 1 glass of hot water. The remedy is harmless. Writes O. R., Sturgeon Bay, Wis.

For Laxative—Take 1 pound Raisins, 1 pound Figs, and 1 ounce Senna, all ground together with 3 tablespoons of Olive Oil. Children are eager to take this. Writes Mrs. M. G. B., Selma, Ore.

Here is a recipe which should be in your columns, for I know it is good for Constipation and has helped many: Make a tea from Rhubarb Root and drink 1 cupful before retiring. You may put sugar in it as it is quite bitter. Writes Mrs. D. K., Merrill, Wis.

Take a tablespoonful of Senna Leaves, pour on a large cupful of boiling water, and let it stand for 2 hours. Wash and drain 24 prunes, strain the Senna, pour over the prunes, cover and let it simmer on stove until the prunes have taken up all the Senna juice. Then place in jar, eat 3 or 4 prunes before going to bed, also drink a cup of water after this. You cannot taste the Senna very much on the prunes. This is a very good remedy for Constipation. Writes E. A. P., Fort Dodge, Iowa.
Editor's Note—This should be very good.

Good for Constipation — Silkweed Roots, boil till water is black and drink a cupful during the day. Writes E. B., Garretts Bend, W. Va.
Black Root made and used in the same way is a good Laxative. Writes Mrs. R. M., Hazel, Ky.

For Constipation—1 ounce Senna Leaves, Licorice Bark and Cascara Bark. Boil all together, drink tea when needed. Writes G. S., Rockford, Ill.

A Recipe for Constipation—Make a tea from Peach Tree Leaves, and drink three times a day. Writes Mr. J. B. M., Spartanburg, S. C.

Old-Fashioned Fruit Laxative — 1 pound Prunes, ½ pound Figs, and the same amount of Dates and an ounce of Senna Leaves. Remove pits from fruit and chop altogether, mold into bars or small sticks and dry. Dose—a piece the size of a hickory nut for an adult, less for a child. This formula will keep all winter. Writes Mrs. M. P., Cleveland, Ohio.

Boneset Tea is a good remedy for Biliousness. Writes C. N. R., Woodhull, N. Y.

For Billiousness, take Black Root, made into a tea, and it will soon have you feeling fine. Writes Mr. P. W., Salem, Mo.

CONVULSIONS

I would just like to say a word about Skullcap. My daughter would have Convulsions almost every month, and I ordered a box of Skullcap and she hasn't had one since she has been taking it. Writes E. J., Orange, Va.

For a Baby with Convulsions—Put feet in hot water with plenty of Mustard added, or give a Mustard bath. Writes K. L., Winchester, Va.

For Convulsion in Children—Take Skullcap and steep a teaspoonful in a cup of hot water, strain, sweeten, give to the child all it will drink each day. It cured my grandson when everyone thought there was no hope, and also a neighbor's child. Writes Mrs. C. T., Barnesboro, Pa.

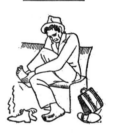

CORNS

Make a salve of Castor Oil and Soda for Corns. Submitted by Miss S. W., Cowan, Tenn.

For Corns and Callous on the Feet—Massage with Castor Oil once or twice a day and it will cause the corn to peel off in layers and leave a soft smooth skin, and the same with the Callous. Writes O. C. C., Marietta, Ga.

Sweet Gum Bark boiled into a strong tea and used on Corns will remove them. Writes N. R., Rammer, Tenn.

CRAMPS OR COLIC

Is generally due to Constipation, undigestible food, abnormal quantity of bile in the intestinal tract, etc. Symptoms are: Often intense cutting, twisting, pinching pains.

The Herb Doctor's choice of botanicals are: Fennel Seed, Anise Seed, Cardamon Seed, Chamomile Flowers, Wormwood, Sage, Cramp Bark.

Anise—A few drops of Anise Seed in hot water is good for colic; it may be sweetened too. Writes Mrs. G. E., Pt. Pleasant, N. Y.

Will send you a recipe for Leg Cramps: Take Olive Oil and rub in good under the foot, the arch of the foot, and it sure does the work. Writes G. U., Halsey, Ore.

Squaw Weed is very good for Cramps in the legs. Steep a handful of the herb in a cup of boiling water, and take a few sips through the day, or just chew the herb, and swallow the juice. It is also good for a woman after childbirth; if the flow stops, then drink this tea as hot as you can stand it, or if flowing too much, drink it cold. Writes Mrs. C. L. M., Palestine, Tex.
Editor's Note—Squaw Weed was used by our native Indians for this very purpose—that's how it got its name.

For Cramps, bathe the feet in Wintergreen Leaves, with a handful of common Salt, using the water just as warm as the flesh will stand, but don't wipe the water off; just let it dry. This was given me by an Indian woman 86 years old and a wonderful woman. Writes N. W., Alma Center, Wis.

A tea of the root of Devil Shoestring will cure any case of Colic, too. Writes R. E. H., Newton, N. C.
Editor's Note—Devil Shoestring Root has no outer bark. Would therefore suggest the use of the whole root.

Chew Calamus or Sweet Flag Root for a bad case of Colic. Writes R. B., Holly, Colo.

For Cramp Colic in an adult, chew a piece of Ginseng about 2 inches long; it is very good. Writes Miss E. B., Rocky Mount, Va.

Colic—Chew the roots of Bull Nettle and swallow the juice. The sufferer will be relieved in a few minutes. A heaping teaspoonful is sufficient for one chew.

Take a handful of Willow Twigs or Bark to a pint of water, boil strength out of it and add Sugar to sweeten. A little of this is of service for Colic in low intestines, and the lower part of abdomen. One dose is generally enough. The dose is half pint for adults and less for children, and take every 30 minutes, and there will be no return of Colic. Writes J. W. W., West, Va.

A small bag of Sulphur placed in bed will keep your feet from Cramping. Writes Mrs. A. E. A., Lincoln, Mich.
Editor's Note—By what secret power, I wonder.

For Cramp Colic—Chew a small piece of dried Calamus Root. Writes Mrs. O. C., White Water, Mo.

For Cramps in Stomach or Diarrhea—Take the Smartweed and make a tea and drink a swallow at a time throughout the day until relieved. Writes Mrs. J. A., Ft. Recovery, Ohio.

Cramping Pains caused from childbirth. Use equal parts, German Chamomile Flowers, and Valerian Root, mix well and then use into a strong tea, drink hot every 30 minutes. It surely should do the work, as I have found it of service. Writes Mrs. M. P., Alabama City, Ala.

Eat a piece of Calamus Root to stop Cramps. Writes Mrs. H. T. B., Potosi, Mo.

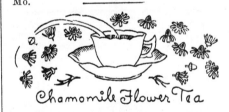

Chamomile Flower Tea

Cramps—Here is a recipe for Cramps and ailments of the stomach, also for Colds when you can not sleep. I am sure anyone will find it useful. Two teaspoonfuls of Catnip. Pour on 1 cup of boiling water, and let stand for a few minutes. Then drink contents hot, sweetened with sugar to suit yourself, at bedtime. Writes Mr. W. D., Matawan, N. J.

Samson Snake Root is good for Colic and Summer Complaint. You can get a piece, that is large pieces, also break up smaller, or obtain just tiny pieces, and swallow as you would a pill or tablets. Writes Mrs. P. B., De Funiak Springs, Fla.

CROUP

For Croup—Mix Pulverized Alum with strained Honey and give a teaspoonful every 30 minutes. It saved my child's life, and about 2 doses did the work. Writes Mrs. N. B., Ravenscroft, Tenn.

Having read your articles in the Almanac on Croup prevention, I thought I would tell you of my experience, for I have had wide experience with it in my family.

My child was taken sick, that was when we lived in Lansing, Mich., and we called a Dr. T., who was the head of the hospital. My wife remarked when he came next morning that the child had Croup last night. Dr. T. said, ''Croup is nothing. When the baby takes it, get cold water, not ice water, wet a cloth so it will not drip and put it on the throat and in a few minutes the Croup will be gone.'' That looked out of reason to me, and I said, ''Doctor, what has that to do with it?'' He explained that the blood is rushing to the throat and that will stop the rush of blood to those parts, and the croup should be gone in a few minutes. I tried it since with good results. So don't let your child suffer for the want of just cold water applied to the throat. Writes M. A. M., Rush, Ky.

Editor's Note—I doubt if this would have much effect on membraneous croup. Pineapple juice is my remedy.

I am sending a recipe for Croup that mother always used. I have known it to cure when all else failed: One teaspoonful (level) crushed Blood Root, ½ cup Vinegar, 4 teaspoonfuls Sugar. Heat this to the boiling point, strain and give from ¼ to 1 teaspoonful every half hour. Writes Mrs. B. N., Clay, W. Va.

Editor's Note—I cannot recommend this—Blood Root is very irritating and vinegar is not so good. Fresh pineapple juice is far better and absolutely harmless. The canned juice is no good. Better call a doctor. I read every one of these recipes and will not let one get by that I cannot approve.

Black Snake Root in a tea and sweetened to taste is very good for a child with Croup. Writes W. L. C., Louisa, Ky.

Editor's Note—All herb teas are made by placing a heaping teaspoonful of the herbs or herb mixture in a cup of boiling hot water. Let stand until cool and it is ready for use.

Croup—Take Marigold and make a tea, drink a third of a cupful till relieved. This was never found to fail. Writes J. K., Capehart, W. Va.

CUTS, SORES AND ULCERS

Here is a recipe that cured an old chronic Sore on a man, and it is also good for beasts: Take a pound of Red Oak Bark, put in a gallon of water, boil all the strength out, strain, and boil the ooze until it becomes thick. Use as a salve and spread on white cloth and apply to sore. It will draw and heal. Writes L. L., Wawrika, Okla.

Wash for Old Sores—I want to write you about the good merits of a real common plant that grows all round here called Cheese Plant. A certain friend of mine had a bad accident several years ago, cutting himself on the shins of his leg with glass. It was so sore that his leg got brown, bluish and open, running all the time. He tried all kinds of salves, including Sayman's, a very good salve. He was very stubborn about changing but at last I got him to bathe his leg in boiled up Cheese Plant, covering the sore entirely with the solution as hot as he could stand it, two or three times, and when it lost the pain, it started getting brighter in color and ready to heal up. Writes H. S., Sheboygan Falls, Wis.

As to Soap making, for several years I have gathered Bouncing Bet or Soap Flower, steeped it until the strength was out, strained it and added a ½ bar of good brown Soap, set it on the back of the stove until thickened and it made the nicest soft soap one could wish. You can use it as I did when I burned my two toes, tender as our eye, but I washed with the soap in the water, then poured pure Ironite over this, put thin cloth over it, put on my shoe and went about my business, that of looking after other people's ills.

I am sending this recipe for making the salve which I found such a necessity during the Civil War. I made the salve where I saw the need of it without cost for countless numbers, and all thought it wonderful. Take the Dwarf Elder Root and place with one teacup of Hog's Lard, about two large handfuls of the root, 1 tablespoonful water and a small lump of Rosin, the size of a bean. Put all in frying pan with low fire, keep stirring and turning, and when the bark is a nice brown, then strain as it is ready for use. Writes Mrs. M. H. G., New Orleans.

Here is a remedy that I did not see in your booklets: Take White Pine Bark and boil it into a strong tea, and apply to any kind of a sore, and it should heal it. Writes E. B., Cloverdale, Ala.

White Pine Pitch at 2 oz. for 25c made into a salve is an excellent remedy for healing Open Sores. Writes Mrs. O. F. E., White Cloud, Mich.

For Old Sores—Take Bitter Sweet Root Bark, boil in pure sweet lard. It is very healing. Will heal deep old sores where other remedies fail. Writes Mrs. J. M. Y., Laingsburg, Mich.

I want to send you a recipe for Varicose Ulcers. I had one last year and just bathed it in a weak solution of White Poplar Bark tea and then dusted on Slippery Elm powdered. The Slippery Elm acts as a poultice and draws out all the infection and heals up while you do your work, and you will not have to go to bed with same. Writes Mrs. G. W., Arcola, Sask., Canada.

Here is a recipe that we think is extra fine. It has cured Sores and Ulcers where nothing else did. Take a pint of Mutton Tallow, put in pan or skillet, cut up in small pieces Yellow Root and cook until it is a golden color. Perhaps a pint of fat would need two-thirds pint of the root. When done, strain and it is ready for use. It is fine. Writes Mrs. C. B., Sardis, Okla.

Sores—Make a strong tea of Red Oak Bark and bathe affected parts while the tea is hot. Writes Mrs. T. C., Keener, Ala.

An Obstinate Sore in the mouth may be healed by touching it with a lump of Alum 2 or 3 times a day. Writes Mrs. J. D. Mc., Lake Charles, La.

For drawing heat out of any chapped place, use the common Plantain Leaves, for they are very good, and are good for Burns, too. Writes Mrs. M. O., Chickamauga, Ga.

For an Old Running Sore, ground Flax Seed Poultice put on fresh every morning and evening until well, is very good. My leg was rare for about 2 years and almost eaten to the bone, when this helped. Writes W. S. N., Narrow, Ill.

My husband cut his knee open nearly to the bone, and the company he worked for wanted him to go to the hospital, but he would not until he used the salve he knew I always made and had on hand, for it is good for everything. Cuts, etc. This salve is made by getting the Balm of Gilead Buds and using together with pure Hog's Lard, frying down. Pine Pitch can be used in it too, for both are very good. Writes Mrs. J. N., Long Lake, Wis.

A Salve for Inflamed Sores—Take a pint of the buds of Balm Gilead, place in ½ lb. of sweet Cow Butter or Butter without Salt, fry till buds are brown and crisp, strain through a cloth and place in vessel it is to be kept in. It is fine for Cuts, Burns, and Leg Sores. Writes Mrs. W. D. J., Grayson, Ga.

Take Wood Betony, fry in Hog's Lard or unsalted Butter, and use this salve on Sores and Cuts. It will take out inflammation and cure. Writes A. J. R., Easton, Pa.

I have not seen anything about Charcoal for healing Open Sores in your "Almanac," so I am sending on this recipe. One Christmas I burned my finger on the top and it became a large blister. As I had to have my hands in water so much the blister came over and the skin rubbed off. It hurt awful, but I just tried to keep it dry as possible and put on Powdered Charcoal. It also healed my sister's bed sores after she had been an invalid for some time. Writes L. T., Marshfield, Wis.

Old Sores—For Old Sores and Inflammation, Catnip and Yeast Bread, boiled till a mush, bound on, will heal. Writes Mrs. L. L. E., Lyons, Ind.

I am sending you a recipe for a good salve for all kinds of Sores. Take a large chunk of Butter and put in it some Calendula Flowers and boil them in the Butter. Then when boiled strain through a cloth and put in quite a bit of Camphor to make it strong. Crush the Camphor before adding it. Let the salve harden and it will be ready for use. Writes Miss R. G., Balfour, N. D.

Here is a Remedy for Bed Sores—Dust the sore with Talcum Powder and use wool under the patient instead of cotton. A doctor said that if this is used a patient could lie in bed for years and not get a bed sore. Writes Mrs. M. J. B., Ypsilanti, Mich.

I am sending you a recipe for soreness and swelling of a wound caused by a nail or wire. Take the bark of Black Walnut, put the bark next to the flesh and bind it on. This sure draws, as we have tried it. Writes Mrs. F. B., Olney, Ill.

Fever Sores—To 1 pint of water, add ½ ounce of Clover Blossoms, and boil half an hour. Apply to the affected parts several times a day. Writes Mrs. M. T., Harrisburg, Ark.

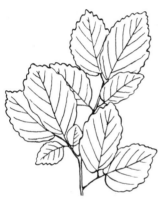

WITCH HAZEL

For Old Sores—Boil a large handful of Witch Hazel Bark in a pint of water until very strong, strain the tea and make a poultice by stirring in Wheat Bran until thick. Wet the poultice with the liquid. One woman had what three doctors called cancer of the hand, and advised her to take radium treatment. This poultice cured her. Writes Miss T. G. C., Basham, Va.

For Old Sores or Cuts—Take a pinch of dry Hops, add a pinch of tea, pour enough water (boiling) over them to saturate well. Let stand a while, but not long enough to cool, pour off water, place Hops and tea in a thin muslin bag, press out surplus water, so it won't run over the patient's face or clothes, bind on sore as hot as can be borne, renew occasionally. Used this when I cut myself in shaving and nothing would heal it only this remedy. Writes Mr. J. S., Arcadia, Ind.

Editor's Note—I believe if you would just soak the Hops in hot water and apply you would get the same results.

I am sending you a recipe for salve. Peel the root of Devils Shoestring, take equal parts of it and pure Hog's Lard and fry until brown. To add more peeling makes it stronger. This will cure any old sore, cuts and bruises, as I have never known it to fail. Writes R. E. H., Newton, N. C.

Old Chronic Sores—Take Sweet Apple Bark and Elder Bark, as much as you can hold between the thumb and first finger, also a cup of parched Oak, grind them, and then boil all together, putting in a cup of Hog's Lard and boil down to a salve, apply freely to sore twice daily. Writes A. H. C., Paris, Ark.

Healing Salve—Here is an herb that I have noticed which is not given much space in your book. Take a handful of Bitter Sweet, place in a frying pan with 1 pound of Beef Tallow, and fry for 15 or 20 minutes, drain off Tallow and add 10 drops of Carbolic Acid, and stir before it cools. This makes one of the best healing salves I ever used. Writes Charley C., Veedersburg, Ind.

Here is an ointment that I have used for years and my grandparents before me. I am now 62 years old and have never heard of anything as good as it. Take a large handful of the Balm Gilead Buds and 2 or 3 tablespoonfuls of fresh Lard, unsalted. Place the buds in the Lard and leave on the stove until all the strength is drawn from the buds, place in a tin box, and use on any fresh Cut and note how it will heal. Writes F. E. H., Glen Gardner, N. J.

Fever Sores—A wonderfully quick way to banish Sores is to wet the place with water or Olive Oil, then pack on as much Cornstarch as will stick. If the Sore has developed over night, the Olive Oil and Cornstarch will soon remove the swelling and discomfort. Writes Mrs. C. E. H., Bradenton, Fla.

For Running Sores—Soak Bay Leaves in cup of hot water for ½ hour, then bathe the sores with the water, when somewhat cooled off. Apply the soaked leaves to the running leg sores over night or keep Bay Leaves on for 24 hours, do this every night until cured.

DYSENTERY

This is a disease which is frequently fatal in summer and autumn. The first symptom is usually a sensation of heaviness and weight about the anus, soon followed by a desire for a stool. Or, there may be diarrhoea for a day or two, then the evacuations become more tedious, scanty and attended with straining and a desire to continue the effort, as if the evacuation could not be completed. The evacuations consist of mucous, mixed more or less with blood. Before and during evacuations there are violent cutting pains, pressing pains in the bowels, often very severe. In some cases there is violent fever; in others there is little or none.

Treatment—First wash out the bowels with Citrate of Magnesia, Salts or Castor Oil. Take Bismuth subnitrate tablets (price, 50c), 2 every half hour. This is not a medicine—merely a protective coating for the bowels. After the disease has run its course a weak tea of Blackberry Root as an astringent may be taken—this tea can gradually be taken stronger. The patient should keep quiet, avoid exercise or labor of any kind, lie down, and confine himself strictly, during the whole course of the disease, to a porridge made of milk and flour, well cooked, or to farina gruel, rice-water and boiled rice. No vegetables or fruit can be allowed; nor meat nor meat broths. Absolutely no sugar should be taken; even a small amount will aggravate the condition.

The Herb Doctor's choice of mild Astringents and Demulcents are: Blackberry Root, Wild Alum Root, Yarrow, Bilberry Leaves, Iceland Moss, Marshmallow, Wild Strawberry Leaves, Red Raspberry Leaves, Bayberry Bark, Benne Leaves, Butternut Bark, Columbo, Cheese Plant, Matico, Persimmon Bark, Rhubarb, St. Johnswort, Sumbul, Water Pepper, Water Avens Root.

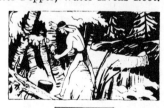

I recently cured myself of the worst Dysentery I ever had with one teaspoonful of Sassafras, Calamus, and Life Everlasting, steeped in 3 cupfuls of water. This did not leave me constipated either, as most do. Writes V. C. M.

Make a tea made of Pennyroyal, Ginger, put in kettle a large bunch of Pennyroyal, say a box, and only 6 small pieces of Ginger Root, and boil until strong, strain. Put this in 2 quarts, boil down to 1 quart, strain, add a teacupful of Honey and 1 of brown Sugar. Drink as often as you can until you drink the quart up, and you will find it very good for Bloody Flux. Writes Mrs. T. T., Dahlonega, Ga.

For Running Off the Bowels or Flux take a dose of strong hot Black Pepper Tea. This is an instant cure. Writes Mrs. F. N., Parks, Neb.

Try this for Flux in Children—Take a handful of Sweet Gum Bark, boil down and then put a little of this in their drinking water. Writes Mrs. L. C., Paris, Ark.

For an adult a teaspoonful of Ginger drunk in a cupful of water is good for Diarrhoea. Writes C. H. B., New Liberty, Mo.

I want to call your attention to Persimmon Bark for Diarrhoea. It is the finest you can use to check and regulate the bowels, so you can add it to your recipes. Steep and drink the bark as you would water. Writes R. D., Marlin, Texas.

Blackberry Root tea will cure Diarrhoea when all else fails. A cupful is all that is needed in most cases. Take a handful of the cut roots, boil in water enough to make a cupful. Boil for 1 hour, cool and drink. Writes Mrs. A. W., Meigs, Ga.

Wild Sage is very good for a child with Summer Complaint. Writes A. H., Peoria, Mo.

Blackberry Root—A favorite and valuable remedy for Cholera Infantum, Diarrhoea, Dysentery, and Relaxed Condition of Intestines in children.

Take Sampson Snake Root, make a tea and drink it through the day, a large swallow at a time, also at bed time. This is a very good remedy for Flux. Writes G. T. H., Trenton, Tenn.

My little girl, 1½ years of age, was taken with Diarrhoea and Vomiting, and I had her to two doctors and they both failed, but I tried the Blackberry Root Tea, and she began to get better and soon was well. Writes Mrs. L. L., Okeechobee, Fla.

Diarrhoea — Raspberry Leaves and Bayberry Bark, half ounce of each. Simmer in one and half pints of water for 20 minutes. Dose: Wineglassful every 2 or 3 hours. Cinnamon can be added if desired. Writes Mrs. E. F., Hugoton, Kan.

For Diarrhoea—Take Pennyroyal and make a tea of it and this has proved very good. I use the whole plant, with the exception of the roots. Writes Mrs. J. T., Colfax, Ill.

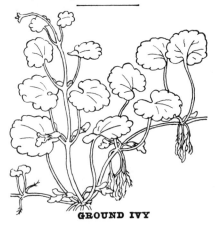

GROUND IVY

Boil a small handful of Ground Ivy and a small handful of Blackberry Root together, strain and sweeten the juice and give to teething babies as it is excellent for Diarrhoea. I tried it and it gave quick relief. Writes Mrs. L. G. R., Port Homer, Ohio.

Editor's Note—Diarrhoea must not be checked too suddenly. I would not use more than 1 teaspoonful to a cup of boiling water for babies.

For Diarrhoea—Take the root of Rhubarb. Make into a tea and take this during the day. This is a sure cure. Writes J. K., Turtle Lake, Wis.

Cranesbill, known also as Wild Alum and Crowfoot, is good for Diarrhoea. Take small doses of the crushed root or a decoction, 2 times a day for 3 days, discontinue for 3 days, and in the meantime take a mild Laxative. If not cured or very much better, repeat taking the remedy until desired results are obtained. Writes P. M. B., Corry, Pa.

For Bowel Troubles, use White Oak Bark, ½ cupful, 3 times a day until they are checked. Writes Mrs. E. M. S., Bernice, La.

When my boy was 18 months old he took Summer Complaint and 4 doctors gave him up. I went to a neighbor's one morning a. d he asked me how the boy was and I told him that he wasn't any better. The old man told me to get some Horsetail Grass and make him some tea, which I did. He got well, and I cured many people since then with this herb. Writes Mrs. W. H., Winnebago, Neb.

For Colic or Summer Complaint: Take 2 ounces of Elecampane Root, and boil down, use 1 tablespoonful every hour, and am sure the results will be beneficial. Writes I. W. W., Easton, Pa.

Here is a recipe for Summer Complaint which was given me by my old grandmother, and it has been used with good results in hundreds of cases. Take the leaves of the Horsetail Grass and steep into a tea. Drink one-third cupful every 4 hours until relieved. Writes Mr. L. W., Udall, Kan.

Take 2 tablespoonfuls Cinnamon, ¾ cup hot water. Let it simmer for about 40 minutes, drink as hot as can be borne, twice a day, eating only such as toasted bread, soft boiled eggs or oranges, and this should prove very good for Dysentery and Diarrhoea. Writes C. S., Allentown, Pa.

Summer Complaint—Here is an old remedy for Summer Complaint for children, which my mother used time and time again without fail. Take Meadow Blossom, also known as Life Everlasting, make a tea and let the child drink instead of water or other drinks. Writes E. L., Dillondale, Ohio.

Chronic Diarrhoea—Take equal parts of Cloves, Cinnamon, Peruvian Bark, all ground, and take 1 teaspoonful mixed with cold water, and drink. Three doses will generally cure the worst cases. Writes A. F., Muskegon, Mich.

Diarrhoea—A friend of mine told me that green Diarrhoea in babies could be cured by procuring Chamomile Flowers, making a tea of it, and in this tea, put some Baker's Chocolate (the unsweetened kind), and after mixing thoroughly, give to the baby about 2 or 3 spoonfuls every 1 or 2 hours. This, she said, saved her child while teething and that it could be used with safety. Of course the younger the child, the more diluted the tea must be. Writes Mrs. C. A., San Antonio, Tex.

Editor's Note—The Chamomile Flowers are harmless but chocolate should be used sparingly.

Sulphur made up with Sweet Cream is good remedy for the Flux. Writes L. W., Coldwater, Miss.

Arrow Root Tea is a fine help to anyone suffering from Dysentery and Diarrhoea. Other plain articles that often are of service are Peruvian Bark and Chamomile Tea. Writes Mrs. J. D. S., Golden City, Mo.

We have found Elder Flowers in a tea fine for Diarrohea and have known it to check babies in severe cases. It is also good for Hives. Writes Miss E. F., Lancaster, Ohio.

A sure relief for Dysentery or any kind of Bowel trouble. Make a tea of Comfrey Root and drink during the day. You will be relieved of the pains and misery. Writes Mrs. J. R. C., Greenville, S. C.

Diarrhoea—Take a dozen or more of Ragweed Leaves, and boil in a pint of water and drink a half saucerful 3 times a day. This will cure the worst kind of running off bowels. Can sweeten if desired. Writes Mrs. J. M., Corydon, Ind.

Editor's Note—Diarrhoea should not be checked too soon—rather remove the cause. Try Golden Seal and Elm Bark instead.

For Diarrhoea—Mix together 1 large teaspoonful of Cinnamon and 1 of Sugar, put in a cup and fill with boiling water, stir well. Drink all as hot as possible. Mostly 1 dose cures but repeat if necessary. Writes J. K., Summerville, Pa.

Summer Complaint—Take a handful of dry Raspberry Leaves, steep in half cup of water, drink a saucerful every 2 hours, and it will prove excellent for a child with Summer Complaint. Writes Mrs. D. T., Battletown, Ky.

Take a handful of Burdock Roots, make a tea and drink every 2 hours. It will prove excellent for Summer Complaint. Writes W. M. J., Coal Creek, Tenn.

Cinquefoil Tea is fine for Summer Complaint in children. Writes W. C. D., Bluefield, Va.

Wild Sage is very good for a child with Summer Complaint. Writes E. A. H., Peoria, Mo.

A tea of Rosin Weed is good for the Summer Complaint. Writes L. W., Coldwater, Miss.

For Summer Complaint, take a pint of boiling water, and a tablespoonful of ground Allspice, cover until cool, give 3 times or 4 times, a tablespoonful a day until the bowels are checked. Writes B. Q. S., Lakeview, Ohio.

Wild Alum Root—A powerful astringent and one of the best remedies for Diarrhoea, Chronic Dysentery, Cholera Infantum, Hemorrhage, etc. Improves the appetite and digestion and promotes nutrition. In Diarrhoea in children the decoction may be given in milk, which covers the taste. Produces sweating and applied externally to stop bleeding.

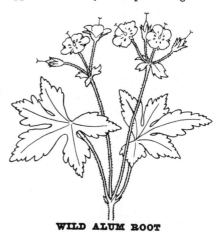

WILD ALUM ROOT

Here is an Old German Recipe for Diarrhoea or Summer Complaint—Take a handful of Pepper Grass and steep it in a pint of boiling water. Take a teacupful with each meal or after. I was under the care of a doctor when I first used this and I have used it ever since. It beats all doctor's stuff, and it is worth its weight in gold. Writes Mrs. E. S. M., Reading, Pa.

For Bloody Flux take a cupful of each of the inside bark of White Oak, Black Oak, Sweet Gum, and a cupful of the root of Blackberry. Boil into a strong infusion and sweeten with Honey. Take a swallow several times a day. Writes Mrs. D. H. H., Haleyville, Ala.

I have always believed in herbs and their uses so I will send you a recipe which I have tried and which I know will never fail for Flux. Take a handful of Sweet Gum Bark, and a handful of the Blackberry Roots, boil to a tea. Drink a cupful 3 times a day. Writes M. S., Louisville, Ky.

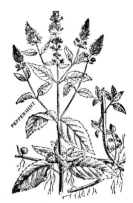

Dysentery—One tablespoonful Rhubarb Root, 1 teaspoonful Baking Soda, 1 teacup boiling water, and just a little Peppermint. Dose: One tablespoonful 3 times a day. Writes Mrs. C. H., Pilger, Neb.

I am sending you a recipe for Summer Complaint for children, which has been a life saver in our own family, two different times. Take 1 tablespoonful of whole Flax Seed, level and steep in a small cup of boiling water, and let stand 30 minutes, well covered up. Then take the liquid from this, 1 teaspoonful every hour for 3 doses, but not more than 1 teaspoonful, then ½ teaspoonful every 3 hours. Be careful to take but 1 or 2 doses of the ½ teaspoonful and then watch the bowels very closely and in a few hours the child will begin to improve and be well soon. Writes Mrs. E. M. V., Cornelius, Ore.

Editor's Note—I would add a little fresh lemon juice, it will surely improve this preparation.

For Summer Complaint, take a handful of Peach Tree Leaves, boil 15 minutes, in a pint of water, and drink in place of water. This recipe I have used with good results and it is harmless. Writes M. P. H., Waters, Ark.

For babies in their second summer for cutting teeth, take Plantain Leaves, make a tea and also give for Diarrhoea, it is fine. Writes R. S., Blaine, Ky.

Diarrhoea—Take 1 teaspoonful Raspberry Leaves in a cup of hot water, let steep 15 minutes, strain, sweeten and drink. Take this much 2 or 3 times a day. Writes Mrs. I. F., Ahsahka, Idaho.

Chewing the root of Ironweed will surely cure Diarrhoea. Writes M. N. D., Keo, Ark.

I am enclosing a sample of Bloody Flux Weed. It is used for Bloody Flux. It will cure it when everything else fails. Take about 1 handful to a pint of water and make a tea and drink a saucerful at a time. It has been known to cure very bad cases of it. (Sample was Woundwort.) Writes I. M., Sublette, Ill.

Here is one of the best recipes we have for Diarrhoea. Take Strawberry Leaves and use 1 teaspoonful into a pint of water, boil for a few minutes and for an adult, use 2 tablespoonfuls, but do not sweeten as it may have a tendency to inflame the bowels. To children give according to their ages, but I have found very good for chronic diarrhoea, dysentery and flux of the worst kind. Writes A. R., Florence, Kan.

Editor's Note—There is nothing growing that is more harmless than Strawberry leaves.

Does everyone know that a small plant known as Rupturewort, made into a tea and drank frequently is a sure cure for Diarrhoea. It is very palatable and infants take it as readily as any drink. This is an old Indian cure and may be relied upon. Writes Mrs. D. L., Fleming, Ohio.

The tea of Cinnamon Bark will cure all Bleeding Bowels. Writes Mrs. M. G. B., San Bernardino, Calif.

A recipe for Flux which saved my wife's life. Take Blackberry Root and make a strong tea. Drink this 3 or 4 times through the day. Also use Slippery Elm Bark in water, made weak, and this you can take in place of water you would otherwise drink. Writes G. A. G., Campbellsville, Ky.

For Diarrhoea—Take Allspice and boil in water, take when cold ½ teaspoonful of the spice to a half cupful water. Writes Mrs. F. E., Munday, Tex.

For Diarrhoea—Wild Strawberry is excellent and I have used it for years. Writes W. H. T., Ingersoll, Ont., Canada.

I had Chronic Diarrhoea, and used many remedies without relief, finally I tried equal parts of Wild Cherry and Wahoo Bark and made a syrup with Sugar. One and one-half pints cured me. Writes J. H. S., Arbaugh, Ark.

Recipe for Diarrhoea—Just chew a few leaves of Ragweed. For Flux make a tea of Flux Weed and usually one dose is sufficient. Writes M. C. P., Layette, Ohio.

DIABETES INSIPIDUS

Diabetes Insipidus is characterized by an excessive flow of urine. It is due to various causes, such as tumors, nervous diseases, malaria, cold and dampness and injury. The immediate cause is dilation of the renal vessels. Other symptoms are constipation, headaches, voracious appetite, skin dry and harsh, loss of memory and nervousness.

Treatment—Consult a specialist. Keep bowels open.

Oranges and grape fruit are excellent to combat acidosis. Abstain from sweets, pastries and eat plenty of fresh and cooked vegetables rich in minerals and chew them into liquid before swallowing.

The Herb Doctor's choice of botanicals containing organic minerals are: Horsetail Grass, Mormon Valley Herbs, Asparagus, Spinach, Globeflower Bark or Root, Huckleberry Leaves and Walnut Leaves.

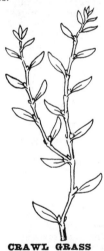

CRAWL GRASS

Here is another recipe for you. I met a man who years ago suffered from Diabetes. He went to his physician for treatment and then someone told him to use Horsetail Grass Tea. At the end of the week the doctor was pleased, but the man had not used the medicine from the doctor at all. But he did use it then for a week and the doctor was disappointed for the man was worse. Then this man gave up the doctor and continued to use the Horsetail Grass Tea, and for years the Diabetes never bothered him again. Writes W. A. W., Pottstown, Pa.

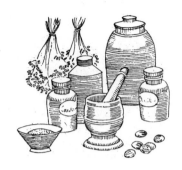

DIABETES

—Myrtillin Comp
   Huckleberry Leaves
   Globe Flower, bark of root
   Mistletoe
   Sassafras
   Licorice
   Juniper Berries

A mild Diuretic and Tonic. Excellent to diabetic patients as a substitute for tea or coffee.

   Bugle Weed Comp.
   Bugle Weed
   Couch Grass
   Mistletoe
   Star Root
   Althea Root
   Cheese Plant

A scientific compound of mild Diuretics and Demulcents.

   —Palmetto-Mistletoe Comp.

The original formula contained only Palmetto Berries and Mistletoe to be used in place of tea or coffee in cases of diabetes and kindred ailments.

   1 ounce Palmetto Berries
   2 ounces Mistletoe
   2 ounces Globe Flower Root
   2 ounces Cheese Plant
   1 ounce Sweet Fern

Place a teaspoonful in a cup of boiling water until cool. Drink 1 or 2 cupfuls a day.

This tea will show an improvement in patient's condition after 2 or 3 days —but it must be taken for a long time to get maximum results.

The Crawl Grass you offered me last year is very good, for I have found it a sure remedy for Diabetes. It took me six months to cure, but I can eat nearly everything now. Writes Mrs. C. L., Mahtowa, Minn.

DIABETES MELLITUS

Diabetes Mellitus, or Sugar Diabetes, is characterized by a constant presence of glucose in the urine, excessive urinary discharge, loss of flesh and strength, pain in the region of the kidneys, burning or itching of the urethra, excessive thirst, dry mouth, tongue irritable and beely red, often cracked, constipation, pale dry stools, occasionally there is diarrhoea. Differs from Bright's Disease by the absence of dropsy.

Treatment—Consult a specialist. Follow same instructions as for Diabetes Insipidus. Abstain from starchy foods. Eat vegetables rich in minerals such as lettuce, cucumbers, spinach, endive, celery, asparagus, sauerkraut, string beans, tomatoes and radishes.

Mr. H. gave me a box of Horsetail Grass and it has helped me wonderfully. I have Sugar Diabetes pretty bad but one box has helped me more than all the doctors, and although I have doctored a lot and got no relief until Mr. H. asked me to try this grass. Writes Mrs. W. B., Millville, Pa.

Editor's Note—Besides it is absolutely harmless—as are all of our roots and herbs.

Equal parts of Dog Grass, Althea, Uva Ursi, Poplar Bark and White Pine Needles, make an excellent remedy for diabetes. We do not believe it can be excelled. Writes Mrs. G. R., Oak Harbor, Ohio.

Take yellow root, make a tea, drink about 2 cups a day and it will cure sugar diabetes. Writes Mrs. E. G., Cherokee, S. C.

Huckleberry Leaves boiled for an hour or more will make a very good tea for Diabetes. After drinking this tea instead of water for several months there is no trace of sugar in the urine. This test was made one year after treatment. Writes C. C., Chicago, Ill.

Editor's Note—This is an old remedy of our grandfathers' days.

Diabetes Mellitus—Eat fruits, meats. Avoid bread, sweet and starchy foods. Abstain from all liquids during meals. Make a tea by steeping two teaspoonfuls Star Root and two teaspoonfuls Wild Alum Root into a pint of boiling water for 30 minutes.

Dose—One tablespoonful after each meal. This may also be taken as a weak tea, 1 teaspoonful of the mixed herbs in a pint of water, and taken in place of water to quench the thirst. J. D.

DROPSY

I am sending you an old recipe that has been used in our family for Dropsy for 50 years, and has cured when other medicines have failed. I am a nurse and have used it on many patients and it has never failed to clear the system of fluid, no matter what ailment has caused it. I had a patient that bursted and the fluid was draining from the openings and I used this remedy and in 10 days the swelling disappeared and the kidneys and liver were in good shape. Another patient had heart trouble and feet were swollen double their size. She had not walked for 14 months and with two weeks treatment she put on her shoes and in four weeks she left for California alone with the swelling all gone. This is not a cure-all but relieves the other cause by reducing the size of the kidneys, liver or heart and gives them a chance to heal. Steep a half-ounce of Wahoo Bark of Root in a pine of water and take a half cupful at a dose for a few days, 3 times a day. Then reduce the dose to about half that amount until the swelling is completely gone. This is not poisonous and may be taken as much as necessary without harm and with any medicines the doctor may be giving. Writes Mrs. R. V., East St. Louis, Ill.

Editor's Note—Wahoo is an old Indian remedy and harmless.

—Dwarf Elder-Kidney Wort
    Compound.....
    Kidney Wort
    Cheese Plant
    German Rue
    Dog Grass
    Juniper Berries
    Rosemary Leaves
    Sassafras Bark
    Bluet's Flowers
    Dwarf Elder

The main ingredient of this formula is Dwarf Elder, used for ages in the treatment of Dropsical Affections.

A word to diabetic sufferers. I was tested by an expert doctor in this disease and I tested nearly 5 per cent sugar. Used his treatment nearly 30 days with no results. Was advised to go for a regulated diet; reading over your booklets, saw where a lady used Crawl Grass, so I sent for two boxes at once and on November 20th started to use it, and on December 8th was sugar free. Writes J. F. G., Hillsdale, Mich.

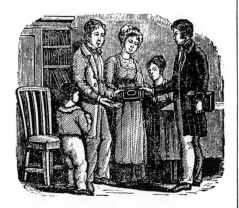

The following is a formula well worth adding to your "Almanac." It has surely helped many a one through this district:

    1 pound Black Walnut Bark
    1 pound Wild Cherry Bark
    1 pound White Ash Bark

Add 6 quarts of water, boil down to a quart, strain, add 1 pound of granulated Sugar, and some other preservative. This is for Dropsy, also Diabetes, and the dose is a wineglassful 3 times a day. This is an old remedy tested with much success, but no good if tobacco is used too strong or for too far advanced cases. Writes L. H., Elmira, Ont., Canada.

For Dropsy—Take Elder Bark, steep in a cup of water, when cool drink a cupful after each meal. Peach Tree Poultice made from the leaves of same is also good to stop swelling and fever. Writes M. B. S., Bessemer, Ala.

Dropsy and Dropsical Swellings—Mix any three or four of the following:

Juniper Berries	Yarrow
Horsetail Grass	Stinging Nettle
Rosemary	Birch Leaves

Use 4 quarts of pure Cider, 1 double handful of Parsley Root, 2 tablespoonfuls Mustard, 1 handful Horse Radish Root, and 1 ounce Juniper Berries. Put the ingredients in a jug and let it stand by the fire for 24 hours, so it is constantly warm and shake the jug often, then strain and keep in a cool place. The dose is a half wineglassful 3 times a day, always before meals, and it surely will help Dropsy. Writes J. A. F., New Madison, Ohio.

For Dropsy—I must say Princess Pine saved my life when I was dying from Dropsy. The leaves were steeped, and drunk by the mouthful, when they were cold. Writes Mrs. C. R., Detroit, Mich.

Dropsy—I had Dropsy in 1899 and cured it in a week by drinking ½ to 1 gallon per day, cold, every time that I wanted a drink of water, instead took a tea made of bark of Poplar. Writes J. R. R., Hot Springs, Ark.

I am sending you a Dropsy recipe:
    ½ gallon old Cider
    1 handful of Parsley, crushed
    1 handful of Horse Radish, crushed
    1 tablespoonful of Juniper Berries

Put in Cider, let stand 24 hours in a warm place before use. Take ½ glassful 3 times per day before meals. Writes W. Mc., Burns City, Ind.

Editor's Note—I don't like the cider undiluted. Why not use half water?

Dropsy Tea—Take the second or inner bark of the Slippery Elm, and make into a tea, using 1 teaspoonful of ground bark (or a few small pieces of unground bark) to 1 pint of boiling water. Boil 5 to 10 minutes, and drink during the day. One pint of this infusion is one day's dose. Continue until desired results are obtained and until you are relieved from the Dropsy. Writes N. N., Sugar Island, Tex.

Dropsy, Burning Urine and Backache. Here is a recipe that has been in use in our family in the old country for generations. Many German families will recognize this recipe. Equal parts of German Cheese Plant, Hollander Berries and Dwarf Elder Root. Take a heaping teaspoonful of this mixture to a cup of water, boil ½ minute and drink 1 or 2 cupfuls during the day. Writes J. S. L., New Orleans, La.

Elder, Dwarf—Very valuable in Gravel, Dropsy, Suppression of Urine and other Kidney and Bladder disorders.

Take the roots of Trailing Arbutus and make a tea. Steep a handful of roots, allow to cool, drink the tea, continue until Dropsy is gone, and it will never return. Writes H. L., Hellertown, Pa.

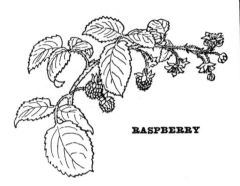

RASPBERRY

DYSPEPSIA—WEAK STOMACH

Thousands of persons suffer from occasional stomach disorders. With some it is but a temporary indisposition, caused by fatigue, or some error in diet, symptoms being loss of appetite, coated tongue, bad taste in the mouth, especially in the morning.

With others, it is a permanent affection, with constant weakness of the digestion so that even the mildest food causes heaviness or uneasiness. There is also constipation and lowness of spirits which mark the confirmed dyspeptic. Sometimes, even the slightest food causes a sensation of fullness of the stomach and a feeling of weight and heaviness, as if a stone lay in the stomach; tight clothes are insupportable and there is tenderness of the part on pressure. Often the food will rise again to the mouth with a taste of sourness. Piles and flatulency are often symptoms.

Treatment—People who suffer from dyspepsia should be careful of their diet. They should eat very moderately, chew the food well, taking plenty of time for meals, and drink no fluid while eating. An hour before each meal take a good stomach tonic.

The Herb Doctor's choice of botanical Carminatives and Tonics are: Gentian Root, Wormwood, Angelica, Juniper Berries, Elecampane, Black Alder, Rhubarb, Wild Cherry, Strawberry Leaves, Red Raspberry Leaves, Balmony.

Stomach and Bowel Disorders—Avoid all animal foods. They give acid reaction. Fruits, nuts and fresh vegetables help to give tone to the stomach and bring the blood back to its normal alkaline condition.

I am sending you a recipe for Dyspepsia. Mix Powdered Rhubarb, Bicarbonate of Soda, Gentian, Peppermint together. Of the mixture you can use a teaspoonful to a cupful of boiling water, and take one hour before meals. Writes M. J. F., Boley, Okla.

Editor's Note—You can improve this formula by leaving out the Soda Bicarbonate.

Flatulence—Eat less starchy foods and avoid rich gravies, pastries, coffee and teas with refined sugar. Use honey instead of sugar. Eat more fresh fruits. Avoid cabbage, Brussels sprouts, onions, dried beans, and peas. Use other green vegetables in salads or steamed.

For Dyspepsia—Take one teaspoonful of the whole Flax Seed twice a day. This is said to have cured cases where saliva would flow from the mouth and the afflicted could scarcely sleep.

For Dyspepsia—Use one-half ounce Centaury and one-fourth ounce Balmony and Ginger in pint of water, and the dose is a wineglassful three times a day.

—Father John's Stomach
    Tea..........
    Thousand Seal
    Juniper Berries
    Milk Weed
    Gentian
    Wormwood Leaves
    German Cheese Plant
    Rose Pink

An old fashioned Carminative and Tonic. Useful in Gastritis, Belching, etc.

Stomach Ulcers—The raw juices of fresh green vegetables taken half a cupful at a time, 3 or 4 times a day, and a little freshly expressed fruit juice at other times, will be all the food needed at first. Afterwards fresh fruit for one meal and a finely chopped and well masticated green vegetable salad twice a day for awhile will be salutary. Later cooked vegetables.

For Dyspepsia—One teaspoonful White Mustard Seed 3 times a day, same dose for rheumatism. Have seen several cases cured, stomach troubles as well as muscular rheumatism. Writes Mrs. J. E. S., Arcadia, Ind.

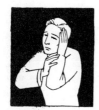

EARACHE

Earache is generally due to a slight cold; it can also result from catarrh or sinus trouble.

Here is a capital remedy for a preparation to be used for earache where one is threatened with mastoid or gatherings about the ear. This, however, is to be applied around the ear or on the side of the face or head, never to be put in the ear, or taken internally. A few drops applied at a time once a day is usually sufficient. Take equal parts of Oil of Cloves, Oil of Hemlock, Oil of Cedar, Oil of Juniper and Oil of Wintergreen, mix a d use as a liniment. This will frequently relieve the pain of toothache and neuralgia of the face. Writes A. O. R., Hewitt, Minn.

For Earache—Take a small wad of sterilized cotton, place on gums back of teeth and bite hard on it for about 15 minutes. Also rub Oil Wintergreen on and around painful ear. The cotton should be put in the mouth nearest the ear that is painful. Warm Olive Oil or Sweet Oil dropped inside of the ear is also good. Several of my neighbors have used this with good results. Writes E. L. M., Long Beach, Calif.

For Earache—Dissolve Soda in Sweet Oil, warm and put a few drops in the ear. Repeat if necessary. Writes Mrs. D. E. J., Smethport, Pa.

Mullein Oil is an infused oil made by processing the Mullein flowers with a bland oil. This oil is used externally as a palliative for irritation of piles, frost bites and minor irritations of the skin. It has been valued as a household remedy for affections of the ear. It allays pain.

Am enclosing a recipe for Bealed Ear. It cured me and I know of a number of others also cured with same. Take Pine Tar; warm till it drops freely; one drop is plenty, and it is absolutely harmless.

Writes A. C., Morris, Pa.

I fail to find anything in your Almanac about the medical value of Hops when used as a poultice. I used them on a child that was going to be operated on for Mastoid trouble and prepared two sacks of Hops. One I kept constantly over hot water in a colander, so as to be kept as hot as she could stand them and changed them when they would get the least bit cool. Next morning her ear gathered and run about a cupful and saved the operation. Another time I used them for a lady that had inflammation in her bowels, and with good results. Writes A. E., Battle Creek, Mich.

For Earache—Pour hot Olive Oil in ear and in a short while the pain will have vanished. Writes M. K., Boston, Mass.

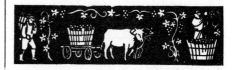

For Ear Trouble—Bake Mullein Leaves in oven in earthen vessel, strain and use the oil obtained for trouble with the ears. Writes S. H. J., Woodville, Wis.

Take Skunk Oil, be sure it is the genuine. Warm three or four drops and put in ear, let run down good, and then put in cotton loose. I have never heard of a case where it did not stop the Earache. Writes A. D. D., Sedalia, Mo.

Here is a remedy that I would like to pass along. For earache, get a small piece of cotton, dampen with Sweet Oil and sprinkle with ground black Pepper and roll it up in the cotton and pack the ear. It is a sure cure as I have tried it. Writes E. E. A., Laurens, S. C.

Take equal parts of Sarsaparilla Root, Sweet Elder Root or Blossoms, and make a strong tea. Divide the tea thus made into two parts; one for internal and one for external use. Take a cup of the tea every two hours while bad, then continue to take four times a day after a seeming cure has been affected, to clear out the system. Bathe the affected parts at least four times a day until all traces of Erysipelas have disappeared. This remedy has effected a cure in a short time, when doctors have failed in years of treatment to do so. Writes J. T. F., Beaver Falls, Pa.

A Sure Cure for Erysipelas—Take Red Puccoon crushed, and add to sweet cream and apply as a salve. Writes Mrs. G. G. D., Coldwater, Mo.

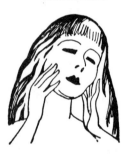

EYES, SORE

Inflamed and sore eyes may be due to a slight cold, eye strain, catarrh, hay fever, etc.

Treatment—Determine the cause and take the proper treatment. Bathe the eyes frequently with a warm tea of Fennel Seed.

The Herb Doctor's choice of botanicals for bathing the eyes are: Eye Bright, Chamomile, Fennel Seed, Cheese Plant, Yarrow.

For Sore and Inflamed Eyes—Make a tea of either the wild or tame Violets, drink freely of the tea which may be sweetened through the day. Then make a poultice of the leaves, and apply to the eyes, for these are very good.

My little girl had something on her eyeball which looked like a small pimple. I washed a whole Linseed and put it under her eyelid. This I did for three nights. Whatever it was the Linseed cleared it away. Writes Mrs. G. W., Ann Arbor, Mich.

I will send you a tried and true remedy. When I was a few days old I caught cold in my eyes. My parents had different doctors who said I would be blind. After trying everything but to no avail an old lady said to let her try her remedy. She got some Mullein Roots, boiled them in water and kept bathing the eyes with the tea, and they soon were perfectly well. Writes Mrs. E. J., Tippecanoe City, Ohio.

For Sore Eyes—Make a weak tea of Golden Seal Root and wash the eyes with it, and it will relieve them. Writes J. W. M., Smithville, W. Va.

Cataract—The root of Devil's Shoe String soaked in water and used as a wash will cut the film called cataract off the eyes of man or beast more effectually than surgeon's knife without pain or risk or apprehension. This was in our daily paper years ago and I imagine it may be of some help to some one. Writes Mrs. M. B., Buffalo, N. Y.

Editor's Note—Better try this with a very small quantity of the root at first and gradually increase the quantity. However, if it appears to irritate the eye discontinue its use.

Use a tea made of Rose Leaves, and add a teaspoonful of salt, use freely. Writes L. E. B., Roxbury, Vt.

We also used to dig Golden Seal and after steeping or soaking in hot water, use the yellow water as a wash for Sore Eyes. Writes S. A. H., Cambridge, Iowa.

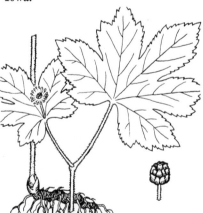

GOLDEN SEAL

Take Sassafrass Pith, soak in warm water, then bathe the Eyes and allow to get well into the eyes, and it surely should prove well for all cases of Sore Eyes. Writes Mrs. L. C., Ornsby, Pa.

For Sore, Inflamed Eyes—Take the dried Elderberry Blossoms, pour over boiling water, and let cool, each night and morning, use as a bath for the eyes, using in an eye cup. This is what my mother used for my father with very inflamed eyes. Writes J. F., Racine, Wis.

Chamomile Flowers made into a tea is fine for a wash in cases of Inflamed Eyes. Writes Mrs. C. T., Los Angeles, Calif.

When my baby was small one of his eyes was inflamed for weeks. It seemed like it would rot out. The doctor's medicine made it worse. I was in California at the time but wrote to Tennessee for some Sassafras Pith which I boiled in a little water until a trifle thick and when it was cold I bathed his eye with it. The eye was well in a few days. Writes R. C. T., South Pittsburg, Tenn.

Editor's Note—You did a very wise thing—be sure to use only the pith of Sassafras as the bark would burn and make it worse.

Use Slippery Elm Bark in a poultice for Sore Eyes. Writes Mrs. S. H. D., Indiana, Pa.

Crushed Golden Seal roots steeped in water is a sure cure for sore eyes of any kind. Writes Mrs. G. G. D., Coldwater, Mo.

For Inflammation of the Eyes—Take the Sassafras Pith, a spoonful into a ½ cup of boiling water and when cold use in eye dropper a few drops during the day, and it works wonders. Writes H. R., Holton, Mich.

Here is how the treatment for Cataract in the eye is done. Take the fresh juice from a cocoanut, and with the eye dropper apply as much as the eye can hold, then apply hot wet cloths (those that have been dipped in hot water) over the eyes. Have patient lying down and keep the towels hot for 10 minutes. One treatment is generally enough. I have never known this to fail. Writes S. H., Valleja, Calif.

Place a whole Flax Seed in the eye, let it stay for a time, and it will aid to remove all small objects from the eye. Writes O. M., Dana, Ind.

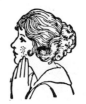

ERYSIPELAS

This is a general or constitutional disease, due to an infection by a germ. It differs from other fevers in the fact that it begins as a local inflammation of the skin, often on the face, and may spread to other parts of the body. The inflamed spot is red, smooth and shines like a piece of polished furniture. There is generally a chill with fever, loss of appetite, dry furred tongue and a lessened amount of urine. Sometimes abscesses occur with the local inflammation and other symptoms of blood poisoning may appear. Meningitis is also a complication of serious importance.

Treatment—Call a specialist.

The Herb Doctor's choice of botanicals are: Strawberry Leaves, Sweet Balm, Elder Flowers, used mainly as refrigerant drinks.

I am sending you a recipe for erysipelas. Take Golden Rod, cut up in small pieces and fry in lard, thus making a salve out of it. My grandmother has cured cases that the doctors gave up with this. Writes T. L. M., Greensboro, N. C.

Place Sassafras Bark in a vessel with water and steep for about 15 minutes, then add a little salt, then thicken with meal and when cool, spread on a white cloth and bind it to the parts. This is a sure cure for Erysipelas. Writes Mrs. O. J. L., Berry, Ala.

For Erysipelas, especially internally, use ¼ to ½ teaspoon doses Sulphur several times daily. Helped my wife when bad in mouth and throat. Writes J. D. C., Aurora, Mo.

My father and I both have Erysipelas and we both were cured. Take Cream of Tartar, and put in a 2 quart fruit jar, and drink several times a day. Then take lemons cut in half and rub on wherever swelling and soreness is. My father's limbs were swollen and I had it in my face. Neither of us have been troubled since. Writes Mrs. W. E. H., Bentley, Mich.

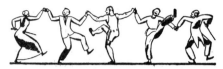

FOOT RELIEF

FEET
(See Bunions.)

The Mistletoe ruins our Oak and Cottonwood trees but it has good points. If one has tired, sore feet, take a quantity of Mistletoe and steep it and place the feet in the mixture and it will relieve them very much, or use it over night as a poultice for callouses. Writes N. L., Porterville, Calif.

For Tired and Tender Feet—Use White Oak Bark in warm water. Soak the feet in it. Writes Mrs. S. M. B., St. Helens, Ore.

Here is a recipe for Sore and Blistered Feet. Take 2 or 3 pounds of Hemlock Bark to a pail of water and boil for 2 hours. Strain and bathe the feet as hot as one can stand, until the water is cool. You will never be bothered with sore feet again. Writes L. M., Gladstone, Mich.

Make a strong decoction of the broad leaved Plaintain Leaves, boil 10 or 15 minutes, let stand and when rather warm, then for Sore or Sweaty Feet, bathe the feet in it once daily for three or four days. Writes W. C., Wheeling, W. Va.

Here is a good cure for Tender, Tired, Sore and Sweating Feet that throw off a strong, offensive odor. Take a big handful of Black Oak Bark and boil in enough water to cover the feet in a dish pan. Boil ½ hour or until a dark color appears, use hot as possible. This will darken or tan the feet and it hardens them. The tan comes off later on. Only one application is needed. I hope this will be useful to many for a weakened foundation is bad for the body. Writes R. F. S., Murphysboro, Ill.

Moisten Powdered Alum and hold on an Ingrown Toe Nail for 10 minutes and it can be cut out without pain. Writes Mrs. A. R. D., Willington, Kan.

For Sore, Tired, Aching, Burning Feet, also Good for Rheumatism—Take 2 large bars of Ivory Soap, shave, put in 3 pints of hot water, in a granite basin, set on back of the stove to melt, but do not let boil. Then take ½ pound Epsom Salts, and put it in ¼ pint of hot water, and set on back of stove to dissolve, but not boil either. When soap is melted and salt is dissolved, set away to cool, when cool mix ingredients together until smooth and light. It is excellent for the purpose mentioned, as it is tried and true. It would be best to use rain water caught in granite, china or glass. Writes Mrs. J. R. E., Wrights, Pa.

Take Mullein and soak in vinegar and put on chilblains and note the great relief. Writes E. K., Gloucester, Mass.

Moisten Powdered Alum and hold on an Ingrown Toe Nail for 10 minutes and it can be cut out without pain. Writes Mrs. A. R. D., Willington, Kan.

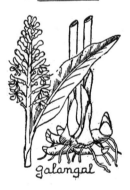

galangal

FELONS

For Felon and Abscesses— Put Pine Tar on cotton and bind on and will draw at once and be ready to open in a short time.

For a Bone Felon—Take Sassafras Root and boil a strong tea and put your finger in as hot as you can stand it, and it will kill the bone felon. I know what they are, and have killed several since I had one with this tea. Writes Mr. A. O., Magnolia, Miss.

Felon—"Procure a good lemon. Cut in half. Make an opening in the center for the sore finger. Place finger in the opening and wrap it with a towel so as to keep the lemon from coming off. Do this when you retire, and remove the lemon in the morning. The lemon has great drawing power and although it will be a little disagreeable do not remove this for at least 12 hours and your finger will be on the road to healing. This has never failed by all who tried this simple lemon remedy."

For Any Kind of Felon.—Yolk of egg and spoonful of table salt mixed, then cooked in shell on top of stove. Place entire yolk on felon hot, prepare to walk the floor all night, but in the morning or 24 hours the felon is dead. My mother's and other's actual experience. Writes Mrs. W. F., Seattle, Wash.

For Felon—Use a Poke Root Poultice. Writes J. S. B., Pittsburgh, Pa.

Make a strong tea of Elecampane Root and place the hand in it. The tea should be as hot as you can stand, and soak the hand for a half hour. Keep adding hot tea as it cools, and two or three applications will take out soreness and bring the felon to a head. Writes F. P. S., Yorkshire, N. Y.

FEMALE DISORDERS

The healthy performance of the functions of the female system is essential to the health and comfort of women. No derangement in these functions can exist for any length of time without drawing the entire life into sympathetic suffering, yet their nature is such as to exclude them, to a great extent, from observation, and often the sufferer groans on for years, the victim of pain and weakness known only to herself.

I wish to tell you all about one wonderful remedy that appeared in your "Herbalist Almanac." I was very weak from flooding spells for the last two and three months at a time. They finally took me to the hospital for an operation but they found me too weak, so I begged to go back home and they finally let me go, until I got stronger. During this time, I read about the Black Haw bark of root, so I tried it and have been up working hard and now it is nearly two years and haven't had another attack since. Mrs. P. H., Chase City, Va.

Use St. Johnswort and make into a salve, and apply this to a Caked Breast. It will sure do the work, and draw the **fever** out.

Flax Seed Poultice applied to the breasts will cure excessive secretion of the milk which often takes place for those that can not nurse their children and have to put them on the bottle. Writes Mrs. J. D. S., Golden City, Mo.

For Inflammation of the Urethra— Tea made from the bark of Red Willow will cure inflammation of the urethra and also sore throat. A harmless remedy. Drink three or four times a day. Writes Mrs. W. A. S., Buffalo, Mo.

A tea of Black Cohosh taken six weeks before confinement makes a shorter and easier confinement. Writes L. W., Coldwater, Miss.

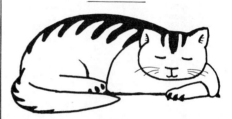

There is one thing you may add to your book if you wish. In excessive flowing, such as childbirth or particularly during change of life, a tea made of Cinnamon Bark will stop the flooding within a day. To be made strong and taken several times a day and stopped as the flooding grows normal. I have tried this and find it successful, and of great value to me. Writes Mrs. L. E. T., Bedford, Ohio.

For Painful and Suppressed Menses— Take a handful of Garden Dittany, pour boiling water over it and make a tea. Drink ½ teacupful while it is hot, go to bed, cover up and you can get up in an hour feeling like a new person. This was my mother's recipe and grew the plant in her garden, using it after it dried. Writes M. R., Anniston, Ala.

I noticed in your "Almanac" about Black Cohosh to be used before confinement. I had a very hard time when my children were born until an Indian squaw told me to take the Indian Squaw Vine and make into a tea and drink this before each meal and the Black Cohosh after meals, which I did, and I was surprised at the results. Writes Mrs. A. W., Dalhart, Tex.

Caked Breast—Two tablespoonfuls of German Chamomile Flowers, 2 tablespoonfuls of pure lard. Mix and fry in a pan very slowly for 1 hour without burning. Then remove from the fire and strain through cloth. This is very effective for caked breast. It may be rubbed on the breast while the salve is still hot for best results. Writes Mrs. J. M. F., Cuba, Mo.

Editor's Note—You should use double the quantity of the flowers.

I also would like to send in a good word for Spikenard. I used it at the birth of two of my children and two without it. I surely would not be without it at this time. Writes Mrs. D. N. H., San Simon, Ariz.

Take Elder Blossoms and fry in lard, then strain. Bathe the Caked Breast, then apply the Elder Flowers you have fried down, and it will ease at once. Writes Mrs. H. J. E., Neodesha, Kan.

For Falling of the Womb—Unicorn Root made into a strong tea and a teaspoonful taken three times a day until you feel better or until you know that you are well. Writes Mrs. E. F., Racine, Wis.

Unicorn Root is surely a wonderful female tonic. Writes Mrs. J. B., Ada, Okla.

Sip Cinnamon Tea if the menstruation flow is too much. Writes Mrs. H. W., Omaha, Neb.

Use Sweet Clover as a tea and drink before retiring and this will stop excessive menstruation. Writes Mrs. P. B. C., Ennis, Tex.

For Menstruation—When you don't flow enough, take Sumach Root, and make a tea. Drink this till the flow is regular, then stop. An old Indian lady said this was what they all used. Writes Mrs. A. B. D., Norman, Okla.

For Flooding—Take ½ pint of fresh sweet milk and a tablespoonful of ground nutmeg, set on the stove and let come to a boil. Give hot as can be taken. Writes B. Q. S., Lakeview, Ohio.

Make a strong tea of Squaw Weed and try for painful menses. Drink as hot as can be borne, and will bring sure relief. Writes A. J. W., Ashland, Ga.

For Change of Life—Make a tea of Black Cohosh and Witch Hazel Bark. Make a tea of equal parts, boil together, and drink in large swallows three times a day. Also use a wash of 1 spoonful Witch Hazel Bark, Red Oak Bark, Life Everlasting, and Persimmon Bark as well as Red Shank. Boil to a strong tea and add a small piece of Alum. This will take all growth away and cure chronic inflammation of the womb. Use a teacupful twice a day with a syringe. Writes A. B., Union Grove, Ala.

I am sending a recipe for home treatment for falling of the womb. Make a strong tea of Black Cohosh, drink a big swallow before each meal. Also use the Red Oak Bark. Mix a half teacupful of the bark with half a cup of dark brown sugar, mix well and take a teaspoonful after eating. It cured me and I have cured several others after doctors failed. Writes A. B., Union Grove, Ala.

I am sending you a remedy highly praised by my mother for women during Change of Life. My mother was down in bed and looked like there wasn't any chance for her. Doctor's medicine didn't help her any and she was spitting up blood by the mouthful. She started drinking a tea made of Chestnut Leaves and was soon out of bed and doing all her work. She also cured my brother of a cough caused by cigarettes with Chestnut Leaves. She is the mother of ten children and all are grown and she is never without chestnut leaves in the house. Writes Mrs. C. C., Pleasant View, Ky.

A boon to women, fine to prevent a miscarriage. Take Tansy Leaves, and make into a poultice. Place a layer on a white cloth, fold together and sew up, then pin the belt around the abdomen, renew the belt fresh, as often as you see required. I have seen this tried with good results. Writes Mrs. V. S., Oneonta, Ala.

For women who suffer much with neuralgia during pregnancy, make a tea of Red Raspberry leaves and drink 2 or 3 cups a day.

For mothers who nurse their babies but have not enough milk, should try steeping Elderberries and drink the juice without sugar. A wineglassful a day is sufficient. Writes Mrs. G. W., Ann Arbor, Mich.

THE OLD HERB DOCTOR

Take Ginger Tea as hot as you can at bedtime and it is good to make you flow, if the flow should be scanty. Writes F. B., Trenton, Ala.

To stop too frequent menstruation, steep a tablespoonful of Alum Root in a cup of boiling water, let cool, then drink. Writes Mrs. J. B. R., Wewoka, Okla.

Wild Ginger Root made into a tea is a sure cure for retarded menses. Writes Mrs. C. B., Lillybrook, W. Va.

Take 2 tablespoonfuls of cinnamon and make a tea of it by adding boiling hot water. Drink this and continue to drink as often as necessary, and it should be very serviceable for excessive menstruation. Writes Mrs. P. B., Utica, Miss.

Make a tea of Sweet Apple Tree bark and use, for it will check miscarriage. Drink the tea warm, as much as needed. Writes Mrs. A. W., Morgantown, Ky.

My daughter was a sufferer for years at her period time. She nearly had convulsions, also flooded so badly she could not be on her feet. She took Blue Cohosh, and it has relieved her of all her misery at that time, also the flooding. Writes Mrs. O. B., Neosho Falls, Kan.

I am sending you one that was recommended to my wife. She tried it and found it good in her case. For delayed, scanty and painful menses, take Life Everlasting, make a tea about color of strong coffee, add a good sprinkle of black pepper on going to bed or as often as needed. Writes H. A. H., Edgwold, S. C.

Ragweed is very good for colic, and painful menstruation. Boil, and drink a cupful and you will soon get relief. Writes F. A., Ritner, Ky.

Take Spearmint Oil and rub on a gathered breast three times a day and will break it up. Also good for any kind of gathering. It takes the pain out right away. Writes Mrs. W. C., Warren, Ohio.

White Oak Bark boiled into a tea and used as a douche is very good for falling of the womb. Writes Mrs. W., Little Rock, Ark.

Periodical Pains—Make a tea of Pennyroyal and drink it three nights before the expected period (before retiring) also bathe feet in hot water as can be borne, adding more as it cools to which a fire shovel of wood ashes has been added. Writes Mrs. G. S., Robstown, Tex.

To mothers who Mrs. Stork has on her calling list, eight weeks before Mrs. Stork is expected, use this simple formula, for it is indeed a mother's friend. Take a large double handful of Tansy Leaves and fry either in Olive Oil or pure Lard. Apply several times daily and especially at night for that tired and aching feeling in the sides. Writes Mrs. L. M., Willow Springs, Mo.

Fennel Seed is considered an excellent remedy for female troubles, strengthening and tightening the tissues of the womb. Will cure falling of the womb. Make a tea by boiling 10 minutes and inject into the vagina, once a day. This is an old family remedy which came from the Indians, and I have used it. Writes Mrs. A. D. R., Jacksonville, Fla.

For Gathered Breast—Take a lump of Beeswax the size of a small egg and add 1 teaspoonful of lard, melt together. Spread on cloth while hot and apply over the breast as warm as you can bear, then cover with warm cloth and keep warm. When cold apply fresh plaster and warm cloth. You will soon get relief and go to sleep. The gathering will burst and be all right. Writes C. H. C., Hutchinson, Kan.

For Gathered or Caked Breast—Fry hops in lard and apply hot. This may be reheated two or three times.

Change of Life—A handful of Plantain and Smart Weed boiled together for a few minutes. After it is cooled it should be taken three times during the day for female complaints and change of life, as it is excellent. Writes S. J. S., Huntsville, Ala.

For a Painless Confinement—Three weeks before confinement, make a tea of 1 teaspoon of Spikenard and fill cup with boiling water. Make the tea in morning and let stand until night, then drink, and make the tea the same way and drink again in the morning, and continue this. Writes Mrs. M. D., Keokuk, Iowa.

Here is relief for Flooding during Menstruation. Dig Black Haw Root, wash and cut in small pieces and boil it a long time until it makes a strong tea. When it gets cold drink a wineglassful three or four times a day. Writes N. H., Troup, Texas.

Editor's Note—The dried Black Haw may be substituted.

Life Root, Ragwort, False Valerian, Squaw Weed are very good for female suffering. Writes Mrs. S. G., Montague, Mass.

To Expectant Mothers—About six weeks before you expect your little one, begin to take a tea made by steeping a tablespoonful of the shredded root of Spikenard or Wild Licorice in a cup of boiling water until cold. Drink this amount during the day. Drink what you can; if but little, drink it—more is better, however. Continue this until baby comes. I have used this and can personally vouch for it in highest terms of praise, having had three little children since I commenced the treatment with very, very little suffering—none, comparatively. It is perfectly harmless and the result sure, speaking from my own experience and that of friends to whom I have given the prescription. It came to me from a dear woman, herself the mother of 14 children, yet still young and vigorous, who has always used and recommended "Spikenard Root Tea." Writes Mrs. L. of Wisconsin.

For one that has taken cold and for some reason fails to menstruate, make a cup or two of St. Johnswort tea and drink it. This never fails unless one is pregnant, then a gallon wouldn't help you. My grandmother used this and gathers the St. Johnswort and used to hang it up to dry. I never knew it to fail. Writes Mrs. J. J. P., Oakley, Ill.

I have looked your book over carefully and can find no recipe any better than this one for caked breast. Pancakes made of Indian corn meal or white flour placed on the breast as hot as can be borne will give certain relief. Writes Mrs. M. L. M., Ripley, Ohio.

For Menstruation—When you don't flow enough, take Sumach Root, and make a tea. Drink this till the flow is regular, then stop. An old Indian lady said this was what they all used. Writes Mrs. A. B. D., Norman, Okla.

Hemmorrhage—For 14 weeks my sister took hemorrhages before confinement, and she ate Nutmeg about every 15 minutes, until flowing ceased, and it saved her life. Writes A. M. E., Kittanning, Pa.

Flooding at Childbirth—Take a tablespoonful of Saffron, steep in ½ cup water, and drink when cool. Writes Mr. B. W., Paisley, Ore.

Try steeping Raspberry Leaves and drinking for Painful Menstruation, also for Pains after Childbirth. Writes Mrs. M. V., Treadwell, N. Y.

A tea made of Rag Weed is very good for Painful Menses. Writes Mrs. C. F., Oak Hill, Ohio.

For Women Who Expect to Become Mothers—Six weeks before confinement take an ounce of Black Cohosh (an Indian Herb), and put a little of it in a quart of boiling water, and allow to steep. Let it stand on the back of the stove and drink a few sips three or four times a day. When this is used take a little more fresh root and steep again. Keep this up for three weeks, then change to Blue Cohosh, and keep up until confinement. This seems to make an easier childbirth. Writes Dr. W. C. W., Placerville, Calif.

Pennyroyal Tea is an excellent remedy for suppressed menstruation due to colds, as also is Mistletoe and Centaury. Tansy is also very good but not very pleasant to the taste. Writes Mrs. E. C. G., Inka, Ill.

Flooding at Childbirth—Mistletoe Tea taken in drinks every 30 minutes, starting when labor starts after the child is born, the tea being kept up until the menses is regulated, is a remedy that cannot be equaled. Writes D. O. D., Memphis.

Falling of the Womb—"The following is considered a very fine remedy for falling of the womb. It must, however, be taken with perseverance and the patient must avoid violent exercise or too heavy work. Steep 2 tablespoonfuls of White Oak Bark in 3 pints of water. Boil for 15 minutes or longer, adding more water as it evaporates. Strain and when lukewarm add a cupful of cold water and use one-half of this as one injection into the vagina. Use twice a day, morning and evening." Writes G. W., Rochester, N. Y.

For Painful Menstruation — Black Haw is an excellent remedy. Boil to a tea and drink it. The first sips should give relief. Writes H. N., Woodland.

Here is an old time remedy my mother used through Change of Life: Take a handful of bark and twigs of Witch Hazel and steep in water, then drink three or four times a day, and it will regulate any one and is beneficial where there is too much flow. Writes Mrs. L. B., Clinton. Tenn.

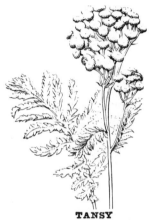

TANSY

For Delayed or Irregular or Painful Periods—This will bring quick relief. Steep 4 tablespoonfuls of Tansy Leaves 15 minutes. Drink hot as possible. Then go to bed, cover up well, and you can use this tea every 15 minutes until relieved. Writes M. L., Gilmer, Tex.

For Gathered or Caked Breast—Fry hops in lard and apply hot. This may be reheated two or three times.

For Weak Men and Women—Dyspepsia and Colic. Ague Root, also called Star Root. Also helpful in restoring activity of the generative organs, also used in cases of a tendency to miscarry and falling of the womb. Writes E. V., Portage, Wis.

Ground Ivy made into a tea will help during the menstrual period. Writes S. B. W., Lancaster, Ky.

Gather Mullein Leaves, saturate in hot vinegar and apply to Caked Breast or Swollen Glands, very hot, cover with flannel, and repeat. Very good. Writes Mrs. W. R., Grand Rapids, Mich.

For Female Troubles—Take a handful of Tansy Leaves, add water, bring to boil and boil down, strain, add lard, and apply this to the stomach, or the part of the body that is affected. Writes M. T., Augusta, Miss.

Women who are afflicted with ulceration of the womb, should use White Pond Lily Root, for it is very good. Unicorn Root is an invaluable cure for falling of the womb, and is specific for restoring sexual losses in all conditions. Writes J. B., Ada, Okla.

Pennyroyal used freely in the form of a warm infusion promotes perspiration and excites the menstrual discharge when recently checked. A large draught of the infusion should be taken at bed time, the feet should be bathed in warm water previous to taking the infusion. Writes Miss M. G., Swords Creek, Va.

Make a tea of Yarrow for Painful Menstruation. The dose is a teacupful three times a day. Writes L. G., Ann Arbor, Mich.

Inflammation of the Uretha—Tea made from the bark of Red Willow will cure inflammation of the uretha and also sore throat. A harmless remedy. Drink three or four times a day. Writes Mrs. W. A. S., Buffalo, Mo.

Stomach Tonic—A very excellent stomach tonic or stomach bitters can be made of the following: One-half oz. of each: Gentian, Angelica, Strawberry, Wild Cherry Bark and Fennel Seed, all ground fine except Fennel. Place these articles in a quart of boiling water, when cool, drink ½ cupful a day, a large mouthful at a time, or same may be placed in a pint of good whiskey and it makes an excellent bitters.

For years I have suffered with a soreness well up in the vagina and around the womb, which I contracted years ago and which doctors said may turn to cancer. I had read of Sheep Sorrel being good though I had never heard of it being used as a douche, but as I already had a 25c box on hand I decided to try it. I was amazed after the third douche to find the soreness very much relieved, and now after about two weeks' use it has almost disappeared. Maybe some other sufferer would like to try it. Writes E. T., St. Louis, Mo.

Menstruation—In the temperate zone the first menses usually appears at about the fourteenth year—in warm climates earlier—and in colder climates later. Menstruation is also subject to variation, depending upon the general health, vigor and development of the person. For a year or two it may be scanty, and not infrequently subject to some irregularities. In healthy women it should appear every 28 days and flow four or five days, varying again according to the constitution and general health of the person. About the forty-fifth year of life it generally ceases, accompanied often with various disturbances of the system. This cessation of the period is termed ''change of life.''

Delayed Menses—When menstruation in young girls is delayed, it is not wise to give medicine to promote this secretion, beyond attention to sufficient clothing, exercise and diet. The clothing should be warm enough to suit the temperature and season, and a wholesome, generous diet should be adopted, avoiding spices, coffee and highly seasoned food. This will generally be sufficient to produce a normal flow.

Theatment—If there are symptoms of its approach, such as flushes of heat, frequent giddiness of the head, heaviness in the abdomen, a hot aromatic Diaphoretic tea should be taken.

The Herb Doctor's choice of botanical Aromatic Diaphoretics are: Sweet Flag, Canada Snake Root, Squaw Weed, Squaw Vine, Yarrow, Elecampane, Mugwort, Mullein, Penny Royal, Ragwort, Rue, Shepherds Purse, Tansy, Thyme, Valerian, Wormwood, Dill Seed, Chamomile and Cotton Root.

The prepared formulas are:
Cotton Root Compound,   Prairie
Mint Compound and   Florida Tea.

Am sending a couple of remedies which I know are very good. Take Pennyroyal and make a tea and drink. It is very good for painful menstruation. Writes Miss H. P., Hawthorne, N. Y.

I want to thank you for the Spikenard Tea, priced at 25c, which I took and it surely helped me. I had two babies before and I suffered so much and after taking the Spikenard I didn't suffer nearly so much with this one. Writes Mrs. L. R., Dixon, Calif.

Editor's Note—Spikenard Tea has been used to promote easy childbirth for ages.

Scanty Menses—Sometimes the menses barely show or are pale in color, or are late in appearing each month. Give the following:
Treatment — Same as for delayed menses.

Suppressed Menses—Sometimes, during the flow or just as it is about to commence, the discharge stops or becomes suppressed from exposure to cold, especially to damp cold. The flow may either cease suddenly or it may come on attended with scanty, irregular discharge, or with severe pain and distress.
Treatment — Same as for delayed menses.

—Cramp Bark Comp.
Gen. Cramp Bark
Swamp Cabbage
Blue Scullcap
Jamaica Ginger
Black Cohosh

Antispasmodic.

—Wildwood Tea...
Gen. Cramp Bark
Alex. Senna Leaves
Eastern Skullcap
German Cheese Plant
Colic Root
Horsetail Grass
Chicory Root

An Antispasmodic—contains no dope of any kind as you can see by the formula. Valuable in Cramps and Spasms.

—Viburnum Palmetto Compound........
Viburnum Squaw Bush
Palmetto Berries
Swamp Lily Root
Beth Root
Mex. Damiana Leaves
German Cheese Plant
Blue Mallow
Bearberry Leaves
Althea
Black Haw
Wild Cherry

An old recognized formula of modern physicians. It is one of the few that are still in use by the (in our opinion) misguided present day physician. It is prescribed primarily for women.

—Prairie Mint Comp.
German Rue
Swamp Lily
Bearberry Leaves
Squaw Weed
Sweet Balm
Sweet Flag
Jamaica Ginger
Prairie Plant
Black Cohosh

Antispasmodic and Carminative. A combination that we prize among our best formulae. Useful in cramps due to the monthly periods of females.

—Squaw Tea...
Tonic—All botanists will recognize these ingredients as the component parts of most of the modern widely advertised female remedies. Yet the ingredients are all of the Indian Origin:

1 ounce Beth Root
1 ounce Crow Corn Root
1 ounce Black Haw
2 ounces Squaw Vine

Steep a teaspoonful into a cupful of boiling water, making fresh every day.

—Cotton Root Comp.
Pennyroyal
Cotton Root
Cheese Plant
Cloves (Powdered)
Rosemary

The properties of this old fashioned formula are diaphoretic and Carminative. It is as harmless as ordinary household tea or coffee.

Change of Life—Cessation of the menses usually occurs between the ages of 40 to 50 years, and is frequently attended with disturbance of the system, such as hot flushes, intense nervousness, paleness, debility, and irregular monthly flow—either too little or too profuse, or colorless discharge. Palpitations and throbbings of the heart are also common. Few women pass this crisis without some of these annoying symptoms.
Treatment—If there is weakness of the heart and fatigue, take a good tonic. Keep bowels open.
Douche is beneficial.
The Herb Doctor's choice of botanical Tonics are: Aletris Root, Cramp Bark, Palmetto Berries, Swamp Lily Root, Beth Root, Black Haw.

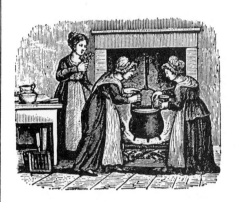

—Mother's Herb Tea
....
Gen. Cramp Bark
Squaw Vine
Yellow Poplar Bark
Star Root
Alex, Senna
Tinn. Senna Leaves
Beth Root
Blue Mallow
Black Haw Bark
German Cheese Plant

Blue and Black Cohosh to any expectant mother 6 weeks before confinement. Get these two herbs and take the Black Cohosh for three weeks and the last three weeks take Blue Cohosh and it will cause a much easier childbirth. Writes Mrs. W. N., Appleton, Ark.

Profuse Menses—Correct the general diet. Try vegetarianism. Fresh vegetables will give your blood more needed calcium.

Painful Menses—Acid forming foods have a tendency to bring trouble at the monthly periods. Meats, fish, poultry, coffee and tea, fried foods, white bread and white sugar are all very acid-forming. Fruits and green vegetables have an opposite effect. Take these with a few nuts and some cottage cheese and vegetable soups made without meats.

Suppressed Menses—Try diet as mentioned under "Profuse Menses."

FROSTBITES AND CHILBLAINS
(See Feet.)

If feet or hands are frozen, thaw them with snow but if they break open take a kettle filled with White Pine Bark or even Needles, cover with water and let boil a long time, then bathe the frostboils in this as hot as you can stand and your feet will get all right. Have tried this myself and know of different people that healed their hands and feet the same way. Writes Mrs. H. S., Westwood, Calif.

For Frosted Feet—Dissolve a tablespoonful of Pulverized Alum and stir it into one-half gallon of very hot water. Sit with the feet in the hot Alum water for thirty minutes. This gives relief at once. Do this three or four nights just before retiring and you will not be bothered with itching feet any more unless you should happen to get another frosting.

For Chilblain—Take 7 onions, fry them in half cup of hog's lard, press out all the grease, keep in tight jar, and apply to feet night and morning. Writes Mrs. D. E., Smethport, Pa.

GALL STONES

Or Biliary Colic consists of concretions in the gall bladder or biliary ducts, derived from the bile. Causes are: excessive eating and drinking, obesity, tight lacing, as an aftermath of fevers, diseases of the liver and stomach.

Treatment—If pain is severe take one or two Tablets. Give Olive Oil freely. Keep bowels open with a hot tea. Eat sparingly and more often. Abstain from meats and sweets. Consult a specialist. Demulcents are often useful.

The Herb Doctor's choice of botanical Demulcents are: Celandine, Calamint Herb, Flax Seed, Boldo Leaves, Radishes.

For Gall Stones—Take Olive Oil night and morning. Sure cure. Writes B. M. L., Plato, Mo.

I cured myself and two others of Gall Stones with Sacred Bark and Sweet Weed. Writes H. C. K., Redfield, S. D.

Gall Stones—"I am sending a remedy for Gall Stones which has cured an old friend of ours. Take a handful of the herb called Shepherds Heart and pour a quart of boiling water on it. Let it steep on the back of the stove for one hour; strain and cool. Drink a wine glassful 3 times a day until cured."

Sweet Weed—Very valuable for gall stones and bladder troubles. A teacupful of the cut root to a quart of water, to which add a cupful or more of best glycerine and enough Anise Seed to flavor it to suit. Dose—2 to 4 tablespoonful three times a day one-half hour before meals. This is a very fine remedy.

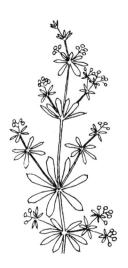

GOOSE GRASS

Gobernadora—Used in rheumatism, being employed for baths and fomentations. Also for gastric disturbances and gallstones. It is much used for pains, aches and sprains and because of its remarkable antiseptic properties is often applied to bruises, sores, cuts and wounds. It can be made into a salve, too.

I have dissolved Gravel three times for myself and Gall Stones for a lady friend when the doctors said nothing but an operation would do any good. I used nothing but German Cheese Plant, and Queen of the Meadow Root. Writes J. W. G., Nampa, Idaho.

Editor's Note—Both of these are absolutely harmless, but I doubt their efficacy in every case.

To facilitate the passage of gall stones, take powdered Goose Grass and powdered Sweet Weed, one level teaspoonful, and swallow in one dose. This will be rather hard on account of the ingredients being powdered, so you may moisten with saliva or hot water or mix with sugar or honey. Take this three times a day.

I have tried several formulas which have done the work and, for instance, the one calling for 10 teaspoonsful Sweet Weed to a ½ teaspoonful of Sacred Bark for Gall Stone. It has helped about six people here, my wife first, whom I used it on. I also want to congratulate you on your Pile Ointment, which is very good. Writes H. J. K., Nashville, Tenn.

I am sending you a sure and tried gall stone remedy that has cured all who have taken it. It dissolves the stones:
One ounce Liver Wort, Dandelion Root, Prince's Pine, Culvers Root, Dwarf Elder Root, one and one-half ounce Burdock Root, one-half ounce Anise Seed and Senna. Steep and boil 4 to 5 hours in water enough to have 2 quarts, strain and add preservative. Dose, one wineglassful 3 times a day not less than 15 minutes and not more than one hour before meals. Writes Mrs. J. B., Ellenton, Fla.

Boneset tea is very good for a person suffering with gall stones. Writes Mrs. P. T., Noxie, Okla.

Gall Stones—Put a generous pinch of Buchu Leaves in a cup, pour on boiling water and take this three times during the day. It is also advisable to take a teaspoonful of Olive Oil every other night upon retiring. Writes Mrs. W. R., Grand Rapids, Mich.

—Powders.......
  Goose Grass
  Elm Bark
  Sassafras Bark
  Boldo Leaves
  Russian Licorice
  Capsicum Berries
This is a combination of botanicals finely powdered. It is pleasant to take and has a tendency to increase and improve the gall fluid, which in itself is often sufficient to dissolve gall stones.

Gall Stones—Take powdered Goose Grass and powdered Sweet Weed, one level teaspoonful, and swallow in one dose. This will be rather hard on account of the ingredients being powdered, so you may moisten with saliva or hot water or mix with sugar or honey. Take this three times a day.

Gall Stones—A most excellent remedy for Gall Stones is a tea made by steeping one cupful of the herb Indian Sage and one cupful Mullein in an earthen vessel containing three quarts of boiling water, until cold. Dose—One cupful 3 times a day.

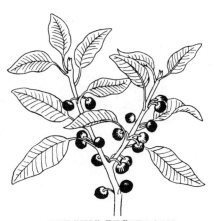

PURGING BUCKTHORN

—Demulcent Tea...
  Buckthorn Bark
  Sweet Weed
  Boneset Lvs. and Flors.
  Cheese Plant
  Flax Seed
  Mayapple Root
  Fennel Seed
  Wallwort
A soothing demulcent, laxative. A tea that will be found useful in various ailments. Often used as a laxative and to facilitate the passage of gall stones.

A Gall Bladder Tonic—Extract juice of a few radishes, mix two-thirds part of the juice with one-third part water, and use two or three wine glasses every other day for about a month. Writes Mrs. H. H., Okemah, Okla.

GOITRE OR BIG NECK

There are a number of different forms of goitre. Each form requires specific treatment. Consult a specialist. Operation should only be resorted to if all other means have proved futile and the system becomes filled up with poison.

keep the bowels open. Walking, deep breathing and sunshine are essential. Eat vegetables rich in mineral salts, especially Iodine.

The Herb Doctor's choice of botanicals containing minerals are Bladder Wrack, Irish Moss, Red Clover Flowers, Spinach, Peach Tree Leaves, Walnut Leaves.

Goitre or Thick Neck—"I have a treatment that has proved successful in the treatment of Goitre, which I am pleased to contribute to your columns. Take 1 cupful of dry wild Red Clover Blossoms. Place in a quart of water and boil down until the liquid when strained amounts to 1 cupful. Add a few teaspoonfuls of brandy or whiskey to keep from souring. Dose, 1 tablespoonful 4 or 5 times a day, provided it does not act too freely on the bowels. If the bowels move too freely the number of doses should be reduced to 1 or 2 doses a day. Best results are obtained if the remedy is taken one hour before meals." Writes Mrs. C. L., Clare, Mich.

I am 76 years old, have practiced botanic medicines for many years, successfully treating many cases and cured cases on which M.D.'s had failed. Here are my tried and true recipes:
Goitre. One tablespoonful Powdered Borax, Alum, Salt, and enough cream to make a paste. Apply every 4 hours. Writes J. R. R., Hot Springs, Ark.

—Red Clover Flowers
    Compound .....
Red Clover Flowers
Buckthorn Bark
Blue Vervain Lvs. and Flors.
Nerve Root
Sassafras, bark of root
Anise Seed
The main ingredient of this formula is Red Clover Flowers. It may be taken freely wherever the therapeutic properties of this article are indicated. The herbal physicians will recognize the value of this formula.

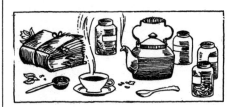

Here is a remedy that I have used when I had Goitre and I had it pretty bad. A friend of mine told me to get a sponge, any kind would do, lay it on a hot lid so that you can scrape it into powder. Do that until the sponge is used up and take one teaspoonful three times a day. Any way you use it do not wash the sponge. I used up 6 medium sponges. They say it takes about a year before the swelling is gone, and I have no goitre now. Writes Mrs. R. C., Geff, Ill.

Editor's Note—I would not be much surprised if this simple remedy cured goitre, for everyone knows Iodine in some form or another is the universal accepted remedy for goitre, and sponges contain iodine and other valuable salts. The sponge placed on a hot stove will naturally turn all the vegetable fibre of the sponge into charcoal ashes and these will then contain the iodine.

Job's Tears are said to be successful in removing a goitre by wearing a string of the seeds. It is also useful for teething babies. Writes L. G. P., Caines, Pa.

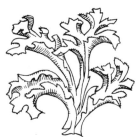

ICELAND MOSS

Goitre—We may be told there is a deficiency of iodine. If that is so, you may find a supply in sea lettuce, dulse, pineapple, green kidney beans and several green leafy vegetables. But gluttony is more frequently the cause of trouble than deficiency of iodine and a fast may do much to clear up the condition.

GRAVEL

The symptoms are scanty and painful discharge of variously-colored urine, and as the stones pass from the kidneys to the bladder, violent colic pains from the region of the kidneys along the course of the ureter—the tube which conveys the urine from the kidneys to the bladder. The pain is usually very severe, coming on in paroxysms and returning from time to time until the stones are discharged.

Treatment—Consult a specialist. Take 1 or 2 Tablets to relieve the pain. Hot foot and seat baths often help to relieve the pain. A change of drinking water and diet are often of value.

The Herb Doctor's choice of botanical Diuretics and Demulcents are: Horsetail Grass, Bearberry, Dog Grass, Carrots, Gooseberry Leaves, Sweet Flag, Buchu, Horsemint, St. Johnswort, Water Pepper, Corn Silk, Plantain Leaves.

For an adult: One pint a day of Sarsaparilla Tea is the "boss" cure for Gravel, and it restores the worn out and wasted system. Writes Mrs. I. L. B., Remus, Mich.

I find that Corn Silk is a cure for gravel when your urinary passages are stopped up. Make a tea of about two tablespoonsful to a cup of boiling water and drink it hot. Writes V. J. W., Anderson, S. C.

Editor's Note—I was just wondering how often the word cure appeared in these recipes. Relief is the better word.

A tea of Flax Seed Meal is said to be a cure for gravel. H. B. A., Walled Lake, Mich.

Gravel Root is fine for Gravel, too. Writes J. H., Searles, Ala.

Editor's Note—All of these herbs are to be made into a tea by placing a heaping teaspoonful of the herbs in a cup of boiling water; allow to cool and drink one or two cupfuls a day.

Plantain, and also White Clover will cure gravel if given a trial. Make into a tea and take often. Writes E. A. H., Peoria, Mo.

Knot Grass—Efficacious in expelling gravel or stone from the kidneys and bladder. Dissolves phlegm.

Use a half saucer of tea made twice daily of Gravel Weed for gravel, and you will surely find it good. Writes L. H., Canann, Mo.

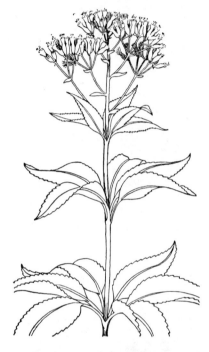

QUEEN OF THE MEADOW
(Eupatorium Purpureum, Aster Family)
Common Names—Gravel-Root, Joe-Pie, Trumpet Weed, Purple Boneset.
Medicinal Part—The root.

Gravel—The diet should be without condiments; no salt, pepper, mustard or vinegar. No animal foods. Plenty of fresh fruit and green leafy vegetables. In addition, one or two cupfuls a day of the freshly expressed juice of raw vegetables, especially radishes.

HABIT BREAKERS

For Tobacco Chewers—I herewith send you a prescription which has never yet failed. Take the inner bark of Poplar and when your friend wants a chew of tobacco let him take a chew of this bark. If he will follow this three weeks, I will guarantee he never will be troubled with a weak stomach, or have any more desire for the filthy weed. Writes Miss R. M. C., Sedgwick, Kan.

Voice Tonic—This is an old Indian remedy and very simple. It consists of chewing the dried herb Indian Balsam, the same as one would tobacco, but swallow the juice. The taste is similar to licorice. The Indian medicine men always carried so much of this fragrant herb with them that it gave them a peculiar not unpleasant odor, similar to the flavor of hickory nuts. It was much used by the Indian auratorist. It clears the voice in a most remarkable manner and seems to create the desire to sing. Singers and speakers should try this herb. It will surely surprise and delight them. It is excellent for hoarseness, sore throat and certain affections of the mouth. These effects are noticed within a few minutes after chewing the herb. Entirely harmless and very beneficial.

The Poplar Bark sure did the work. I haven't taken a chew of tobacco for four weeks, and the Mate, I got, put four pounds on me. I am 68 years old. My former weight was 140 pounds, ranging sometimes to 150. I only weighed 111, now I weigh 115 after using the Mate, and I feel a lot better. Will try it longer. Writes R. S., Cowden, Ill.

Tobacco Habit Remedy—Take about a teaspoonful of Archangel Root, ground fine and place it in your cheek, the same as you would a plug of tobacco, but swallow the juice. This is a good substitute for tobacco, both chewing and smoking, and an excellent tonic for the stomach, and also for some nervous troubles, especially such as are due to using tobacco.

Colombo Root is a good substitute for tobacco and is claimed to stop the craving for tobacco. Writes Mrs. E. C. G., Iuka, Ill.

I am going to try Ginseng Root for a "chew" to quit smoking. I have tried everything without fail, but I saw a man use that root and now he can't stand for one to smoke at his side at all. Writes S. S., Greenwood, Ark.

Editor's Note—It can do no harm—but much good.

I would like to add my recipe to your edition. I find Clover flowers a delicious table drink, full of health giving elements with brown sugar and cream added, also Elder Flowers, especially the fresh ones. I do not crave coffee or tea any more and glad to find something so good to take the place of these death-dealing drinks. Writes Mrs. F. R., Sulphur, Okla.

Here is a Tobacco Habit Remedy—Chew Life Everlasting or Oldfield Balsam. This is better than advertised "remedies." It is also good for throat troubles. Writes L. M., Bogalusa, La.

Anti-tobacco Remedy—Two ounces White Poplar Bark and Gentian, also Licorice, all coarsely ground, one ounce Wild Cherry Bark, Cinchona Bark and Molasses or Corn Syrup, to make a still mass, make into tablets. This to be used as needed and to be chewed and the juice swallowed. Writes L. A., Bangor, Me.

King Tobacco Cure is made of Gentian Root, coarsely ground. Take a pinch of it after each meal or oftener and chew it, swallowing the juice. Writes H. O., Kimball, W. Va.

—Golden Seal Comp.

    Anise Seed
    Fennel Seed
    Golden Seal Root
    Gum Myrrh
    Jamaica Ginger
Tonic. Golden Seal is the principal active agent of this tea.

If Nervous or using too much Tobacco try taking a small piece of Ginseng Root and chewing it, when nervous or about to smoke. The juice should be swallowed. It is perfectly harmless but very good for you. Writes W. O. B., Birch Run, W. Va.

Editor's Note—I'll say it is. But rather expensive. An acre of this plant full grown is worth around $20,000, even in these dry depression days.

HAIR

I tried some of the Peach Tree Leaves made into a tea for making the hair grow and it certainly does the work. Writes J. F. T., Charleston, Ark.

Editor's Note—That's something a smart barber could use to advantage.

To Cure Dandruff—Put one cupful of Sage Leaves in a vessel, pour one quart of boiling water over, boil down to one and one-half pints, add one teaspoonful borax. Wash head with this three times a week, as it's good. Writes Mrs. J. A. E., Mason, W. Va.

A Rinse for the Hair—Make a tea of Chamomile Flowers, using about a handful of flowers to a quart of boiling water. Let it steep about 10 minutes then strain it off, and use it as a final rinse for the hair after the usual shampoo, running it thoroughly through the hair several times over. Allow to dry without using a towel. It is harmless to any hair, and gives it lustre and beautiful tints, especially light brown hair. Writes Mrs. E. M. W., Baltimore, Md.

If you want to keep your hair brown, just wash it in White Oak Bark. A woman told me about this valuable article. Writes M. F., Oronago, Mo.

To Darken Faded Hair—Wash in Garden Sage. Writes S. J. W., Ashland, Ga.

Here is a remedy that will prevent the hair from turning gray. Make a tea of the roots of the common Grape Vine, and wash the hair with it once a month. Some use it two or three times a month for a while, when they discover a tendency to become gray. It is the method in use by the Indians. Writes Mr. M. A., Ogden, Utah.

Editor's Note—This is a new one on me. Someday I'll try it myself. If I don't try it soon I'll have no hair to try it on.

For Coloring the Hair—Here is a recipe as I copied it recently from Dr. Brady's column of the Chicago American: Pour a quart of boiling water over 10 or more Butternut Shucks and let it stand for an hour or so until it is dark brown. Then strain and bottle and keep in a cool place. It will keep for two years without souring. I have found it O. K. for touching up my gray hair. Writes Mrs. Z. A., Chicago, Ill.

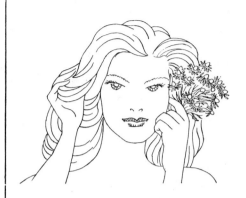

Take a small handful of both Agrimony and Common Sage, place both in a half pound of pure Hog's Lard or Vaseline, put in a vessel, put on stove, stew until herbs are well mixed in, then take off the fire and let cool. After it is cool place enough Powdered Orris Root in it to give it a good odor, strain, and the preparation is ready for use on the hair. To be used every other day, three times a week, apply by rubbing in well with finger tips and then brush good.

Agrimony—Useful for arresting any itching skin, strengthening hair roots, also restoring its color.

Sage—Diaphoretic, and is both stimulating and invigorating to hair and scalp with its coloring effect. The same has been tried and found very helpful as a hair invigorator, scalp cleanser and colorer. Known to the Indian profession, and my ancestors were Indians. Writes G. T. B., Painter, Va.

A Recipe for Gray Hair—Sage Tea; use every other day until color comes back in your hair, and then use twice a week. With continued use will bring in a new crop of hair. Writes Mrs. M. F., Nocon, Texas.

Here is a recipe for all mothers. Oil of Sassafras applied to the head will kill every nit and louse. Writes S. V. T., Thonotassa, Fla.

I want to mention how my grandfather would take bark and twigs from Wild Cherry Trees and wash his hair to keep it from falling out. He would boil the bark down to a strong tea and this surely did preserve his hair. When he died he was eighty years old and had as thick a head of hair as a young man. Writes Mrs. Wm. A. B., Hillsboro, Ill.

Swamp or Tag Alder cut up, steep in 2 quarts of water, boil down to a quart. Apply as you would a shampoo, by using once a month or so. Whenever you wish to wash the head use this. Will color white hair a pretty shade of brown so it will look natural. An old man tried this and was much pleased with results, and also uses it now whenever he sees any of the gray hair returning. Writes Mrs. L. S., Cocolalla, Idaho.

Here is a good recipe for any person that is getting bald. Take a large handful of Peach Tree Leaves and steep them into a strong tea, and rub into the scalp well, and you will soon see new hair coming. Writes E. C., Helena, Ark.

I am using your Peach Tree Leaves at 25c per box as a tonic and my hair sure is growing in new and coming in thick. My friends all even notice it. Writes Mrs. S. R., Evansville, Ind.

HAY FEVER

(Also see Asthma.)

Hay Fever and Rose Catarrh are the names by which a peculiar yearly recurring catarrhal affection is known. The access is sudden, often attended with violent sneezing; also running from the eyes and nose of thin, irritating water; redness and itching of the nose and eyes; general irritability and lassitude. The disease is less in high, mountainous regions, or at the sea. It is aggravated by dust, and by pollen of hay and flowers. Sea bathing is often beneficial, and a sea-voyage often affords entire relief. Treatment—See treatment for Catarrh.

I had the Asthma so badly and I got the Wild Plum Bark and made a syrup of it, like it says in the book. That was last fall I started taking this, and I haven't had a touch of it since. Writes Mrs. J. H. L., Nowata, Okla.

In the fall when the Hay Fever starts, or even before, get the Life Everlasting and make a tea. Take a glassful night and morning and also make a pillow of it and sleep on it. My husband has been troubled with Hay Fever for years and he was pretty bad at first, but an old German lady told me about it and now all I do is make the tea in the fall and he gets relief just as soon as he takes it. A friend of mine had the same trouble last fall, and she could not even sleep at night when I told her about it, and it helped. Writes Mrs. F. R. A., Norristown, Pa.

Editor's Note—This surely is a simple remedy and I am going to recommend it to some of my friends. Thank you.

I have found from experience that a small amount of Slippery Elm with hot water made into a small poultice and applied to the nose as warm as you can stand will give almost instantaneous relief in Hay Fever. Rub some of the liquid up into the nostrils, too. Writes Mrs. L. G., Winfield, Kans.

In regard to Gobernadora, we have used this for the past three years for Hay Fever and it is wonderful; will relieve the most severe case. Writes W. T. S., El Paso, Tex.

Editor's Note—Well—that's good news.

Hay Fever Remedy—Get Crimson Clover, Plantain, Boneset and Spikenard. Mix together same amount of each and take a teaspoonful of the mixture, put in cupful of boiling water, drink 2 cups daily. If not relieved, then use only one-half cup of water instead of a cupful. Writes Mrs. M. L., Elyria, Ohio.

Hay Fever—Take the juice of a lemon in a glass of water morning and evening. Eat four oranges for breakfast and four for supper. Have a large plateful of vegetable salad for lunch. Better abstain from milk until recovered.

Hay Fever—Take the root of Yellow Dock, pulverize it and snuff it up the nostrils. I had the Hay Fever four years and tried different localities but to no avail, when an old trapper told me to try this Dock Root and it proved successful. Writes D. E., Jackson, Wyo.

HEADACHES

(See Nerves and Constipation.)

Headache is a symptom of some disease or derangement of the system. The cause should be determined before any treatment is taken. Eye strain is also a very common cause. Other causes are diseases of the womb and ovaries in women, piles and malaria, anemia, the excessive use of tobacco, exposure to cold, errors in diet, a plug of wax in the internal ear, catarrh of the nose and upper part of the frontal sinus, the inhalation of gas in houses where the fixtures are leaky, sleeping in close and illy-ventilated rooms, etc., etc.

Treatment—Take one or two Tablets to relieve the pain. Then determine the cause and take the proper action to remove same. If of a nervous nature, take Calmative Tea; if due to constipation or disturbance of the digestive organism, take a large dose of Calumet Herb Laxative Tea.

Mustard Seed ground and moistened, then spread on a cloth, place on the patient's abdomen, will cure Sick Headache. Writes M. B., Vannoy, N. C.

To Cure Headaches and Insure Restful Sleep—Fill a pillow with Pine Needles and sleep on them at night.

For Sick Headache, Induced by Bilious Derangement—Steep one part of Senna and Chamomile Flowers in a cup of hot water, to make strong decoction and drink. It has been tried successfully in various cases.

Sick Headache—There are few ailments that are more distressing than a sick headache. The following, while very bitter, will give quick relief: Take one teaspoonful of each of the following coarse ground: Chamomile Flowers, Catnip, Sacred Bark and Turtlebloom. Place in a cup of boiling hot water, and cover tightly until cool, drink the whole cupful at one time. It will seldom be necessary to repeat the dose but if not benefited repeat as often as necessary.

For Sick and Nervous Headache— Take Nerve Root, Blue Scullcap and Catnip; one teaspoonful of each; steep in a cup of boiling water half hour. Drink cold one tablespoonful every half hour until relieved.

For Bilious Headache—Take one-fourth ounce Senna Leaves, Sage, and Crushed Ginger; infuse in pint of water, and take a wineglassful 3 times a day.

For Headaches—Take a teaspoonful of Cinnamon with water. Writes J. W., Clover, S. C.

For Sick Headaches—Drink a cupful of Boneset tea hot, or if needed for a cathartic drink the tea cold. Writes C. H. D., Keisters, Pa.

The best thing in the world for a headache. Make Catnip Tea, sweeten, drink while hot. Writes M. E. S., Timblin, Pa.

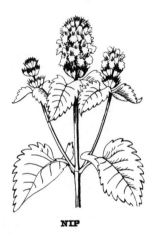

NIP

I have tried Catnip Tea for Headaches and it is wonderful. Writes E. L. T., Veedersburg, Ind.

Sick Headache—Bull Nettle Roots. Make into a poultice and bind to the head, or chew and swallow the juice. Writes Mrs. A. S., Patmos, Ark.

I have tried the Nerve Root, Blue Scullcap and Catnip at 25c per box for Sick and Nervous Headaches. Taken in tablespoon doses it will relieve. Writes M. S., Westville, Ill.

Take half teaspoonful powdered Ginger, same amount of sugar in a half glass of water, and this will relieve Headache in 15 to 25 minutes. Writes O. L. T., Watseka, Ill.

Sick and Nervous Headache—Take equal parts of the following: Nerve Root, 1 teaspoonful; Blue Scullcap, 1 teaspoonful; Catnip, 1 teaspoonful. Steep in cup of boiling water and drink cold, 1 cupful a day. Writes G. S., Tower City, Pa.

For Nervous Headache—Take Butterfly Root and make a tea and drink about a teacupful warm and it will relieve in a short time. Writes A. M., Hartville, Md.

I have been using Catnip Tea for Headaches and I surely think it is wonderful. I also used it for a roaring in my head and it stopped that also. Writes Miss M. S., Ashland, Ohio.

For Headache—Take a small bunch of Balm that is dried thoroughly and put in a cup, pour boiling water over it and set until cool enough to drink, or use when still warm with a little sugar, and it usually relieves headache in a very short time, and is harmless, and it is good to drink at the table with the meals. Writes E. N., Paducah, Ky.

HEART DISEASE

Symptoms—Shortness of breath and weakness upon the slightest exertion, swelling of the feet.

Treatment—Consult a specialist. Keep bowels open. Get plenty of rest. Eat lightly. Breathe a little deeper than usual. Walking is one of the best exercises for this ailment. Avoid smoking and strong alcoholic drinks. Take no liquids during meals.

The Herb Doctor's choice of botanical Tonics are: Hawthorne berries, Mistletoe, Sweet Balm, Cleavers, Corn Silk, Valerian, Lavender Flowers.

Neuralgia of the Heart—Or Angina Pectoris is a very serious ailment. It is attended by an intense pain beneath the breast bone, which usually extends down the left arm and up into the neck. The breath is short, there is a feeling of pressure upon the chest.

Treatment—Call a specialist at once. Avoid all excitement and worry.

Palpitation of the Heart—Palpitation (or fluttering action) of the heart may be due to mental excitement, fright, excessive use of tobacco, alcohol, coffee, or tea; frequently to gas or acid in the stomach.

Treatment—Place the patient in bed and assure him that there is no danger. This will do much to restore cheerfulness and shorten the attack. Apply cold compresses or icebag over the heart. The administration of Aromatic Spirits of Ammonia, 1 teaspoonful in water, is useful.

The Herb Doctor's choice of mild botanical Sedatives and Tonics are: Blue Vervain, Wild Cherry Bark, Lavender Flowers, Valerian.

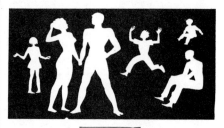

—Heart Tonic Tea.
Lily of the Valley
Black Cohosh
Valerian
Wild Cherry
Gentian
Wild Strawberry
Mistletoe

The ingredients of this remarkable formula speak for themselves.

I received your wonderful book and would like to give you a remedy for the heart. Take Heart Leaf Root and chew them 3 or 4 times a day. Just use two or three roots at a time, and swallow the juice. It is wonderful for weak heart. Writes C. W., Keener, Ala.

Fatty Heart Disease—Or fatty degeneration of the heart. Due to an excessive amount of fat around the heart.

Treatment—Consult a specialist. See instruction under Heart Disease.

I have found that the Mormon Valley Herb Compound has had a tendency to slow the heart action, just as you thought it would. Now I feel that with the constant use of same it will be probably all that will be needed. Writes O. D. T., Mattoon, Ill.

Recipe for Heart Disease—Take the English Plantain which is the common broad leafed Plantain, and make into a tea, and take 3 times during the day. To each cup add a grain of salt, and one-half teacup of white vinegar. Writes W. B. N., Ragged Island, Bahamas.

Editor's Note—I have grave doubts about this, especially the vinegar.

Here is a recipe for you for the heart. It is a good one. Take one ounce each of Tansy, Yarrow, and Wood Betony and scald them in 3 pints of boiling water. When cold, strain and bottle and take a wineglassful after meals and at bedtime. Writes J. F., New Bedford, Mass.

For Palpitation or Pain Near Heart—Put a small quantity of Virginia Snake Root in a cupful of boiling water and drink all such water as is required. In such cases I use it in place of water I otherwise drink for two or three days. Writes E. C., Flat Rock, Ala.

Editor's Note—This looks very good.

My whole family is using the Boteka Leaves and it is doing good for all of us. My boy remarks he can work better, when he takes a cupful in the morning, and I have not had any spells with my heart since. Writes T. C. D., Sharon, Pa.

Editor's Note—I know it's good.

Hawthorn Berries for the Heart—A tea of Hawthorn Berries has a brown red color of fruity odor and a pleasant taste. As it is not poisonous, the dosage need not be so accurate. An average dose of the tea for an adult would be a teaspoonful in water, three or four times a day. The indications for its use are: functional and organic affections of the heart, mitral insufficiency, rapid and feeble heart action, angina, dyspnoea of cardiac origin, and in general the condition known as the senile heart. The writer has used Hawthorn Berries for many years in the above-named conditions, and like other remedies, it frequently disappoints expectations formed as to its utility, but in a large proportion of cases treated the result has established its value as an approved remedy for the conditions to which it applies. It will not take the place of Fox Glove, there is not a plant medicine that will. But it may be depended on within its own sphere of action and it possesses the advantage over Fox Glove that it is not poisonous. Writes Dr. B., Ennis, Ireland.

I have tried Wild Cherry Bark for my heart and it has done me more good than half a dozen doctors. I had palpitation of the heart for eleven years and it beats better now than in that length of time. I suffered so much I would like everyone to know about it that suffers with the heart. Writes Mrs. C. C., Starrsville, Ga.

HEARTBURN
(See Dyspepsia and Stomach and Bowel Troubles.)

Heartburn—Take the inner bark of Butternut tree and make it into a tea; fix it to suit yourself, just as strong as you think you can take it. Steep for about half hour, strain and use. You can repeat if necessary, but I doubt if this will be necessary. Writes M. C. G., Rochester, Minn.

For Heartburn, or Sour Stomach—Use Tansy Leaves, in a glass of cold water, sweeten with sugar, drink a few mouthfuls at a time and it will relieve at once. Writes E. N., Paducah, Ky.

Here is a Good Formula for Heartburn—Chew a small piece of Wild Alum and swallow the juice, and you will get relief very soon. Writes A. L. D., Columbus, Ga.

For Heartburn—Chew three grains of corn and swallow it, and note the results. Writes R. K., Sentinel, Okla.

—Father Bernard's Stomach
    Tea..........
    Italian Sage Leaves
    Stone Root
    Colic Root
    Fennel Seed
    Wormwood Leaves
    Gentian Root
    Juniper Berries
    Wild Strawberry Leaves
    German Cheese Plant
A combination of valuable stomachics. Give tone to the stomach and improves the gastric juice.

Heartburn—The cure must be adapted to the cause. If it proceeds from indigestion a dose of Rhubarb will give relief. If from acidity, eat Magnesia, but if from "wind" use Caraway or Coriander Seeds or take a dose of Composition Powder. This Composition Powder contains a pound of Bayberry Bark, 8 ounces of Ginger and 3 ounces of Cayenne Powder, mix in powdered form, and all mixed well. Writes I. S., St. Petersburg, Fla.

HEART DROPSY

Is a symptom of heart disease, ne-
phritis, liver disease or of a complication of ailments.
Treatment—Consult a specialist. Rest
in bed. Take only milk or liquid diet,
beef juice, soft boiled eggs, fruits and
vegetables.
The Herb Doctor's choice of botanical Diuretics are: Dwarf Elder Root,
Juniper Berries, Cleavers, Birch Leaves.

For Heart Dropsy—Make a tea of
Ground Ivy, and use it for your table
tea and for drinking water. It has
cured when all doctors failed. Writes
I. C., Ela, N. C.

—Lavender Flowers
    Compound.....
Lavender Flowers
Rosemary Lvs. and Flors.
Cheese Plant Lvs. and Flors.
Althea Root
Thyme Leaves
Virginia Snake Root
Properties: Mild Diuretic, Tonic and
Astringent. The herbal physician will
find many uses for this fine combination.

HICCOUGHS

For Hiccoughs—I worked in an office
where an elderly gentleman was employed. An attack of hiccoughs came
upon him. He tried everything including medical treatment but with no relief. It began to look serious for it continued 3 or 4 days. We were afraid for
him. Finally he came back to the office
one day after they stopped. We asked
him how he did it, and he said he finally
succeeded in stopping them by putting
a few drops of Anise Oil in a teaspoonful of sugar and taking it. Hiccoughs,
I understand, sometimes become dangerous. Writes J. W. G., Clare, Mich.

Pineapple juice will cure the Hiccoughs. Writes Mrs. G. H., Metropolis,
Ill.

Pineapple juice is one of the best
things to use in case of Hiccoughs.
Writes F. A. W., Tremont, Pa.

Hiccoughs—A tablespoonful of Pineapple Juice with a little salt is very
good for hiccoughs. Writes T. K.,
Monessen, Pa.

Cure for Hiccoughs—Drink 3 swallows of water slowly while holding your
breath. Writes Mrs. H. S., Westwood,
Calif.

I am sending a cure for Hiccoughs,
which was taken from my mother's
recipe book which was printed in 1840.
Use powdered Rhubarb and prepared
Chalk mixed thoroughly together. Of
this take one level teaspoonful dry on
the tongue and swallow with a glass
of cold water. Writes Mrs. A. P. B.,
Ozona, Fla.

Common Dill Plant—The use of this
in our family will never fade. It has
been handed down these last four generations and I would like all who see it
to give it a trial. Make a tea of the
plant and give in teaspoonful doses for
the Hiccoughs. Writes Mrs. E. F., Racine, Wis.
Editor's Note—Well, this is simple enough—
and harmless enough to say the least.

HIVES OR NETTLE RASH

Are reddish spots, which resemble
mosquito stings, with burning and itching.
Treatment—Keep bowels open.
    Bathe the affected parts
with Medicated Witch Hazel. Use same
treatment as for Prickly Heat.

Make a tea of Catnip and this is good
for hives on the baby. Roasted onions
filled with sulphur is also very good.
Writes H. P. A., Walled Lake, Mich.

I am sending you a good recipe for
Hives. Take an ounce of Bull Nettle
Root and a quart of water, and let it
steep down to a pint, then strain, let
cool, and give by the half cupful a day.
Writes G. M. S., Portland, Ore.

Get the Red Alder Bark and make a
tea and use internally, and you will
find it very good for Hives. Writes
Mrs. E. A., Ball Ground, Ga.

For Hives—Make a tea of Tag Alder,
and give to children. This is a sure
cure. Writes Mrs. R. R. D., Lynn, Ala.

For Hives on a Baby—Make a strong
tea of the Ground Ivy by steeping in
hot water, and sweeten. Give teaspoonful every 10 or 15 minutes or at longer
intervals such as you see fit. It will do
no harm. Writes M. E. T., Palmersville,
Tenn.

Make a tea of Sage and drink freely, will cure worst case of Hives. Have tried it after doctor's medicine failed, and know it to be true. Writes Mrs. G. K., Pittsburg, Kans.

Here is something good for the Hives of little babies. Take a tablespoonful of Catnip Leaves, add this to a pint of water, let boil down to ½ pint, strain, add sugar to suit the taste. This can be given with a spoon or in the bottle with nipple. Give what you think is needed, it will not hurt the baby for I used it and know it is good. Writes Mrs. W. F. D., Rockwell, Texas.

Medicated Witch Hazel—Made from fresh, green young twigs of the witch hazel shrub. About twenty pounds are used to make one gallon—double strength. Best money can buy. Useful after shaving, for sunburn, ringworm, toothache, neuralgia, headaches, muscular pains, and hundreds of minor ailments.

An old tried remedy for Hives. Take an ounce of Ground Ivy, put in 1 quart of water and boil down to 1 pint. Strain and take a cupful a day. Writes F. L. C., Lebanon, Va.

For Hives on small babies, take Catnip and make a tea. Give a teaspoonful three or four times a day. If tried, you will agree it is a good recipe. Writes R. S., Hollowell, Kan.

My complaint was Hives and I had them for years and they almost drove me insane. I spent over $70.00 at one time with 10 results, when a lady told me to make a teacup of Catnip Tea. I did and the hives disappeared much to my amazement for nothing ever helped before. Take a handful of the Catnip and about a quart of water, and boil until you have a teacupful of the tea. I did not put any sugar in it for I was told not to. I took the tea as soon as it was cool enough, and if they return just take more tea. Writes Mrs. T. D., Moulton, Ia.

Try equal parts Sassafras, Stillingia, to twice as much Sarsaparilla. Mix and keep in tight glass jar. Take a teaspoonful steeped in a cupful of boiling water once a day for Hives, and note the results. Writes Mrs. J. H., Hubbard, Minn.

INDIGESTION
(See Stomach and Bowel Disorders.)

Is caused by over-eating or eating food which "disagrees" with the stomach or it sometimes appears at intervals of a few weeks for no apparent cause. It usually is a fixed, violent pain at the pit of the stomach. Sometimes there is nausea and vomiting, the pain is not steady but comes and goes and the region of the stomach is often bloated and tender to the touch.

Acute indigestion is sometimes very serious. Treatment should be started immediately and continued until the patient is entirely recovered.

The patient should remain quiet until completely relieved. A hot water bag at the pit of the stomach will often help.

The Herb Doctor's choice of botanical Cathartics are: Sacred Bark, Turtlebloom, Wormwood, Senna Leaves, Butternut Bark.

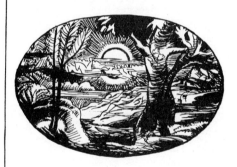

Chewing a small piece of the root of Ginseng will mostly cure a bad case of Indigestion. If too bad, take pieces of the root and pour a least bit of hot water over and let stand a few minutes and give the liquid. Writes Mrs. C. K., Benton, Pa.

Take half gallon Poke Berries, and half gallon Elder Berries, put up or make sour wine of this. Use 3 times a day, and it hardly ever takes over a pint but a quart at the most to cure the worst case of indigestion. Writes L. B., Alligator, Miss.

Take whole Flax Seed not ground, one teaspoonful before retiring for the night. My wife tried this for Indigestion and never had an attack since taking it. Use sufficient, and take until cured. Writes Geo. E. H., Shamokin, Pa.

My father cured himself of Indigestion by chewing Sarsaparilla Root and swallowing the juice. Writes Miss L. J. L., Punxsutawney, Pa.

Purge—A strong purge is made from the root of Blue Flag, even taken in small quantities, especially when fresh. The inner bark of common Elder is a strong purge, too. Write W. J. P., Whitestone, L. I., N. Y.

I suffered so with Indigestion and the doctor told me he had done all he could for it. Why, I was hardly able to walk over three or four blocks without getting all out of breath, and I also had a misery in my chest. I began taking the Life Everlasting in tea. I took a cupful for three days, then waited three days, etc. It is worth its weight in gold. I now work hard again, eat anything I want and can sleep all night. Writes J. F., Annistan, Ala.

About seven years ago I had a bad case of Indigestion. I steeped a pinch of Yarrow Blossoms in a cup of water, and drank a swallow several times a day for 3 days. I haven't had such trouble since. Writes Mrs. O. C., Cadillac, Mich.

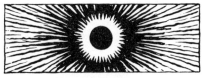

INFLAMMATIONS

Inflammations—Do you know that the little Smart Weed that grows in damp ground is the finest thing to draw inflammation out of a sore? I had boils in my ear and it was swollen until I could get no sleep. I made a poultice with it, a handful with enough water to cover, boil until you get the strength, then thicken with corn meal. Put inside a cloth bag and spread out till it covers the sore spot. Relief comes mighty quick. Writes M. D. G., Cornwell, Ill.

For Inflammatory Conditions—Make a poultice of Elderberry Blossoms and apply on affected parts. Especially good for Blood Poisoning and Boils. Writes N. N., Sugar Island, Tex.

Plantain Leaves—Made into a poultice will draw harder than anything. Writes J. H. T., Greenfield, Ind.

I found in my practice of over nine years the following poultice the best remedy for external application in all manner of inflammation from sciatica to appendicitis and pneumonia: A handful each of Tulip Tree Bark and Mullein Leaves, cut small, boiled 10 minutes in a quart of vinegar. Remove from the stove and add sufficient bran or meal, preferably bran, to take up all the liquid. Place in cloth and pack on affected part as hot as can be borne. Allow to remain until cool (about an hour), then heat again with small amount of boiling water added, and place on the spine opposite the affected part until cool. Have had remarkable results with it. Writes Dr. C. B. T., Mowrystown, Ohio.

INFLUENZA OR LA GRIPPE

(Also see Coughs and Colds.)

The first symptoms are a chill, sneezing and cold in the head, followed by a cough which may be the beginning of pneumonia. Sometimes the throat is sore and ulcers may appear on the tonsils. Aching pains often appear in the back and other parts. There is apt to be considerable fever and much weakness, and the patient is low-spirited.

Treatment—Patient should be put to bed and kept warm. Give whiskey diluted with lemon juice. Should pneumonia develop it will require the usual supportive and stimulating measures. The after-effects of this disease are frequently more to be dreaded than the disease itself. The system is frequently left weakened and debilitated, in which condition it is open to attacks from other diseases and even to recurrence of this trouble. Whiskey will keep up the strength—Diaphoretics and Tonics are often useful.

Call only an experienced doctor.

The Herb Doctor's choice of Febrifuges and Diaphoretics and Tonics are: Boneset, Jesuits Bark, Chamomile, Sweet Flag, Goose Grass.

Boil a handful of Motherwort in two cupfuls of water until you have a cupful, then sweeten and drink this hot upon retiring for the Flu. Writes Mrs. L. McM., Sparta, N. C.

Editor's Note—Looks rather strong to me. Better use a quart of water to a handful and boil it down to a pint.

La Grippe—This will cure the la grippe. Take a double handful of Life Everlasting and put it in a quart of water and boil down to one pint. Take one tablespoonful three times during the day. Writes A. W. P., Mounds, Okla.

I have had La Grippe yearly, and usually lasts one to two weeks, but this year I drank profusely of Boneset Tea (eight cupfuls during the day), and I was only confined to bed one day. Writes S. S., New Britain, Conn.

Editor's Note—You did the right thing.

Influenza Tea—Take a handful of the plant (Desert Mint), place in a vessel, pour a teacupful of boiling water over the contents and let steep. Do not boil, as boiling weakens this tea. Strain, sweeten, drink a cupful before retiring. This is an excellent remedy for influenza. Writes K. M. N., Good Springs, Tenn.

Editor's Note—The sample plant this generous lady sent was Desert Mint, also called Horsemint. It grows in sandy soil and is very fragrant.

During the epidemic I contracted the Flu and could not obtain a doctor. I ordered a strong brew of Boneset tea, mixed with lemon juice and sugar, and in the meantime I wrapped up in a blanket, then drank it as hot as possible. Writes M. E. S., Englishtown, N. J.

Editor's Note—You could not have taken anything better.

I have used more of this recipe this spring with the Flu than ever before. It surely cures the sore throat, the mouth, and it is good for pain in teeth, or any place you want to use it. This may be used as a tea or a wash. The use of it just once will prove its worth. It is Persimmon Bark. Writes Mrs. L. L., Calhoun, Ky.

—Agueweed Comp.
    Ague Weed
    Sweet Flag
    Sassafras Root
    Juniper Berries
    Goose Grass
    Snake Root
    Thyme Leaves

Stimulant and Diaphoretic—This is a combination of Boneset, Thyme, etc., of excellent service in Colds and Fevers where a diaphoretic is indicated. When taken cold in the form of a tea it acts as a general tonic to be used after a siege of fever. Taken hot it drives out the poison through the respiratory system. Take it in time as a preventive.

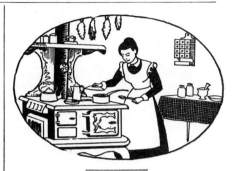

Diaphoretic—Useful in Fevers, Malaria, Ague, Flu, La Grippe, etc. This is truly a great remedy containing botanicals that could be found in the pocket of the Indian Medicine Man as well as the medicine chests of many of the early settlers.

    2 ounces Boneset Leaves
    1 ounce Juniper Berries
    2 ounces Elder Flowers
    1 ounce Wild Ginger
    2 ounces Sweet Flag Root

A teaspoonful used to a cupful of boiling water. Tea should be made fresh every day.

Take equal parts of Boneset, Black Root and Blue Cohosh, make into a tea and try for Influenza. Writes W. L. C., Louisa, Ky.

I am sending a recipe which I hope you will find a place for in your booklet, for it is good and cured my mother of the flu. It contains equal parts of Chestnut Leaves, Pine Tops, Sweet Gum Bark, Butterfly Weed Root and Boneset. Mix in equal parts, and use a teaspoonful to a cupful of boiling water. Writes Miss M. G. B., Fayette, Ala.

La Grippe—Here is the very best remedy I ever saw for La Grippe: Take a heaping teaspoonful of Indian Hyssop and Turtlebloom. Place into a cup of boiling water. Let it steep for 10 or 15 minutes and drink while still hot upon retiring at night. It will cure in 24 hours. Writes Z. G., of Bangor, Me.

Make a tea of August flower and use it as a gargle for common sore throat and drink several cupfuls a day for cold and flu. Writes F. B., Southwest City, Mo.

INSECT CHASERS

I am writing you a recipe for Bed Bugs. I once had Bed Bugs in the house and it seemed as though nothing would get rid of them. One day I was looking for something to put on them and had nothing but a bottle, perhaps an ounce, of Eucalyptus Oil which I tried. I lived seven years in the same house and never saw another Bed Bug, so I always recommend Eucalyptus Oil. Writes Mrs. E. L., Ontario, Calif.

To Keep Ants Away—Put some kerosene in the mop water. Writes Mrs. C. M., Woodland, Mich.

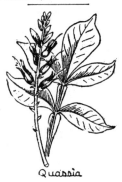

Quassia

For cockroaches, mix together 8 ounces Insect Powder, 8 ounces Borax, 4 ounces Sulphur and one-fourth ounce Eucalyptus Oil.

To help rid the place of ants, cut up Poke Root and scatter it in their runs. Writes Mrs. E. C. P., Scottsville, Ky.

A means of destroying black Beetles and Cockroaches is to strew the roots of the White Hellebore on the floor at night. Next morning, the whole family of these insects will be found either dead or dying. Such is their avidity for this poisonous plant that they seldom fail to eat it when they can get it. Writes H. F., Galveston, Tex.

"The Ohio State Board of Health states: 'Nature has given us a simple remedy for Flies—place White Clover Blossoms in each room.'" Writes I. N. L., Lansing, Mich.

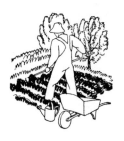

To make a scent to be applied to baits or rat traps to lure the rodents, mix together one teaspoonful Rose Geranium Oil, one teaspoonful Cubeb Oils and 6 teaspoonfuls Balsam Copaiba. This will not destroy or poison the rats or mice. It is merely a lure to use on poisons or on traps.

Another insecticide which is very good for luring insects but is harmless to human beings and animals is made by mixing 33 parts Insect Powder, 48 parts Borax, 12 parts Glucose, sugar or any other sweet substance and 7 parts flour, preferably rice flour.

For Moths—A preventive against moths, and also a pleasant perfume. Take Cloves, Caraway Seeds, Nutmeg, Mace, Cinnamon and Tonka Beans, an ounce of each, then add Florentine Orris, as will equal the other ingredients, put together, grind the whole until powder and put in little bags among the clothes. Writes D. J. D., Corfu, N. Y.

Here is a recipe for Roach Powder, which is good, and may find space in your next "Almanac." Three teaspoonfuls Corn Syrup, 1 teaspoonful Powdered Borax, and 2 teaspoonfuls of sugar, mix in a pan, and when well mixed, it is ready for use. Writes C. A. C., Tulsa, Okla.

A good insect powder can be made by mixing seven parts Insect Powder (Pyrethrum flowers) and three parts Quassia in a fine powder.

Another good insect powder is made by mixing 8 ounces Insect Powder with 8 ounces powdered Quassia, 1 ounce Cedar Oil and one-fourth ounce Pennyroyal Oil.

KIDNEYS

(See Bladder Trouble.)

The symptoms are pain in one or both sides above the hip, and toward the spine, in the region of the kidneys and thence usually extending forward and downward with frequent desire to urinate, and scanty hot discharge and numbness along the inner side of the thigh on the affected side. There is fever and sometimes vomiting.

Treatment—Rest in bed and application of hot water bag to seat of pain often give relief. Keep bowels open and give soothing Demulcent drinks. The diet must be light.

The Herb Doctor's choice of botanicals are: Cheese Plant, Marshmallow Root, Corn Silk, Dog Grass, Cubeb Berries, Wallwort, Horsetail Grass, Sassafras, Speedwell, Bearberry Leaves.

Kidney Troubles—Use three parts Corn Silk, Wild Cherry, 2 Red Raspberry Leaves, 1 Swamp Lily Root and 1 Rocky Mountain Grape Root. Mix, and then put 1 tablespoonful in a quart of boiling water, let stand 3 hours, strain and take wineglassful 4 times a day. Writes Dr. L. E., New Lexington, Ohio.

For Bladder Troubles, Scalding Pain and Catarrhal Discharges—And perhaps pus and blood there is nothing better than tea of Marshmallow Leaves. One heaping teaspoonful to a cupful of boiling water. Drink freely. It is marvelous how quick the pain leaves and the urine gets clear again. Writes Mrs. L. P., San Francisco, Calif.

Editor's Note—Marshmallow leaves are one of our finest soothing demulcents.

When the kidneys are inactive in man or horses, give Caraway Seeds. Writes Miss G. N., Whiting, N. J.

Watermelon Seed Tea will make the kidneys act. Writes Mrs. J. W., Columbus, Ga.

Here is a good remedy for Kidney and Bladder troubles. Fill a half gallon fruit jar full of Spignet, then fill it full of boiling water, drink two cups a day. This is harmless but a sure remedy. Writes F. H., Valley, N. C.

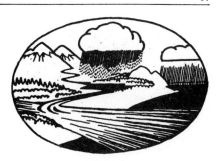

—Pale Face Kidneywort Comp.

This is a mild soothing demulcent tea useful in gravel, burning urine and inflammation of the bladder.

1 ounce Sassafras
4 ounces Horsetail Grass
2 ounces Cheese Plant
1 ounce Elecampane
1 ounce Bull Nettle
1 ounce Gravel Plant

Steep a teaspoonful of the mixture in a cup of boiling water until cool. Drink one or two cupfuls per day.

—Fr. John's Kidney-Liver Leaf Compound....
Kidney-Liver Leaf
Seven Barks
Blue Chicory Root
Senna Alexandria
Red Clover Flowers
Boneset Leaves and Flowers
German Cheese Plant
Sassafras Bark of Root

This is a very mild diuretic, containing Boneset and Kidney-Liver Leaf which gently stimulates the liver.

Kidney Tea—Mild Diuretic—A tea that will prove valuable to those suffering from weak kidneys, dropsical affections, incontinence of the urine.

1 ounce Sassafras Root
1 ounce Dwarf Elder Root
1 ounce Cheese Plant
1 teaspoonful Lily of the Valley Root
1 ounce Juniper Berries

Steep a teaspoonful of the mixture in a cup of boiling water until cool. Strain and drink one to two cupfuls per day.

For Dysentery drink a strong tea made of Red Oak Bark, and it will prove fine. It is also good for Bowel Trouble among chicks. Writes Mrs. J. T., Holmesville, Mass.

Broom Corn Seed is good for the kidneys, boil into tea, and take. Writes N. R., Rommer, Tenn.

For the Bladder—A sure remedy. Take the bark of Slippery Elm Bark, soak it in cold water, and drink it instead of the water you would otherwise take. I have known it to cure when other remedies have failed. Writes J. S., Edgefield, S. C.

Editor's Note—Elm Bark is a fine demulcent. All demulcents are soothing to the urinary passages.

I had a Kidney trouble for some time, had such smarting and sometimes bloody urine, but I just took Elder Flowers and made into a tea. Drink a good swallow three or four times a day. Writes Mrs. A. M., New Florence, Mo.

My mother had a bladder affection and she made a tea of Scouring Rush and Juniper Berries, and took it off and on for 6 years but she was cured. She made the tea and drank it just whenever she noticed her troubles and did not take continually. Writes Mrs. G. C., Austin, Texas.

Take Cherry Bark about two handfuls to a gallon of water for bad kidneys, and drink as often as you please. It is harmless and will do no harm, and I have seen pretty bad cases of kidney troubles cured with this. Writes J. F. W., Sullivan, Mich.

A friend of mine in Pittsburgh had kidney trouble quite badly. She had doctored with specialists who seemed to help her case very little. I told her to steep Buchu Leaves. She did so and found they were fine. She was much benefited and said they helped her more than all the doctor's medicine. Writes E. J. C., Buffalo, New York.

A Good Kidney Remedy—Take one tablespoonful of Juniper Berries, cut up and pour over four cups of water, boil down to two cups, drink one before going to bed. This has been a great help in our home. Writes N. N., Chicago, Ill.

Editor's Note—I don't doubt this a bit. Juniper Berries are fine for the kidneys and stomach.

A soothing tea for the Kidneys. German Cheese Plant, Quack Grass Root, Dandelion Root and Silk of Corn. Take two ounces of each and steep together, and sweeten. To keep this also put in four crushed cloves. (This makes one quart.) Writes A. W., Gobles, Mich.

Uva Ursi is fine for the Kidneys. It is harmless. Make a tea and drink a cupful at night. Writes Mrs. W. A. F., Vanleer, Tenn.

I have also used the Marshmallow treatment for kidney trouble and have received benefit from it already and I have been using it only a few days. Writes Mrs. J. R., Ririe, Idaho.

Editor's Note—Keep it up and you will be delighted. I use it myself occasionally.

Retention of the Urine—Take what Queen of the Meadow Roots you can hold between your thumb and fingers, place in a quart of water, boil slowly for fifteen minutes, pour off while hot, take about half a teacupful every three or four hours until entirely relieved. This I know from my own experience to be a sure cure for retention and scalding urine. Writes M. B. Taylor, Iceledo, Ark.

Editor's Note—It appears to me you should use at least a full 25c size box of this root to a quart of water to get any results, as it is harmless.

When the kidneys do not act, take a handful of the Peach Tree Leaves, make into a tea and drink one-half cupful and they will then act quickly. Writes W. F., Summerland, Wis.

Here is a sure cure of weakness of the kidney and bladder. Cook one pound of Seven Barks Tea in three pints of water, down to one pint and take a tablespoonful three times a day. That is what my uncle used to cure him. Writes Mrs. D. C., Louisville, Ala.

Editor's Note—"Cure" is a strong word to use; "relief" would probably be better.

One tablespoonful Flax Seed, also Slippery Elm Bark put in a quart of water, boil down to 1 pint, drink teacupful twice a day for one week and it will help bladder and kidney troubles. Writes L. B., Maysville, Ky.

Editor's Note—This makes a soothing demulcent.

For anyone that cannot make their urine, give Parsley Herb. Of the tea, give the baby only 2 or 3 teaspoonfuls, while for the adults, use one-half cupful. I just had a friend who was sick and doctors wanted to tap him, but this is what helped him. Writes Ed. V., Portage, Wis.

Here is a recipe for lame back, caused from strain or colds: Chew the Queen of the Meadow Root, swallowing the juice. Writes J. T. C., Braintree, Mass.

Each summer when we husk our sweet corn we save all the silks and dry them thoroughly. These we place in an air-tight can or jar and when needed we take a small amount and make a tea of them. This is good for any kind of kidney trouble. A cupful of this tea will regulate the amount of urine—if too much or too little. This can be taken any time. Writes Mrs. R. L. C., Thompsonville, Mich.

Editor's Note—And it is absolutely harmless.

Parsley Root is very good to increase the flow of urine. Chew and swallow the juice. Writes M. S., Fresno, Ohio.

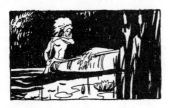

For Weak Kidneys—Drink a cup of strong Sassafras Tea every night. Writes Mrs. E. N., Roseboro, N. C.

I have also found that there is nothing better than Bull Nettle Root for bladder troubles. Writes M. L. W., Tennille, Ala.

Painful Urination—Take two tablespoonfuls of Yarrow, put in one quart of boiling water and boil five minutes, then let stand on back of the stove for one-half hour, stirring frequently. Drink one cupful half hour before breakfast and supper. This is good for painful urination, weakness of the bladder, for it has cured me of these, where all patent medicines, and doctors of this city, failed. Writes Mrs. M. B., Bedford, Wis.

Editor's Note—This can be improved by adding Cheese Plant and Cubeb Berries in equal parts.

Irritated Bladder—Two tablespoonfuls Flax Seed Meal in a half gallon of water, boil down to a quart, let stand and drink all before retiring. Sweeten if necessary and repeat every night until relieved. A positive cure for burning bladder. Writes S. E. G., Atlanta, Ga.

Perhaps you did not know that Nettle Root was so good for the bladder? I have had people use it with wonderful results. Writes C. F., Summit, N. J.

Chronic Kidney Troubles, Etc.—"I wish to contribute a remedy for chronic kidney trouble, such as scalding urine and congestion of the kidneys. It is an old Indian formula and tried and true: 2 teaspoonfuls Button Snake Root, 2 teaspoonfuls Unicorn Root, 1 teaspoonful Rock-brake Root, 1 teaspoonful Robins-Rye. Take 1 large teaspoonful of the mixed roots and steep for half an hour in a quart of hot water. Dose— One teaspoonful three times a day." Writes C. F., Allegan, Mich.

Juniper Berries — These eaten or steeped are good for all kidney and bladder troubles. Writes Mrs. G. E., Pt. Pleasant, N. Y.

This is used by many people in the south for kidney troubles. Bake the seeds of Watermelon, beat them up into a pulp, from which a tea, made in the ordinary way should be made. Then an occasional drink of it keeps the kidneys in good shape. Writes M. G., Hemlock, N. C.

Use Watermelon Seeds for kidney and bladder for they are very good. Take a handful and boil in a little water and drink a cupful with a little sugar. One cupful is enough for about three days. This can be taken when the back aches, too. Writes Mrs. J. T. D., Cedar Rapids, Ia.

For urinary troubles, to increase the flow. Use a tea of Elder Roots. Writes J. H. S., Arbaugh, Ark.

Give your child Cinnamon Bark to eat if it has a weak bladder and it will cure.

To one cup of Bran add four cups of cold water, simmer for 10 minutes (do not boil), strain and use as a drink between meals. This little remedy has proved very successful in extreme Kidney troubles. Even when the kidneys have been bleeding badly, in such cases give Bran Tea every hour for 24 hours. Writes F. G. R., Melbourne, Victoria, Australia.

Editor's Note—This is a fine remedy, no doubt. But it could be greatly improved with the addition of a little German Cheese Plant and Lemon juice.

I want to thank you for your wonderful remedy. I have tried the Peach Tree Leaves for Kidney trouble and it surely did some good. I can't say enough about it. I got some of the people to using Yellow Dock and they say it did the work. Writes A. M. B.,

Tea made of Peach Leaves and drunk as faithfully and in place of tea or coffee is a sure cure for kidney trouble. Writes K. R. R., Oakland, Md.

Here is a recipe for obstruction of the urine, gravel deposits in the urine, pains in the back. Use half ounce of Marshmallow Root, Pellitory, Gravel Root, Parsley Piert, and Wintergreen. Boil all in one quart of water slowly for five minutes, strain, add to the liquid two ounces of honey and mix well. The dose is a wineglassful 3 times a day. Writes Thos. C., Medomsley, So. Durham, England.

Use a tablespoonful of Marshmallow in one quart of water, boil until the root is tender, strain, and use. It will cleanse the kidneys, for I have used it for years and it never failed. Writes Mrs. L. B., Westville, Ind.

Cockleburr and Corn Silk makes a good kidney medicine. Writes J. H. T., Greenfield, Ind.

To keep kidneys in good condition before childbirth, take one teaspoonful of Slippery Elm Bark to one cup water. When cold drink one-half cup a day. I have great faith in this recipe and would advise beginning before the third month. Writes Mrs. R. V., Angelica, N. Y.

Editor's Note—Yes, and German Cheese Plant and Spikenard are also very good.

Inflammation of the Kidneys and Bladder Troubles—Take three tablespoonfuls of Buchu Leaves and six of Indian Sage. Pour over one quart of boiling water, let stand eight hours. Drink four tablespoonfuls four times a day. In severe cases one-half teacupful every three hours until relieved.

Sassafras Bark made into a tea will cure inflamed bladder. Writes Mrs. C. T., Los Angeles, Calif.

I am sending a remedy for bladder troubles which I have tried and it gave relief. Use Oil of Juniper; taken ten drops on a lump of sugar at bedtime. In 48 hours take eight drops, then 48 hours later six drops, then another 48 hours use four drops, the next 48 hours two drops. This is a ten-day cure, and while relief comes quickly, it will take the ten-day limit that will be required for complete subsidence of the difficulty. Writes Mrs. A. G., Stouffville, Ont., Can.

Editor's Note—Be sure to get Oil Juniper Berries, as the oil of Juniper wood is not for internal use.

Take the leaves of Wild Carrot and make a tea and drink as often as you want water, and it is a sure cure for kidney troubles, and has even helped gallstones. Writes J. M., Blacksburg, Va.

For kidney disorders and nerves we use a tea of Oregon Grape Root and Pipsissewa, and they are both great medicines. Writes H. H. S., Marial, Ore.

For children that can not urinate. This is an honest recipe and from true experience I will say my mother used it, and it is a help for any other mother. Take plenty of Parsley Root and put in an enamel vessel and pour boiling water over and let child sit over the parsley fumes until urinating. Do not have it too hot; if the water is too hot, allow to cool. Writes C. R., Bellevue, Pa.

Dandelion Roots dried and steeped, is excellent cure for weak kidneys or bladder troubles. Writes Mrs. G. B., Bellevue, Idaho.

For Kidney Troubles—Take a handful of Queen of the Meadow Roots to a quart of water, boil for a few minutes and drink throughout the day.

While still another one for kidney troubles is to take Horse Radish Root and Egg Shells and boil for a few minutes. Writes M. B. Gilmore, Ky.

For Bladder Troubles—Pour one pint of boiling water over 2 tablespoonfuls of whole Flax Seed, add 2 teaspoons of Cream of Tartar. Drink this quantity each day, one-half in the morning and one-half in the evening. Add a little sugar if it cannot be taken without. This will help anyone within 24 hours. Writes Mrs. J. C., Middleboro, Mass.

Painful Urination—Take two tablespoonfuls of Yarrow, put in one quart of boiling water, and boil five minutes, then let stand on back of the stove for one-half hour, stirring frequently. Drink one cupful half hour before breakfast and supper. This is good for painful urination, weakness of the bladder, for it has cured me of these, where all patent medicines, and doctors of this city failed. Writes Mrs. M. B., Medford, Wis.

Editor's Note—This can be improved by adding Cheese Plant and Cubeb Berries in equal parts.

For one that cannot urinate, give a tea made of Watermelon Seed. I know this is good for I have tried for myself as well as my children. Writes C. A. W., Cobalen, Ill.

The greater part of the kidney and bladder remedies bring forth an increased action of these; many need more of a soothing demulcent to get any real relief. I have found that a tea or extract made from Corn Silk, Cheeseplant, Asparagus Root, more nearly approaches a true relief. Take three times a day after meals. Writes S. P., Muscatine, Iowa.

Lame Back and Kidneys—Have tried this many times, and always got relief without fail. Take the leaves and roots of Trailing Arbutus, make a tea of this, drink about 1 pint a day and keep up until relieved. Writes C. D., Brookville, Pa.

I don't think Plantain is appreciated enough. I sprained my ankle very badly, could not walk on it for two weeks. I gathered the fresh green Plantain and bound it on for two days and nights and the leaves were crisp when I took them off each time which was night and morning, and the ankle got all right. I also cured my son's hand with it. I have used a lot of it dried for kidney troubles, and it is very good, too. Writes Mrs. W. W., New Westminster, B. C.

This is a remedy that I have not seen in your book. A remedy for people who can not urinate. Steep Peppermint, a tablespoonful to a cupful of hot water, like you would tea and drink it hot. Writes Mrs. E. A., Tripoli, Wis.

Use one-half cupful Sassafras Tea, which has been prepared from the Sassafras Bark, twice a day, and you will not have urinary troubles. Writes A. M. L., Vermillion, S. D.

Editor's Note—All herb teas are made by placing a teaspoonful of the herb or bark in a cup of boiling hot water, the same as you would make ordinary household tea.

A tried and true remedy for inflammation of the neck of the bladder in women, of which the symptoms are inability to hold the urine or a continuous desire to urinate, with a burning, scalding sensation when passing the urine, the pain of which extends up the arms, is made by steeping a handful of Elder Flowers in a pint of water, let cool and use as a douche twice a day. Two or three applications are usually sufficient. Writes Miss L. S., St. Charles, Mo.

Retention of the Urine—Here is a good and sure remedy, which will work the kidneys in 15 minutes. Boil Watermelon Seeds and drink the tea. Writes Mrs. M. F., Hot Springs, Ark.

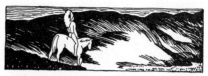

Birch Bark Tea is useful in kidney troubles. Writes Mrs. C. S., Pleasant Ridge, Pa.

If you should learn of anyone suffering from bladder trouble do not hesitate to recommend Parsley Root, for it is wonderful. I know it has done so much for me and it will no doubt do as much for others that may be suffering in a like manner. Writes J. S. L., New Orleans, La.

Take one box of Boneset Tea and one ounce of Buchu Leaves and three pints of boiling water, make a tea and drink a wine glass full 3 times daily. Good for kidney trouble. It helped my husband more than doctors ever did. Writes Mrs. E. G., Grafton, Ohio.

Pumpkin Seeds are excellent for kidney trouble. Put the seeds in a container and bring to a boil, then strain and take the tea immediately. Writes Mrs. W. M., Manitowoc, Wis.

Kidney Troubles—Use three parts Corn Silk, Wild Cherry, two Red Raspberry Leaves, one Swamp Lily Root and one Rocky Mountain Grape Root. Mix, and then put one tablespoonful in a quart of boiling water, let stand three hours, strain and take wineglassful four times a day.

I am writing this all for the benefit of other folks. Juniper Berries made into a tea given to my old mother three times daily, a small cup each time has cured her of a very unpleasant smelling discharge. The urinal analysis indicated pus on the kidneys and this caused the discharge. Writes Miss F. S., Valley Stream, N. Y.

I am writing you regarding my case of bladder irritation and would certainly recommend the Wild Alum Root and Jezebel Root to anyone ailing with chronic cystitis. Try it and be convinced. I drank the teas nearly eighteen months and for nearly three months now I have been in good health as far as the bladder is concerned. Writes L. H., Brooklyn, Iowa.

Take a handful of Corn Silk and steep this in a quart of water and drink the water. This is a good formula for bladder troubles. Writes J. F. S., Cleveland, Ohio.

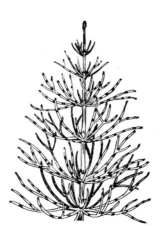

Horse Tail Grass—Highly prized for kidney and bladder troubles; steep two teaspoonfuls in a cup of boiling water. Drink cold two to four cups a day. Children half this quantity. Also very valuable in blood vomiting, bloody or difficult urine. Putrid wounds and ulcers should be washed daily with this tea. This is a very valuable herb.

For Flux or Diarrhoea—Take Dollar Leaf Vine (Pyrola) and make a tea of the leaves and vine; sweeten and give as often as necessary. I have given this to a baby when it was passing blood and it cured. It is also good for adults. Writes A. M., Hartville, Md.

LEUCORRHOEA OR WHITES
(See Female Complaints.)

The symptoms are a discharge of mucus from the genital organs, variously colored and of different degrees of consistency. It is usually white or yellowish; sometimes reddish; mostly mild, yet sometimes burning; causing soreness of the parts. It is usually most profuse immediately before and after the menstrual period and may continue during the entire menstruating life of the female, and is known even in young girls. Sometimes the discharge is slight and only trifling, while at other times it is copious.

Women subject to these ailments should carefully guard their feet and abdomen from sudden changes or extreme cold; take moderate exercise in the open air; avoid coffee, exciting drinks, spices or highly seasoned foods.

Treatment—Take a hot douche every night.

The douche should be taken very slowly (20 minutes) to give the heat and medicinal virtues time to act; and should be taken while lying flat upon the back if possible. In severe cases the douche should be taken twice daily.

The Herb Doctor's choice of botanical astringents and tonics are: Wild Alum, Horsetail Grass, Thyme, Mormon Valley Herbs, Mistletoe, Blessed Thistle, Golden Seal, Rue, Bearberry Leaves, Peach Tree Leaves, Water Pepper and Helonias Root, Black Haw, Beth Root, Palmetto Berries, Swamp Lily Root, Cramp Bark.

Take Slippery Elm Bark and soak in water, drink the water. It will cure Diarrhoea and Flux. Writes C. A., Cuervo, N. M.

Take White Oak Bark enough to make 2 quarts of liquid and pour boiling water over and let set until lukewarm, and then use as a douche for Leucorrhoea. It is very good and entirely harmless. Writes Mrs. D. H., Hoquiam, Wash.

Comfrey Root made into a tea is good to stop Leucorrhoea. Writes S. H., Vallejo, Calif.

Leucorrhoea—Leucorrhoea and inflammation of the female genital organs. Specially recommended as a douche for ladies, who are on their feet constantly.
   ⅓ teaspoonful Golden Seal
   ⅔ teaspoonful Cranesbill
Steep in one pint of water, use very warm. A small piece of Alum may be added. Writes L. E. McD., Rock Island, Tex.

A Recipe for Whites—Take Red Alder, put in a pitcher of water, let it steep, then drink this whenever you are wanting a drink. Writes Mrs. J. A. S., Crossville, Ala.

Leucorrhoea—"This recipe has been recommended to me by an Indian herb doctor and I have found it very efficacious. Take Beth Root and break into small pieces. Place 1 teaspoonful of the roots into a cup of boiling water. Let it remain until the water cools and drink just before bedtime every evening." Writes I. S., Lafayette, Ind.

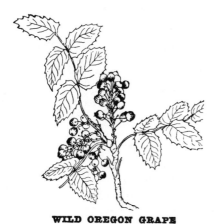

WILD OREGON GRAPE

LIVER TROUBLE

The Rocky Mountain Grape grows in reckless profusion in many districts on the Pacific Coast. The root of it has no equal as a liver tonic. A tea made from it and taken before retiring for the night will overcome that weariness which is too often but the result of a sluggish liver; and produce a feeling of health and vigor. Sufferers from rheumatism of many years' standing have been cured by its use. As a laxative it should be taken before breakfast, but taken in the evening it quickly restores the tone to the liver and will give immediate relief in acute indigestion or gas on the stomach.—From the "Torch Monthly," Vancouver, B. C.

Jaundice — Liver Troubles — Quicker progress will be made towards health on a fruit, nut, cottage cheese and vegetable diet.

Liver Troubles—Three parts Licorice Root, 2 Sweet Weed, Dandelion Root and Yellow Root, mix well with one part Black Root. Dose, one tablespoonful in a quart of boiling water, let stand all night, next morning, strain and take a wineglassful 3 times that day, half hour before each meal. I have cured several cases of gall bladder troubles with this, too. Writes Dr. L. E., New Lexington, Ohio.

Liver Tonic—Those suffering from sluggish liver will be very thankful for this valuable formula:
1 handful Liver Leaf
1 handful Horehound
1 ounce Mayapple Root
1 ounce Sacred Bark
1 ounce Cheese Plant
Steep a teaspoonful in a cup of boiling water until cool; strain and drink one or two cupfuls during the day.
Author's Note—This tea is very bitter, but it may be improved by adding a 25c size of Licorice Root, or a handful of Fennel Seed.

Liver Troubles—Equal parts of Mayapple, Black Root Sacred Bark and Licorice Root, and Sassafras Bark of root, mix and use one teaspoonful to a cup of boiling water makes an excellent liver medicine. If you have any liver trouble whatever, just try this tea. Writes I. C., Chicago, Ill.

A Good Liver Remedy—Use Mayapple Roots, and take as much as you can hold in one hand and steep in a quart of water, boil down to a pint, put in 2 cups of sugar so it will keep, and take one tablespoonful morning and night, but if you find the dose too strong then use just one teaspoonful, and it will be fine for I have used with good results. Writes Mrs. N. A. D., Terre Haute, Ind.

A strong bitters or tea made from the Peach Tree Leaves taken in moderate doses 3 or 4 times a day for jaundice and liver affections. While a cold infusion made of the leaves and given in tablespoonful doses every hour is good for inflammation of the bowels and stomach. Writes J. A. M., Yates Center, Kan.
Editor's Note—Have received quite a number of similar reports on this remedy.

For Torpid Liver or Gall Stones:
1 ounce Dandelion
½ ounce Mandrake
½ ounce Sarsaparilla
½ ounce Blackberry Root
½ ounce Buchu
1½ ounces Gentian
1 handful of Hops
Add four quarts of water to the above ingredients and steep four hours. Strain before bottling and add a preservative.
Dose—One wine glassful before meals, if too laxative reduce dose. Writes E. A. Warner, Angelica, N. Y.

LOCKJAW

I am sending a recipe which is valuable for lockjaw. Put Saltpetre in water as hot as you can stand to wring flannel cloths out and put on the jaws covering with another flannel or heavy towel. I have known this to cure where the doctor gave the patient up and laughed at the lady for wanting to try the Saltpetre, but her daughter is living today. Writes Mrs. A. A. T., Bayard, Ohio.

For Lockjaw from a Nail—Just cook Garden Beets and poultice. If put on in time, will never get sore. Writes M. R., Pueblo, Colo.

Lockjaw—I am sending you an Indian remedy for Lockjaw: Take a plug of strong chewing tobacco, soak it in hot water; split it and bind on the pit of the stomach, the patient lying on his back. This will make him sick at the stomach and jaws will open. If necessary, repeat the next day, soaking same tobacco. Writes Mrs. O. J., Wainfleet, Ont., Canada.

Editor's Note—I know this would have no effect on me, unless I swallowed some of the juice.

In this as in every other serious ailment one should lose no time in calling a specialist—and while waiting—there is no harm in trying some of the recipes given in these pages.

EPILEPSY FITS OR FALLING DISEASE

Epilepsy occurs in more or less severe forms. It is a serious ailment and should not be treated with so-called patent or secret medicines containing bromides and other powerful drugs which often do more harm than good.

Treatment—Consult a specialist. Take no medicine of which the ingredients are a secret. Country life, plenty of fresh air and nourishing food and sunshine will do more than any medicine.

The Herb Doctor's choice of mild botanical nervines are: Nerve Root, Valerian, Blue Vervain, Blue Scullcap, Gentian, Angelica, Swamp Cabbage Root.

Epilepsy and Fits—Eat a piece of Swamp Cabbage Root the size of a pea 1 hour before breakfast every morning. Keep this up for 6 months or longer if necessary until cured.

LUMPS OR SWELLINGS

Take Solomon Seal, and use it to bathe any kind of a lump or swelling. It is excellent for both man and beast. My father used it on a cow's udder, when there was inflammation and caking of the milk. When the horse had a lame leg, he would bathe it, then bandage and keep the cloths wet with this Solomon Seal. He walked miles to give it to a man whose leg had been severely jammed, and to a woman · who had sprained her knee. In such cases, he always bathed the injured part first, and then bandaged, keeping the cloths wet with the Solomon Seal. He also used this for inflammation in the breast of a woman, and it always gave relief, and our family has great faith in its virtues. Writes Mr. H. D. W., Costigan, Me.

Editor's Note—The Solomon Seal Roots should be ground fine if the dried root is used. To one part of the root take about 4 or 5 parts water. I believe the fresh undried roots would give better results. We cannot furnish undried roots and herbs for the reason that these articles would rot or get moldy before they reached our customers.

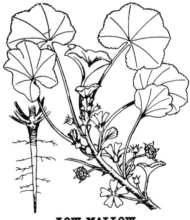

LOW MALLOW

Inflammation and Swellings—Here is a simple remedy for inflammation and swellings: bathe the affected parts with Quack Grass. Take Quack Grass, cut and dried, steep it and use the liquid to bathe the affected parts. Fine to take down swelling and soreness. Writes Mrs. N. M., Manson, Wis.

Editor's Note—Yes, and it is also fine as a tea taken internally, especially if used in equal parts with German Cheese Plant.

White Swelling—Here is a cure for White Swelling: Take Bears Grass Root, beat, boil, and make a poultice. Keep on until swelling is out. Writes Mrs. A. E. L, Teague, Texas.

Lump in the Chest—Use an ointment made of Bittersweet Root. Steep one package in a cupful of water until the strength is all extracted. Boil down, add 3 tablespoonfuls of pure Lard, then cook for an hour or more. When cool, rub the affected part for 10 or 15 minutes gently, and 2 or 3 times a day. This removed a lump as large as a hen's egg which was very painful. The ointment is splendid for any sore.

White Swelling—This is a very old recipe and has been tried and has always had good results. It is a remedy for White Swelling and is called Lily Root Salve. Use a handful of the Yellow Lily Roots, and a cupful of Lard, also Resin, the size of a hen's egg, and the same amount of Beeswax. After these have been melted together, strain through cloth, and apply. Writes C. L., Stoyestown, Pa.

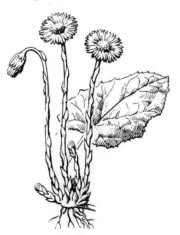

Coltsfoot

LUNGS—CONSUMPTION

In these ailments, fresh air, sunlight and the proper nourishing food can do more than medicine. Keep bowels open.

Eat plenty of vegetables and food rich in vitamines and mineral salts. Take Coltsfoot Tea as an expectorant to relieve the coughing spells.

There are a number of ailments for which no recognized cure has been found yet the patient lives his full span of life by arresting the ailment with common sense living methods.

The Herb Doctor's choice of botanicals for relieving coughing spells and to aid expectoration are: Coltsfoot, Mullein Leaves, Horehound, Holy Herb, German Cheese Plant, Marshmallow Root, Elm Bark, Linden Flowers, Nettle Leaves, Wild Cherry Bark, White Pine Bark, Sundew, Thyme.

Try using Slippery Elm Bark into a poultice for White Swelling, for there is nothing better. Writes Mrs. J. C., New Castle, Ind.

I am sending you a recipe for T. B. cure taken from the New York Sun, which appeared twice in the last five years. M. A.-T. B. Hospital treat patients with raw eggs and milk taken as a drink every day often. I know of three people cured. Have heard that this is the only thing that grows tissue back on the lungs, if taken early in first stages. Writes R. B., New York City, N. Y.

Editor's Note—This is a good treatment and could be improved by letting patient drink a tea made of Coltsfoot

This is an old Indian recipe for the lungs: Take a handful of Balm of Gilead Buds and put in a pint bottle. Cover the buds with alcohol, if obtainable, if not use water, and let stand one-half day. Strain off the buds and put alcohol back in the bottle and fill up the bottle with strained honey. Dose —take one-half teaspoonful on the start and when you can stand a teaspoonful, then it will soon tell, you will soon feel better. Take about 3 bottles. It is certainly wonderful medicine. Writes D. B., Le Roy, Mich.

An Indian chief told my father that a tea made by taking 2 teaspoonfuls of Coltsfoot would cure Bleeding Lungs, and it did. Writes C. L., Ypsilanti, Mich.

Chew Sang Root or make into a tea and drink, for it is very good for Weak Lungs. Writes Miss E. N., Cowell, Ark.

For All Lung Troubles—Red Sassafras, Willow Bark, Calamus—a double handful of each and two sticks of Licorice, or the powdered or cut article equivalent to this. Cover with water, simmer 8 hours, then strain, add sugar, and let simmer to a quart of medicine. Dose—One tablespoonful 3 times a day. Writes A. T., Iron City, Tenn.

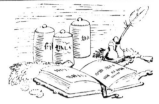

—German Breast Tea,
Coughwort Leaves
Nettle Leaves
Fennel Seed
Juniper Berries
Blue Mallow
Black Mallow
German Cheese Plant
Yerba Santa
Iceland Moss

Another of the Benevolent old Pastor Kneipp's cherished formulae slightly improved with certain Indian botanicals. Try it for Congestion in the Chest.

—Floral Breast Tea
    Linden Flowers
    Blue Mallow Flowers
    Black Mallow Fowers
    Mullein Flowers
    Saffron Flowers
    Calendula Flowers
    Red Clover Flowers

A truly remarkable tea, composed entirely of flowers recognized by all herbalists for their demulcent and emollient properties.

Demulcent and Expectorant—The ingredients of this remedy were all used by the Indians of North America and the knowledge handed down to their pale face conquerors. The Indians themselves probably had but little use for a remedy for lung troubles.

2 ounces Mullein Leaves
1 ounce Pleurisy Root
1 ounce Inner Bark White Pine
1 ounce Cheese Plant
1 ounce Coughwort
1 ounce Canada Snake Root

Steep a teaspoonful of the mixture in a cup of boiling water until cool; strain and drink one or two cupfuls per day.

—Wahoo Pleurisy Root
    Compound.....
    Pleurisy Root
    Coughwort
    German Cheese Plant
    Wahoo Bark
    Wild Cherry Bark
    Bluets

A very fine combination of Amercian Botanicals, most of which are of Indian

La Grippe—Our family doctor said for us to use Wormwood for la grippe and influenza. Better than Quinine, and don't leave the after affects. We have used it in our home now for the past 40 years. Writes C. A. B., Cazenovia, Ill.

Editor's Note—Boneset tea is also very good for this purpose.

Place a piece of Camphor Gum in a little sack and pin it to your underclothing or wear around the neck, and it will keep the flu away and help you from having colds. When the sack is empty re-fill. Writes M. F., Miltonvale, Kans.

A cup of hot Horsemint Tea before going to bed is a sure thing for the flu. Use a handful of the dried herb to a cupful of boiling water. Allow to steep but do not boil. Writes S. H., Vallejo, Calif.

For Bronchitis, Lung and Throat Troubles—Here is the best remedy I ever used. Two handfuls Wild Cherry Bark, Inner Bark of White Pine, 1 large handful Indian Turnip, 1 of Horehound, and 1 of Bull Nettle. Put all in gallon of water and simmer down to 3 quarts or until the strength is out, then strain and add 1 pound of Honey. Take a wineglassful 3 times during the day, and 1 on retiring. Writes G. L. D., Idal, Tenn.

Here is a good remedy for Kidney and Bladder troubles. Fill a half gallon fruit jar full of Spignet, then fill it full of boiling water, drink two cups a day. This is harmless but a sure remedy. Writes F. H., Valley, N. C.

Here is a recipe for lame back, caused from strain or colds: Chew the Queen of the Meadow Root, swallowing the juice. Writes J. T. C., Braintree, Mass.

For Consumption or Lung Troubles, Mullein is very good. Cook for an hour in 3 quarts of water, strain and drink no other water. Make fresh every day. This is a sure cure unless the lungs are too far gone. Writes Mrs. E. S., Rockford, Ill.

Coughs, Catarrh and Lung Troubles—One ounce each of Elecampane, Horehound and Comfrey, as well as Hyssop, to these add 1 pound brown Sugar and a quart of water, boil slowly down to a pint, strain and bottle. Take a teaspoonful every 2 hours. Writes Mrs. A. T., Atlantic City, Wyo.

I am ordering 4 more boxes of Coughwort, as this sure done me good. The doctor gave me up to die but thanks to your medicines I am able to get up and work a little now. Writes M. McC., Norwalk, Ohio.

Editor's Note—Coughwort is excellent for weak lungs.

For Consumption, get the inner bark of White Pine and chew it. A man I know said he used this when a young man that was nearly gone, and he died this year about 90 years old. Writes E. L. M., Oxford, Mass.

This is a good recipe for Lung Troubles, that has been tried and is good. An ounce of Elecampane Root, Horehound, Spikenard Root, and Comfrey. Boil in 1 quart of water, then strain. Put back on to boil, with 1 pound of strained Honey and a quart of Cider Vinegar. Boil down to 1 quart, take a tablespoonful 3 times a day. Writes Mrs. S. G., Stanberry, Mo.

Common Mullein—This has cured a number of cases of Consumption, after they had commenced bleeding at the lungs, and had the hectic flush on the cheek. Steep this herb strong, and sweeten with sugar, and drink freely. The medicine must be continued from 4 to 6 months according to the nature of the disease. This is also good for the blood, as it strengthens the system and builds up strength. Writes M. B. E., Fletcher, W. Va.

I was taken down with Bronchitis, which turned into Consumption of the Lungs. I doctored for 1 year and then the doctors said they could do me no good. A friend recommended Coltsfoot or Coughwort, which grows all over the fields. I used to go out and pick it and dry it myself. Take a large handful of the plant and place into 3 pints of water. Boil down to 2 pints; strain and cool. Sweeten with Honey if desired. Drink a wineglassful the first thing every morning and upon retiring at night. I took it 90 days and was entirely cured. This was 30 years ago and I have good lungs and a good developed chest. Writes J. L., Old Forge, Pa.

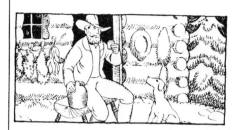

A party I know who had Consumption took Balm of Gilead Buds and mixed them with Honey and Alcohol or Whiskey; drink it. This is a sure cure. Writes J. H. T., Greenfield, Ind.

To Cure a Consumptive Cough—Take 3 pints of rain water, half pound Raisins, chopped fine, 3 tablespoonfuls Flax Seed, sweeten to a syrup with Honey and boil down to a quart. Then add a drop or so of Oil Anise. Take a tablespoonful 8 times a day. Writes H. E. H., Mystic, Conn.

Editor's Note—I would also add a big handful of Coltsfoot Leaves.

Spitting of Blood—Make a strong tea of Witch Hazel Leaves and to a half pint of it add tea prepared from equal parts of Sage and common Nettle. Dose—A wineglassful every half hour until bleeding stops. Writes R. L. J., Hot Springs, Ark.

A tramp told this simple remedy to a woman that was so weak with T. B. that she couldn't walk:

1 quart boiling water
1 handful Swamp Cabbage Root
1 handful Sage Tea
1 handful of Horehound

But if you add too much Horehound, it may make it too bitter. If you desire you can boil it down, and add Rock Candy to thicken it. Dose—One tablespoonful 5 or 6 times a day. Writes K. M. P., Belleville, Pa.

Severe Coughs and Bronchial Troubles—Take an ounce of the following: Horehound, Irish Moss, Flax Seed, Boneset and Licorice, and place in a pan, with a gallon of cold water. Put this on the back of the stove and let it simmer slowly until reduced to one-half gallon. Strain and bottle. Dose—One wineglassful 3 times a day. Add Sugar if desired. This is one of the best home remedies for such purposes. Writes A. B., Canton, Ohio.

A tea of Butterfly Weed Root will stop Bleeding Lungs, and Horsemint will cure Chills when all others fail. Writes Mrs. A. V., Witts Springs, Ark.

Testimonial—Mr. Anton Markovitz of 501 Third Street, Versailles, Pa., was taken to the McKeesport Hospital in April afflicted with Pneumonia and Pleurisy. After a stay of 3 weeks, he was dismissed with remarks of the doctors that he could not live more than one to four days, that he had Consumption in the last stage.

After being home with his family, Mr. J. G. Staudenmayer, of Versailles, Pa., supplied him with dried Bull Nettle of which I, his wife, made him a tea which worked wonders.

After using this tea for 4 days the fearful cough broke and at the same time an immense quantity of black mucous slime or impurities came from his throat and lungs. By continuing using Bull Nettle he became perfectly cured from his Consumption.

His Kidney and Bladder Trouble was cured by using tea from Cheese Plant and Horse Tail Grass.

Today the man, with the last stage of Consumption, is working again for the National Tube Co., at Versailles, Pa. Sworn and signed by himself, Anduc Markovitch, and wife, Anna Markovitch. Sworn and subscribed to this the 20th day of Sept., 1927. W. H. Clay, J. P. (Seal)

Editor's Note—I received the above affidavit, but I cannot explain how Bull Nettle could have much effect on a case of consumption—unless, as expressed elsewhere—this root may contain certain vitamines that are doing the work. However, I would not care to recommend it for this purpose until I had more reports on it.

Take Wild Cherry Bark and make a strong tea. Boil for one-half hour. Strain and put in an equal quantity of strained Honey and boil until mixture is thick like the Honey was when it was put in Cherry tea. Put up in bottle or fruit jar. Take 1 tablespoonful 3 times a day or oftener, if the cough is bad. It is harmless and I have known it to cure genuine T. B. when it was in the last stage. Writes L. M. O., Paroquet, Ark.

Take Wild Cherry Bark and boil to a strong dose and thicken with Honey. Will cure Lung Trouble. Take 4 swallows a day, and should cure Consumption if taken regular. Writes R. R. H., Forest City, N. C.

Editor's Note—Wild Cherry Bark is an excellent expectorant, and useful where indicated. I doubt its efficacy in consumption.

Weak Lungs—I am the person you referred to over the radio. Was completely cured of my lung troubles, which I neglected to tell you at the time we met in Harlingen, Texas, was Consumption. I told you I had weak lungs. That tea of Coughwort and this climate did the trick. Mostly I thank you for the tea. Coughwort is one herb I recommend to anyone suffering from Consumption.

At this time I have taken 6 boxes of Coltsfoot. When I began to take it I had been in bed 4 months. All the doctors had given me up and had said I couldn't live 2 weeks. They took me out of the hospital. They said one of my lungs was gone and the other was just about gone. I was so weak I couldn't turn myself around in the bed. My mother sent for the Coltsfoot and made it into a tea. I took it for one week and got up and sat in a chair, but I couldn't walk. When I did get able to walk I weighed 76 pounds, and after I had taken 6 boxes of the Coltsfoot tea I weighed 110 pounds. I sure believe in it. I took Pneumonia fever and it turned into Tuberculosis, and I had an abscess on my left lung. I am now better than I ever was. Writes P. B., Danville, W. Va.

Try using the flowers and leaves of the Basswood and making a tea, for it is good for Lung Troubles and Light Colds. Skunk Oil (50c per ounce) is very good, too, and is simply rubbed in around the chest and neck. Writes L. W., Athens, Wis.

Red Clover Tea is good for Cough and Lung troubles. Writes Mrs. E. C. G., Iuka, Ill.

Chest Troubles—One handful Horehound, same amount of Garden Rue, 2 pounds coarse Sugar, boil in 2 quarts water down to 1 quart. Dose—Three tablespoonfuls early every morning.

My mother used herbs when I was a girl. She cured my father of a sickness the doctor called Bleeding of the Lungs. She steeped Lobelia and sweetened it. He would drink a small saucer of it. The dose she used was a tablespoonful to a pint of boiling water, just so it is not too strong. She used to give it to my sister and I for colds too. Writes Mrs. R. W. T., Lansing, Mich.

For Weak Lungs—Drink Catnip tea, regularly as you would use tea or coffee. Writes Mrs. H. S., Cocolalla, Idaho.

Lung Troubles—I have found nothing as good as Mullein alone by boiling the leaves to pieces in enough water to cover them, adding brown Sugar and then using. Writes J. R. R., Hot Springs, Ark.

I am a great believer in herbs—have taken lots of Mullein for Colds and I know a man that had terrible Hemorrhages of the Lungs, and the doctor gave 6 months at the most to live, that was entirely cured by taking 3 glasses a day for a year. It surely is wonderful for taking pains out of the chest. I put a little Lemon and Honey in it and take it hot, 2 or 3 times a day, when I have a cold, and they never amount to very much. Writes E. L. G.,

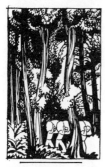

Take equal amounts of Wild Cherry Bark, Dogwood Bark, Burdock and Black Haw, and take a large cupful to a quart of water or amount of water needed, and boil into a tea, then use a tablespoonful 3 times a day, and you will find best ever for Malaria. Writes Mrs. C. M. R., Benton, Ark.

Ague—Take 2 ounces of Sassafras Bark. Place in a pint of water and boil for 20 minutes. Add a pint of best whiskey and let it cool. Dose—A tablespoonful 4 times a day for adults. Writes A. T. M., Fruitland, Ga.

—Florida Tea.......
    Sweet Flag Root
    Jamaica Ginger Root
    Juniper Berries
    Clove Buds
    Cubeb Berries
    Sassafras Bark of Root
    Senna Alexandria Leaves
    Oregon Grape Root
    Cassia Bark
This is an excellent diaphoretic if taken hot. Useful in Fevers, Ague, and to break up a Cold.

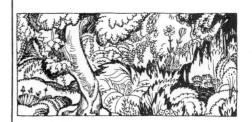

MALARIAL FEVER

There are two kinds of malarial fever, the intermittent and remittent. In the intermittent form there is a severe chill followed by fever and profuse sweating, after which the fever entirely disappears. These attacks may come on only every other day, or they may appear every third day. In remittent fever, the fever does not entirely disappear, but rises and falls within well-defined limits.

The parasites which cause malarial fevers feed upon and destroy the red-blood cells, and this accounts for the pale, sallow complexions of people who live in malarial districts and have had the disease, which is known as "ague." It is known that these parasites are transmitted to human beings by mosquitoes which breed in stagnant water. A person suffering from malaria should always sleep in a screened room, as mosquitoes biting him and sucking his blood may then transmit the disease to others.

Treatment—In the chronic type of this disease, generally known as "malaria," "ague," etc., the patient should have regular daily action of the bowels, wholesome food, fresh air and exercise; these are better than medicine. A Febrifuge with Antiperiodic and tonic properties is often useful.

The Herb Doctor's choice of botanical Febrifuges and Tonics are: Ague Weed or Boneset, Cinchona, Sweet Flag, Galangal, Elecampane, Agrimony, Elder Berries, Five Finger Grass, Sage, Blue Vervain, Wood Sorrel, Yarrow, Hops, Juniper Berries, Lovage, Sweet Marjoram, Blessed Thistle, Cloves, Jamaica Ginger and Wild Ginger. Any selection of two or three of the above may be mixed in equal parts and a heaping teaspoonful of the mixture taken to a cup of boiling water.

MEASLES

Is generally a mild, although under certain conditions, it may become a dangerous disease. It begins like many fevers, with headache, backache and chills, a redness of the eyes and soon a hoarse, loose cough, which is characteristic of the disease. The rash appears first on the face in clusters with a reddish blush, deepening and increasing as it comes out. There is generally fever.

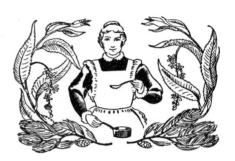

Treatment—Patient must be kept quiet and in a darkened and well-ventilated room. Great care must be taken to prevent the patient from catching cold. A hot Botanic Tea is excellent as a diaphoretic to bring out the rash. Hot Lemonade is also good.

The Herb Doctor's choice of botanicals are: Elder Berries, Elder Flowers, Lovage, Sage, Tormentil, Birch Bark, Yarrow, Tansy, Holy Herb, Marigold, Saffron and Bistort.

Measles—A tea made of Pennyroyal and Ginger is a sure remedy for Measles. It will break out Measles when they are hard to break out. Put enough of the herbs in a pint of boiling water to make a strong tea, and put in it a teaspoonful of Ginger. Drink hot. A cup of this tea every 3 or 4 hours until the Measles break out quickly. Writes M. B., Clever, Mo.

Measles—Make a strong tea of Spicewood, by pouring boiling water over it. Drink hot as you can stand and it will break the Measles.

To Break Out Measles—Boil about 3 tablespoonfuls of Rosemary in a quart of water, boil down to a pint, sweeten and drink a cupful at going to bed. This will break them out after they have gone in the second time and is harmless. Writes Mrs. J. L. L., Murry Cross, Ala.

To cure the Measles Cough, drink a tea made of Red Clover Blossoms. Writes Miss L. S., Bradford, Ont., Canada.

Elder Flowers will break out Measles and will check the Fever. Writes E. M., Byron, Ill.

Editor's Note—Yes, they will—and so will the berries. I used them on my own children years ago.

Make a tea of Elderberry Blossoms, drink hot. Very good for Measles. Writes Mrs. E. G., Grafton, Ohio.

For Measles—Buy a carton of Saffron Blossoms, make a tea of them, add juice of 1 Lemon with Sugar and let the children drink all they want. They will like it, as it tastes like lemonade, and it certainly brings out the Measles beautifully. Writes Mrs. A. J. C., Vining, Minn.

Catnip and Elder Flowers in tea is very good for Measles. When my five children had them I gave them these teas alternately, and I saved a doctor bill. I called our family doctor and told him what I was doing and how they were, and he said it was just fine. Writes Mrs. L. W., Plymouth, N. H.

Editor's Note—Another good man.

A recipe to break out Measles: Take a handful of Ground Mustard Seed, put in a pan of warm water and bathe all over in this and in no time you will be broke out good. Writes R. B., Elizabethtown, Ill.

When I had the Measles I caught cold with them. Mother made me a hot drink of Catnip tea, and when I asked for water she gave me hot Catnip tea. It brought the Measles all out again and in a week I was well and better. Writes E. P., Fort Dodge, Iowa.

MILK LEG

For the Swelling that goes with Milk Leg, make a strong tea of Mullein Leaves and bathe the affected parts. Writes Mrs. A. W., Saltville, Va.

A mild tea of European Centaury can be taken in cases of milk leg or phlebitis as a mild tonic.

MOLES

I had a Mole in the edge of my hair
and when it turned white it was very
plainly seen. I had another on the
other side of my forehead, so I decided
to massage them very tenderly with
Castor Oil (6-ounce bottle) 50c) and
after a while they were gone, but of
course it took some time to get rid of
them. Writes Mrs. C. K., Utica, N. Y.
Editor's Note—Very good, if it works only half
the time.

Take Wormwood, German Chamomile,
Rhubarb Root, Dandelion Root, and
American Sarsaparilla, of equal measure, and a little Cinnamon and Cloves.
Pour over water to make a tea, and
st ep 5 or 6 hours, set it away to cool,
then strain, add Sugar if desired. Take
a mouthful at mealtime and this will
build up the stomach and nerves and
is very good for all old people. Can be
made up fresh every day, or the entire
lot at a time just as you desire. Writes
Mrs. E. L., Chatfield, Ohio.

NEURASTHENIA OR NERVOUS PROS-TRATION

Too much worry and care commonly
due to too much excitement, too many
parties, and excesses of all kinds. The
symptoms are: Irritability, despondency,
fear, sleeplessness, physical exhaustion,
poor appetite, spells of dizziness, trem-
bling, palpitation of the heart, backache and headache in the back of the
head.

Treatment—Absolute rest is essential.
Plenty of fresh air and deep breathing
is beneficial. Avoid flesh foods. Drink
milk. A good Nervine is often useful.

The Herb Doctor's choice of botanical
Nervines are: Fragrant Valerian Root,
Blue Vervain, Chamomile, Scullcap,
Wood Betony, Lady Slipper, Catnip,
Comfrey Root, Sage Leaves, the latter
very mild.

Hysteria—Food should consist of
fresh fruits, nuts, fresh vegetables,
vegetable soups, with no meat, fish or
poultry. Avoid condiments, salt, pepper, mustard and vinegar. Nightly take
a few laxative fruits such as figs,
prunes, dates.

—Old Style Nerve Root
  Compound....
Nerve Root
Fragrant Valerian
Chocolate Root
Nepeta
Wild Strawberry Leaves
Sassafras Bark of Root
German Cheese Plant
Bluets
This is a fine Old Style Stimulating
Tonic for the Nerves. The main in-
gredients are recognized for their value
by modern physicians as well as by the
old herbal practitioners.

—Dr. Brown's Nerve Root
  Compound....
Nerve Root
Eastern Scullcap
Mex. Damiana
Gentian Root
Hop Flowers
German Cheese Plant
A mild Nervine—useful in nervous
exhaustion.

—German Celery...
Celery Seed
Nepeta Flors. and Lvs.
Hungrn. Chamomile Flors.
Blue Mallow
A mild Antispasmodic and Tonic.
Pleasant to take. Useful in many cases
of nervous headaches, etc. A very mild
tea and absolutely harmless.

—Celery Compound.
Celery Seed
Angelica Root
Gentian Root
Sacred Bark
Marshmallow Root
Bearberry Leaves
Juniper Berries
German Cheese Plant
A well known compound. Advertised
so extensively it needs no comment.
Properties: Carminative, Tonic and De-
mulcent.

Nerve Exhaustion—One ounce Motherwort, Scullcap and Gentian. Boil the
ingredients for 10 minutes in a quart
of water, when cold strain, and take
wineglassful about an hour before each
meal.

Neurasthenia—Alkaline foods are
needed, as found in fruits and fresh
green vegetables. All kinds of meat
are acid forming. Vegetarian diet is
corrective, especially vegetable salads.

We are very thankful for the change that we see in our grandson. He rests so good at night now and before he started taking Skullcap he was so nervous some nights that he hardly got any sleep. I do hope that he will keep improving. Writes Mrs. V. T., West Unity, Ohio.

Squaw Vine as a Nerve Tonic is very good, and you can use a tablespoonful every night. Writes J. H., Searles, Ala.

I am sending you a recipe for All Kinds of Nervousness and St. Vitus Dance, which it will cure. Take 1 box each of Scullcap Leaves, Lady Slipper Roots, Fever Few, and place in a quart of boiling water, let it boil until but a pint remains and then add another pint of cold water. Then strain through a clean cloth and take a wineglassful before meals and at bedtime. Be sure to make tea in earthenware. This will also help Paralysis. Writes O. L., Muncie, Ind.

Nerve Tonic—½ ounce Catnip, ½ ounce Boneset, ½ ounce Scullcap and ½ ounce Valerian. Steep in a quart of water, take ½ wineglassful 4 times a day. Writes L. H., Montpelier, Vt.

Celery for Nervousness, or even take a teaspoonful of the Celery Seed to a pint of water, boil 3 minutes, strain and flavor. Dose—One-half teacupful 3 times a day before meals. Writes E. V., Portage, Wis.

Nerve Exhaustion—One ounce Motherwort, Scullcap and Gentian. Boil the ingredients for 10 minutes in a quart of water, when cold strain, and take wineglassful about an hour before each meal.

Sleepless Nights—For sleepless nights, we steep Hop Tea, take a pinch of Hops for 1 cup, steep same as any tea, and it has proven good. Writes Mrs. J. B. G., Drummond, Wis.

Nervine, Nervous Breakdown—Take a teaspoonful of Lady's Slipper Root to a large cup of water. Make a tea and drink in small doses throughout the day. Will give quiet rest, and is also good for St. Vitus' Dance. Writes Miss L. G., Ann Arbor, Mich.

Asafoetida helps my nerves better than anything else I have taken and our friends think so too. Writes S. H., Vallejo, Calif.

For Insomnia—One-fourth ounce Scullcap, Valerian, Gentian, and Hops. Scald 1 ounce of the mixed herbs in a pint of water, and take wineglassful of it, too. Writes T. C., Medomsley, England.

A Tried Recipe for Nerves—One ounce of Ginseng, 1 ounce of Ladies Slipper and 1 ounce of Black Snake Root. Put all of these into whiskey or brandy, if you can get it, if not water; let stand 2 days before using, giving time for roots to penetrate liquid. Dose—One tablespoonful 3 times a day, the third dose at bedtime.

I am glad to send you this recipe as it may be a help to someone, for St. Vitus Dance. Make an infusion of Black Cohosh, 1 ounce to a pint of boiling water, strain and cool. Give a teaspoonful 4 times a day. Writes N. F., Columbus, Ohio.

I want to tell you about Catnip Tea. I have been using it for Nervousness, and it worked fine for me. I was hurt where the nerves cross on the back of my head, and since then I have had to use Nerve medicines, and Catnip is the best I have found. Writes Mrs. L. D., Wis. Veteran's Home, Wis.
Editor's Note—And it is absolutely harmless, but it must be fresh, last-season crop. Herbs over a year old are worthless.

Nervousness—This is a good recipe for Nervousness, as I have tried it myself:
  1 ounce Valerian
  1 ounce Scullcap
  1 ounce Catnip
  ½ ounce Coriander Seed
  1 dram Cayenne Pepper
Pulverize and mix. Take a teaspoonful of the mixture in a cup of boiling water with a little Sugar and Milk added. Repeat when necessary. It calms the nerves without deadening their sensibility. Writes S. B. M., Southwick, Mass.

I could not sleep at night, but after using the Squaw Vine, at 25c per box, I surely can sleep now. I want to give praise where credit is due, so I am writing you. My mother is using it too, and it is good for female troubles. Writes A. W., Marvell, Ark.

A good remedy for Sleeplessness or Insomnia: Take a large handful of Thyme and make a tea of this and drink just before retiring. This is a very soothing tea, good for tired and overworked nerves. Writes Miss G. S., Shelby, N. C.

Ladies Slipper Root made into a tea should be very good for Insomnia. Writes M. O., Hominy, Okla.

For St. Vitus Dance—My sister's boy could not hold his feet or hands still for one minute and this recipe cured him:

    1 ounce Scullcap
    1 ounce Fever Few
    1 ounce Lady Slipper

Take half of each one, put in quart jar, fill with boiling water and seal. Let this stand for 2 hours, then take a wineglassful 3 times a day. Writes Mrs. E. C., Canton, Ohio.

I also find Catnip Tea very good for the Nerves and Sleeplessness. Writes Mrs. C. F., Oak Hill, Ohio.

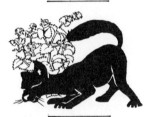

My husband had a partial stroke of paralysis. I gave him a teaspoonful of the whole Mustard Seed, either Black or White will do, every few hours until his face looked flushed. He couldn't speak to be understood, and his speech came back and remained so until death, when his age was near 86 then. Writes Mrs. R. G., Putnam, Tex.

A pillow made of Hops will produce a quiet, peaceful sleep.

I want to say that I have used Catnip and Red Clover Blossoms and find it good for my nerves. I have told others about it. Writes C. A., Winfield, Tenn.

A good household nervine can be made by taking one ounce each of Blue Vervain, Blue Scullcap and Boneset; mix them together and use a heaping teaspoonful to a cup of boiling water —let it stand until it cools, the same as you would make ordinary household tea. Drink the cupful during the day, a large mouthful at a time.

The seed of Common Dill is warming, stimulating and quiets the nerves. Writes Mrs. J. C. A., Wilburton, Okla.

Take a double handful of Princess Pine and put it in a crock and pour boiling water over it, let cool and strain and start taking it the next day. Dose, a wineglassful three times a day before meals. This is very good for the nerves. I relieved a girl 15 years of age with this remedy. Writes R. H. M., Danville, Pa.

I do not believe you know half the value of your Swamp Cabbage Root or Skunk Cabbage Root which ever you call it. I got it for my nephew and use some of it myself, and I found that when I used it I could sleep all through the night, otherwise I would lie awake nearly all the night. Writes I. J. B., Chicago, Ill.

For Nervousness take a cupful of very strong Catnip Tea. A sure cure. Writes Mrs. C. C., Arbough, Ark.

I have found this of good help in overcoming sleeplessness. Take Hops and put into a sack, and place under the head and in a short time one is able to go to sleep. Writes Mrs. J. O. G., Chicago, Ill.

I want you to accept the following prescription which I have proved to be sure and certain for St. Vitus Dance, Hysteria or Nervous Complaints in any form: Mistletoe, Scullcap and Valerian. One handful of each to a quart of boiling water, take 1 wineglassful 3 times a day. Writes G. L., Pittsburgh, Pa.

Editor's Note—This should be good.

For Strengthening and Invigorating the Nerves—

    1 ounce Juniper Berries
    1 ounce Weed Bugle
    3 ounces Chamomile Flowers

Steep 1 tablespoonful in half pint of boiling water and drink during the day. I have found that by adding Blue Scullcap to the mixture it improves it. This recipe was taken from my grandfather's book which was published in 1855. Writes E. E. L., Andover, Ohio.

For Sleeplessness and Nervous trouble, I can highly recommend Catnip, Blue Scullcap and Blue Vervain herb and leaves. Take a small pinch of each herb and place them in a cup of boiling water, and cover the vessel until the tea cools, then drink 1 cupful during the day. Save ½ cupful of the tea to drink upon retiring. Writes J. S. L., New Orleans, La.

For fright and to prevent its severe developments. One ounce Valerian Root, 1 ounce Ladies Slipper Root, ½ ounce Violet Blossoms and leaves, and ¼ ounce Dandelion Roots. Mix thoroughly and to a half quart of boiling water, add 1 tablespoonful of the mixture, drink 3 times a day a teacupful at a time, which may be sweetened to taste. Writes A. Z., Ashley, Pa.

Palsy—Maiden Hair Fern will help palsy and stops shaking also. Writes Mrs. A. V., Louisville, Ky.

St. Vitus Dance—I have a remedy for this distressing nervous ailment which I wish to pass along, as I have known it to cure two severe cases of 14 and 16 months' duration. Make a tea of the dried herb of Blue Scullcap by steeping 2 tablespoonfuls of the powdered or crushed herbs into a pint of boiling water. Dose—A half wineglassful 4 times a day. This is a sure cure, also excellent for sleeplessness and other nervous troubles.

Insomnia—This is fine for those of a nervous temperament who are so often troubled with sleeplessness. Also valuable in Hysteria and Delirium Tremens. Take 1 ounce of each of ground Blue Scullcap, ground Angelica, and ground Catnip. Place in a quart of boiling water, cover tightly and allow to cool. Drink 1 cupful during the day, and 1 upon retiring at night.

Take the inner bark of Dogwood and make a tea of it and drink for it will cure Neuralgia. Writes Mrs. O. W. H., Russellville, Ala.

Editor's Note—You cannot get good results from bark that has been on the shelves of a drug store for years.

I have a good recipe which I wish you would pass on to others. I suffered a long while with Neuritis of the arms and used Black Snake Root, 1 teaspoonful in half glass of water night and morning, the first day, then 3 teaspoonfuls the second day, 4 teaspoonfuls the third day and so on until 8 teaspoonfuls can be taken. Keep up until relieved. Writes Mrs. I. P., Delta; Ohio.

Editor's Note—Black Snake Root tea is made by steeping 1 ounce in a pint of boiling water, until it cools; strain.

Here is a home remedy. If you are very nervous and have broken sleep, drink a cupful of Sage tea before retiring and it will help you get a good night's sleep. Writes C. R. L., South Bend, Ind.

NEURITIS

Is an inflammation of a nerve. It may affect the entire nerve and its branches or only a single branch. Exposure to a severe cold wind is the most common cause. Other causes are injury, strain, or severe pressure, and the aftermath of severe illness. The most important symptom is a peculiar shooting pain.

Treatment—Determine the cause. Avoid exposure to cold and dampness. Rest the part involved. If the pain is severe take 1 or 2 Aspirin Tablets. Some get relief by applying ice packs, others by applying a hot water bottle.

The Herb Doctor's choice of Antiperiodics and Nervines are: Black Snake Root, Fragrant Valerian, Chamomile Flowers, Mormon Valley Herbs.

I was awfully nervous, and after taking Catnip I can rest and sleep good. Writes Mrs. E. R., Durand, Wis.

I have used Star Root and it has helped me wonderfully. I also used Scullcap for nervousness. It is the best medicine I have found for nervousness. Writes Mrs. F. C. H., Elkview, W. Va.

Been using your Rocky Mountain Grape for Neuritis. Have never had a touch of it since. Writes Mrs. R. P., Jamul, Calif.

Neuritis—My husband's nerves were all dead, and, in fact, he was given up by doctors. I made a tea of Nerve Root and Red Clover, which he took for about 6 months. I also put hot cloths on him and rubbed the afflicted parts with Oil of Wintergreen. He has not been bothered since. Writes Mrs. O. P., Robindale, Minn.

For the Treatment of Neuritis—Here is a recipe from a cousin of mine that is a high class chemist. To a ½ cup of hot water, add 5 drops of Oil of Wintergreen and a teaspoonful of Baking Soda, stir well, take once daily for 3 days, discontinue for 3 days. If no relief, proceed as before until permanently relieved. Writes W. C., Wheeling, W. Va.

Editor's Note—It is very difficult to get the genuine Oil of Wintergreen

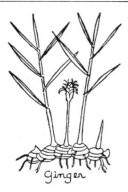

Ginger

—Cohosh Wild Root
Compound.....
Black Cohosh Root
Sweet Fern Twgs. and Lvs.
German Cheese Plant
Juniper Berries
Wintergreen Leaves
Fennel Seed
Mayapple Root
Rosemary Leaves
Marshmallow Root

The first ingredient of this formula—Black Cohosh—is often one of the main ingredients of remedies for Muscular Rheumatism. ————

NEURALGIA

In this ailment the pain generally affects one side of the face. Exposure to cold is a common cause of Neuralgia. Often decayed teeth or teeth in which the nerve has been taken out are the cause. Malaria is also a cause.

Treatment—Determine the cause and use the proper treatment. Apply Euca-Mint and take one or two Aspirin Tablets. Keep the bowels open.

The Herb Doctor's choice of Stimulants and Antiperiodics are: Canada Snake Root, Rocky Mountain Grape Root, Jamaica Ginger, Galangal, Chamomile Flowers, Celandine, Juniper Berries and Black Cohosh.

Neuralgia—The leaves of the common garden weed, Cheese Plant, which the children call the seeds of "Cheeses" and often eat, steeped in a tea, and drank a little at a time, also the leaves bound on the face, will quiet the nerves and often produce sleep, cure pain from Neuralgia after one has suffered for hours. Writes Mrs. W. McC., Ashtabula, Ohio.

For Neuralgia Pains—Beech Leaves should be used; take a quart of the leaves and steep them. Then make a corn meal mush and put the mush in a cloth bag. Then dip the bag in the liquid of the leaves and keep dipping and keep hot, and soon the pain will ease. I know it is good for I have used them when nothing else would help. Writes O. P., Nicholson, Pa.

Horse Radish grated and mixed with Vinegar, the same as for table purpose and applied to the face, is a simple cure for Neuralgia. Writes S. J. B., Port Washington, Ohio.

My wife has been sick with Neuralgia for 4 years and could not do anything, but since she has used the Blessed Thistle according to the recipe in your Almanac, she is getting along fine, and can do all her house work also out of door work. Thanks to you. Writes B. M., Picayune, Miss.

Take the leaves of Bull Nettle and make a tea and drink. Make a poultice of the leaves and lay on the affected parts. Will cure the worst case of Neuralgia. Writes J. E. P., Siloam Springs, Ark.

I prescribe Catnip to everyone who is nervous and complains of sleepless nights and also as a hot drink before retiring when there is a cold in the head. Writes Mrs. G. W. G.,

Neuralgia Cure—Take Lady's Slipper Roots and make a tea. Drink in small doses throughout the day. Will give quiet rest, and I have never known it to fail. Writes W. M. J., Coal Creek, Tenn.

Thistle Leaves cut in small pieces is a sure cure for neuralgia. Steep and drink the tea several times during the day and also upon retiring. Writes Mrs. L. S., Cocolalla, Idaho.

It is said that neuralgia is caused from lack of iron in the blood, and the pains are a prayer for iron. Writes G. W., New Sheffield, Pa.

My neighbor smokes dried Sumach Berries in a clay pipe for neuralgia. Writes J. M. C., Utopia, Ont., Canada.

To relieve Neuralgia I take a cupful of hot Boneset Tea before retiring. My father has always given us this tea when we were bothered with common colds. Writes Miss R. F., Gladys, Va.

Thistle Tea for Neuralgia cure. This tea is made by pressing a vessel full of the common Thistle Leaves, filling with water, and boil down one-half. Take a wineglassful of this tea twice a day. This is sure a great formula for Neuralgia. Writes Wm. H. B., Asquith, Sask., Canada.

NIGHT SWEATS

Take four heaping tablespoonfuls of dried Sage to about a quart of boiling water. Let this steep until cool. Take each night about a teacupful of this tea for three nights. Then skip a night or two. You may sweeten the tea if you desire. Then repeat this again. Keep this up till you get relief. It won't be long till you will notice the effect. I had night sweats bad and got so weak I took real nervous chills. I tried so many doctors and they all failed to cure them, until an old friend told me this and it sure did the work. Writes Wm. E., Cape Girardeau, Mo.

Cold Sage Tea, once a day for 3 days will surely stop the night sweats. Writes M. C., Trenton, Tenn.

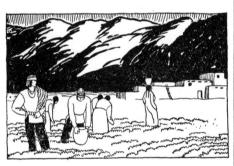

Drink cold Sage Tea to cure night sweats, while the hot Sage Tea will produce sweats. Writes Mrs. R. S., Mansfield, Ohio.

Sage Tea cured several people of night sweats. A cupful can be taken at bedtime, and I have found it cured in three nights. Writes Mrs. W. W., Fremont, Neb.

For Night Sweats—Make a tea of the Sweet Fern, drink several times a day before going to bed. A doctor ordered this for me when my lungs were bad and I was in bed a month from being so weak when it helped. Writes Mrs. A. G. D., Watervliet, N. Y.

I have found the Garden Sage which is mentioned several places in your literature is very good for night sweats. A handful to a pint is used, and drink a cupful before retiring, and will cure the worst case of night sweats. Writes O. L., Berry, Ala.

A tea from inner bark of Hickory, well boiled, drink hot, for night sweats. Writes John L. W., Florence, Miss.

Take inner bark of Birch, a handful to a pint of boiling water, allow to remain for 20 minutes, and drink cold before going to bed and it surely will help night sweats. Writes J. W., Munising, Mich.

Four tablespoonfuls of Sage, one quart of water, boil ten minutes, strain and when cool take in place of water. It is a sure cure for night sweats. I know what this did for me and many more, so I am glad to tell it to all. Writes Mrs. C. D., Knox, Pa.

—Sage-Mullein Clover

Italian Sage Leaves
Low Mullein Leaves
Red Clover Flowers
Bearberry Leaves
Palmetto Berries
Bluets
Gentian Root

Properties, Mild Tonic and Carminative.

NOSE

Foreign Bodies in the Nose—You may list this little hint in your Almanac if you desire. If a child gets a kernel of corn or a bean fast in the nose, place the palms of the hands flat over the child's ears, cup your mouth over its mouth and blow. I have found this to do the work when most everything else failed. Writes Mrs. T. A. S., Fontanelle, Iowa.

I am sending a recipe which has helped me and I hope it may be of some benefit to others. Take the Bark of Wild Cherry and a pod of Red Pepper and put this in a pitcher and pour hot water over it, cover and let stand until cold. Help yourself if your nose is inclined to bleed. Writes W. T. N., Johnson Springs, Va.

Editor's Note—I know this would be much better without the Red Pepper. Wild Alum Root is still better.

For nosebleed, use the dried leaves of Witch Hazel, powder them, and snuff into the nose, for a pinch drawn up the nose or on a wound will stop bleeding. Writes S. N. T., Worcester, Mass.

Here is a recipe that helped me. Take Hops and diluted Vinegar, heat and wring cloths of the hot vinegar and then apply hot for Headaches. Writes M. W., Harrietta, Mich.

—Prairie Plant Comp..
Wild Alum Root
Prairie Plant
Buckthorn
Indian Sage
Fennel Seed
Flax Seed
Cheese Plant
Marshmallow Root

Mild astringent, carminative, possessing at the same time emollient and laxative properties.

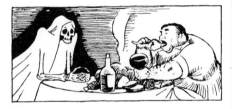

OBESITY

Obesity, or overfatness, is generally due to overfeeding, especially foods rich in carbohydrates, and lack of exercise.

Treatment—East less of foods rich in carbohydrates such as bread, cereals, sweet potatoes, nuts, milk, cream and all sweets. Take long walks.

The Herb Doctor's choice of botanicals containing organic minerals are: Horsetail Grass, Mormon Valley Herbs, Sassafras Bark, Poke Berries, Chickweed and Bladderwrack. This latter is probably the most effective and worst tasting of the lot.

For Obesity—You may eat anything except potatoes with this treatment:
1 ounce Sea Wrack
1 ounce Sassafras
1 ounce Pipsissewa
1 ounce Wintergreen
½ ounce Epsom Salts
Juice of 6 lemons

Steep the herbs one hour in 1½ quarts hot water, strain, and add the remaining ingredients, cover the herbs while steeping and if the water evaporates too much, add more. Shake well and the dose is one tablespoonful upon arising and after each meal and before retiring. It is perfectly harmless and it helps in more ways than one. It thins the blood, stimulates the circulation, and helps the kidneys. Writes N. S., Potlatch, Idaho.

Editor's Note—If it does all those things it must be good. At least, I know it is harmless.

—Sassafras Comp..
Sassafras Root
Elder Flowers
Rosemary Leaves
Rocky Mtn. Grape Root
Chickweed
Poke Root
Horsetail Grass

Mild Carminative, Tonic and Astringent. As harmless as ordinary household tea. The ingredients are well known to Herbalists. Sassafras, Poke Root and Horsetail Grass are some of the ingredients of numerous so-called obesity treatments. Our object in presenting this formula is to save the over-fat people the exorbitant cost of the various obesity treatments.

—Saline Herb Tea..
Gulf Wrack
Celery Seed
Angelica
Nerve Root
Horsetail Grass

A rather unpleasant tasting tea—but very useful to the experienced herbal physician. May be taken freely. On account of its saline nature—it is supposed to create abnormal thirst—and if this thirst is not satisfied—cause fat people to become thinner. The only sure remedy we know of for reducing is bending down exercises and walking. This formula is presented to expose the simple ingredients of these so-called obesity treatments which are often sold at exorbitant prices.

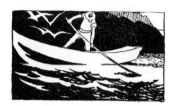

Gathering Bladderwrack

I am also using your Bladderwrack for obesity, my weight being 230 pounds, and I am getting good results. Writes Mrs. O. S. R., Goldsboro, N. C.

I must pass on to you what Mrs. G. wrote me about the wonderful results obtained from Indian Chickweed.

Mrs. G.'s letter reads: "Today I never found myself in better health. All my heart troubles have vanished, and I have reduced 30 pounds of bulky weight. The fat has disappeared. Thanks for the wonderful results of your herbal tea. No poison—no mineral—no narcotics. I am absolutely well. Take this as a send-off of one who faithfully stuck to herbal preparations to secure health and happiness." Writes A. G. B., St. Louis, Mo.

Editor's Note—I cannot understand how any one can get thin without the proper exercise. Oh, well! miracles sometimes happen.

Indian Chickweed—Used chiefly for overfatness. Is harmless and beneficial.

PELLAGRA

I am sending you a recipe for pellagra. A lady used this and it cured her. The doctor gave her up, for her hand was cracked open. Take Queen's Delight, and put it in a fruit jar with enough water to cover. Close the jar and let it set in water, bring to boil, also the water in the jar. Drink this in place of water and also use as a wash. Writes A. B. D., Norman, Okla.

Pellagra—Gather Yellow Root (Golden Seal) and wash the roots, cut them fine. Place in glass or earthenware and drink the water instead of clear water. Can leave set on stove and steep. This has, to my knowledge, cured cases where doctors had given up. It is also good for any stomach troubles. Writes Mrs. M. O., Nashville, Tenn.

Here is a recipe for pellagra. Take one cup of tea a day made of Yellow Dock Root and a teaspoonful of Golden Seal. Writes Mrs. A. L., Fallsville, Ark.

Editor's Note—You can expect no results of herbs that are over a year old.

Pellagra—My sister had pellagra, and she used this remedy. Sulphur and Cream of Tartar mixed well in equal parts, and she took 3 times a day. She also got some Poke Root, and bathed in the solution of it, as well as took a little of the tea internally. Writes B. G. D., Walnut Grove, Miss.

Here is a recipe that I have used with good results for pellagra: Make a strong tea of Yellow Root and drink two or three cupfuls daily. Writes L. R. S., Waynesville, N. C.

Here is one that is good for all mankind. Get Yellow Root. Make it into a tea. Drink two or three cups during the day. Or if you prefer you may chew the root. This is a sure relief for pellagra. I have used this with 100 per cent results. Writes P. M. T., Piedmont, S. C.

For Pellagra—Take one tablespoonful of Black Haw Root, one tablespoonful of White Oak Bark, one tabespoonful of Sampson Root, one tablespoonful of Dogwood Bark, three pounds of Brown Sugar and three quarts of water. Boil together down to one quart. Dose—Take one tablespoonful before each meal. I have used this with wonderful results. Writes J. G. D., Rembert, S. C.

—Yellow Dock Clover Compound..
Yellow Dock Root
Red Clover Flowers
Stillingia Root
Poke Root
Prickly Ash Bark
Rocky Mt. Grape Root
Elder Flowers
Marshmallow Root
German Cheese Plant
Tinn. Senna Leaves
Sassafras, Bark of Root
Am. Sarsaparilla Root

A mild alterative. A scientific blend of twelve different botanicals in which Yellow Dock predominates. A very fine tea. All patent so-called "Blood Purifiers" are composed of one or more of these various botanicals. Yellow Dock is one of the botanicals richest in organic iron.

PILES

(See Constipation)

This disease is well known. The piles may swell, burst and bleed profusely, forming what are known as bleeding piles. The loss of blood rarely weakens the patient. In some cases there is little discharge of blood, but frequent discharge of mucus attended with much irritation and violent itching. When there is only a slight attack, there is only itching of the parts.

Treatment — Apply Pile Ointment after each stool and at night before retiring. This ointment is soothing to the inflamed parts. To receive permanent benefit and to relieve the congestion which caused the piles, take a good demulcent tea.

The Herb Doctor's choice of botanical demulcents are: Sweet Weed, Flax Seed, Wallwort, Mullein, Cheese Plant, Agar Agar, Pilewort, Sweet Marjoram, Dwarf Elder, Chicory.

Pile Remedy—Balsam Copaiba, 7 drops on sugar, three times a day. Then Gum Benzoin in a strong infusion, three times a day, both these should be taken alternately. Writes Mrs. C. G., Hallstead, Pa.

I will give you a recipe for piles, which my grandfather used for years, too. Take Witch Hazel Bark, make a tea and drink it, and it certainly will cure piles. Writes W. E. B., Winona, W. Va.

Black Root cured me of the worst case of hemorrhoids. I was going to be operated on when an old lady gave me these roots and they cured me. Then she had me take Red Clover Blossoms also. Writes Mrs. A. C., Seattle, Wash.

A Cure for Piles, Sores, Etc.—Gather the buds of Balm of Gilead, put a little water on them and boil until soft. Then warm mutton tallow and mix in. For piles make a little cone and insert and for other sores soften with a little Olive Oil and apply. Writes Mrs. R. R., Ashtabula, Ohio.

Piles—Mash up Blue Flag Root and boil down. Add lard enough to make a salve. This cured my daughter when doctors failed. Writes Mrs. C. B., Concord, Tenn.

Take pure hog's lard and Sweet Clover, boil down and strain and let cool, then pour into any jars or tin ointment boxes which you may have for salves, and use this for piles, cuts and any sores. Writes W. H. D., Enterprise, W. Va.

For Piles—I find that a piece of Stone Root carried around in the pocket will cure or relieve nine out of ten suffering with either kind of piles. This Stone Root is also used for the kidneys by using 2 ounces of it scalded with a pint of boiling water, leave to steep and take a tablespoonful 3 or 4 times a day.

Editor's Note—This one has me stumped.

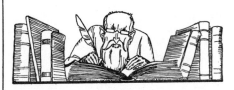

Try this for Hemorrhoids—Use four ounces of Cocoa Butter, and melt, then add three or four good sized cloves of Garlic which you have ground up fine. Let cool, and form into suppositories the size of a thimble. Use one after each evacuation of the bowels and upon retiring. This cured my husband in less than two weeks and have had no trouble since. Writes Mrs. M. L. P., Denver, Colo.

Here is a good recipe for piles. Take a half ounce of Yellow Dock, soak in hot water, apply to piles, and you will find it serviceable. Writes J. C., Mason City, Iowa.

Recipe for Fistula—Sweet Gum Bark and Mullein. Cook down with lard and make an ointment or salve. My father used this remedy for fistula and it gave quick relief. Writes S. S., North Garden, Va.

Piles—For Bleeding or Protruding Piles apply frequently equal parts of Glycerine and Witch Hazel. I have known this to give quick relief in several cases. Writes Mrs. C. A. S., Borger, Tex.

Here is a tested recipe for piles: Take a Buckeye and stew it in old bacon grease and strain, and apply like a salve. Writes M. E. R., Levee, Ky.

Here is a Recipe for Piles—A sure remedy if the people will continue taking it and not quit when they feel better. An old doctor told my father about this 50 years ago. He said it should be taken for one year and it would cure and it surely did the work and he never had them since. Put one package of Horehound in 3 pints of water and boil down to one pint, strain and add a small cupful of sugar and then boil to a syrup. Put in a glass fruit jar and take 1 tablespoonful before each meal. Writes M. B., Unionville, Ind.

Editor's Note—Almost too long.

Here is a recipe for piles. **Take one-**half ounce of Origanum Oil, one-half ounce tincture of Iodine, and 8 ounces of pure lard. Heat lard and put others in so it will stay mixed. It is instant relief. I have used it and given to others with good success. Writes W. F. L., Garnett, Kans.

More than ten years ago my brother suffered from hemorrhoids, which were so bad at times that he was compelled to stay home from work. He finally went to an herb doctor who had been recommended to him, who gave him Solomon's Seal, to be steeped in milk, one pint each night for three nights. He experienced results almost immediately, and after the third night he had permanent relief. That occurred more than ten years ago, and he has had no return of the trouble since. Writes B. M. S., Pittsburgh, Pa.

Carry a Buckeye in your pocket for piles. I had piles bad, when a friend told me he was bothered the same way until he began carrying the Buckeye, and did not have them since, and that was over 20 years ago, so I got a Buckeye, too, at once, and have not been bothered since that and it was 3 years ago. Writes W. J. T., Ashburn, Ga.

Editor's Note—This sure is a simple remedy. It reminds one of that Bible quotation, "As you believe," etc.

A good remedy for blind, itching or protruding piles: Boil Red Oak Bark down to an ooze and put with pure hog's lard and make into a salve, then use. Writes Mrs. V. M., Union Point, Ga.

Here is a valuable recipe for piles, as I know several who have used it and found relief. Make a salve by frying Mullein Leaves in fresh unsalted butter and use locally. Writes Mrs. M. J., Porterville, Calif.

Nut Gall used with Lard as a salve is very good for piles. Writes Mrs. M. D., Keokuk, Iowa.

Take Nutmeg, grate fine in pure hog's lard, about half and half, and apply and it will take the inflammation out of piles overnight. Plantain Leaves fried in pure lard also make a good healing salve.

Take Elder Bark, one handful, the same amount of Spicewood and fry with lard until brown, then take the bark out and add a lump of Rosin the size of a walnut, and fry again until the rosin dissolves. Then allow to harden and use as any other pile ointment for piles. This is known to be good where others failed. Writes A. M. B., Blairsville, Pa.

Take 2 ounces of Oil Wintergreen and a lump of Hog's Lard, the size of a hen's egg. Warm them together, and make a salve and cure for piles. It is a sure cure, for it has cured me and they never returned. Writes C. W., Indiana, Pa.

Steep a tea of the Burdock Roots in the Spring and Fall of the year and drink a wineglassful three times a day, and you will never be bothered with piles. Writes Mrs. E. H., Clinton, Iowa.

Editor's Note—Here is another new one on me —and well worth remembering. Burdock Roots are absolutely harmless.

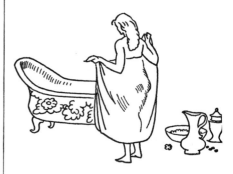

A salve for bleeding piles. Take two large handfuls of Peach Tree Leaves and fry in two tablespoonfuls of lard until the leaves are black and the lard is dark. Strain and let cool. Apply as you would any other salve. Writes Mrs. J. B., Canton, Mo.

Piles—The following is an excellent treatment for piles. Steep a tea of the herb Lousewort and take a swallow several times a day, which is apt to effect a cure, but about a teaspoonful of a tea made by steeping a handful of Hazelnut Burs in a pint of boiling water into the rectum, several nights in succession, and I believe they will cure to stay cured. Writes A. O. R., Hewitt, Minn.

Author's Note—Taste this tea before injecting into the rectum and if it puckers your mouth very much dilute with the warm water, or it will be too strong and contract the rectum too much.

Having found this of service, will also contribute it. For piles, take the White Oak Bark, one pound to two gallons of water, boil for three hours, strain, and boil again until it becomes a thick extract, then mix with an equal quantity of tar, simmer together until union takes place when cold. Apply with finger each night until well. Writes Carl B., Walnutport, Pa.

Editor's Note—I would improve the above by the addition of a pound of lard as tar becomes sticky unless mixed with some kind of grease.

My grandmother told me of this recipe to cure piles in their worst form, and I have known her to make the salve for her neighbors who suffered terribly for years and after using it have never heard any more complaints.

Take Buckeyes and peel off the outside hull and slice the kernel, and fry in any kind of fresh grease. Apply this both before and after stool. Writes R. L. W., Winston-Salem, N. C.

For piles take low Mullein Leaves, cover with hot water, and sit over it as it allays pain. Writes W. A. Y., Boiling Springs, Pa.

PIMPLES

I have been drinking tea made from Red Clover Flowers and think it is the best blood purifier. I had pimples and blackheads all over my face and since I started taking the tea I don't have as many and in a little while I think my face will be cleared of all of them. Writes A. C., Smithfield, Pa.

Take about a pound of the twigs of common Smooth Alder, and boil them for about one hour in a gallon of water. The water is applied to them. Also a good tonic is made from the bark by boiling longer, and taken internally. Writes W. J. P., Whitestone, L. I., New York.

I took some Chamomile Tea for pimples. It has made a very decided improvement. Writes Miss B. D. P., Great Falls, Mont.

For Pimples of the Face—Make a brine of Epsom Salts and pat on the face with Cotton and let dry on before going to bed. Do this until the pimples are dried up. Writes E. E. S., Myricles, Mass.

Editor's Note—Not bad if it works.

My son's face was broken out with Pimples, like a lot of young men at his age (18 years old). He had tried several tonics that were recommended to him but nothing helped. He finally began drinking one cup of Chamomile Tea each day and within two weeks' time there wasn't a trace of a pimple on his face.

For Rheumatic Pains I use a tea made of Wormwood, Red Clover and Catnip. One teaspoonful of each to a cupful of boiling water, let cool, strain and drink one cupful a day. I have used nothing else but this tea for rheumatic pains. Writes Mrs. C. M., Lakemore, Ohio.

PLEURISY

This comes on suddenly, with a chill, fever, and sharp, stabbing pains, called stitches in the side. The pains are made worse by coughing, pressure, or deep inspiration. There is also a frequent, dry cough, parched tongue. The patient lies on the back or affected side. If the lung is involved, the sputa or expectoration will be adhesive and streaked with blood.

Note—This disease is of a serious nature and should be treated by a physician. Under conditions where no physician can be obtained, give at once a good botanic tea. Apply hot, wet cloths to affected side and give a hot footbath. Great care must be taken to avoid exposure and not to go out too soon.

The Herb Doctor's choice of botanical Expectorants and Diaphoretics are: Pleurisy Root, Wahoo Bark or Root, Horehound, Coltsfoot, Blessed Thistle, Nettle Leaves, Holy Herb, Angelica, Bryony, Holly Leaves, White Pine, Lungwort, Wild Cherry Bark.

Pleurisy, Shortness of Breath—Make a tea of a teaspoonful of Pleurisy Root or Butterfly Weed and a cupful of water. Drink a teacupful on and off during the day in swallow doses. This remedy also assists digestion. Writes Miss L. G., Ann Arbor, Mich.

Pleurisy—Nothing better than a piece of Saltpetre, the size of a pea, taken once a day, will usually relieve or cure after the second dose. Writes Mrs. S. C. Y., Freedom, Me.

Pleurisy Pains—Use a teaspoonful of Sulphur at meal times, 3 times a day. Writes H. S., Mounds, Okla.

Editor's Note—Sulphur seems to be a great household remedy but I for one would much prefer Pleurisy Root in a case of this kind.

—Wahoo Pleurisy Root
   Compound.....
Pleurisy Root
Coughwort
German Cheese Plant
Wahoo Bark
Wild Cherry Bark
Bluets

A very fine combination of American botanicals, most of which are of Indian origin. Any physician should recognize the value of this tea.

Here is a very simple remedy that is good for piles. Fry the Cheese Plant in lard or unsalted butter, strain and leave set until cold. It is very good and I trust that it will help some one. Writes Mrs. J. R., Traverse City, Mich.

Pulverized Slippery Elm as a poultice cures piles. I have tried it mixed with boiling hot water, as hot as you can bear on. Writes Mrs. M. G., Adams, Mass.

Here is a recipe for an ointment we have used for piles:
  ¾ pound Lard
  ½ pound Resin
  ⅛ pound Beeswax
  ½ ounce Oil Amber
  ½ ounce Oil Spike
Writes Mrs. C. H. F., Clyde, Kan.

Take one tablespoonful of Powdered Sulphur in one pint of milk each morning or evening. This has cured me of protruding, itching and bleeding piles. Writes J. B. K., Timblin, Pa.

Editor's Note—Use only the purest Flowers of Sulphur.

Pile Remedy—Balsam Copaiba, 7 drops on sugar, three times a day. Then Gum Benzoin in a strong infusion, three times a day, both these should be taken alternately.

PNEUMONIA

This is a disease of dangerous character. It may affect one or both sides of the chest, the double form being the more serious. It comes on often unnoticed at first after a cold, with restlessness, a chill, and fever, and occasionally is well seated before its true character is known. There is a deep-seated dull pain or oppression under the shoulder blades, side, or breast; frequent short coughs and expectoration of sticky, adhesive matter of a green, yellow or rust color, usually tinged or mixed with blood. The breathing is oppressed, short and hurried. The skin is hot over the ribs and armpits; the nose is dry, eyes are tearless. There is great thirst. The speech is interrupted and hurried in bad cases. The pulse varies—sometimes rapid and full, at others hard and wiry, or quick and weak. The urine is reddish, scanty and sometimes burns and the patient lies on the affected side or on the back.

Note—This disease is of a serious nature and should be treated when possible by a physician. Put the patient to bed and give a good botanic tea. Rub the chest with Triple Strength Mustorine No. 142 and apply a hot water bag, or cloths wrung out of hot water, to the chest, cover with dry flannel if the oppression is severe.

The patient must be kept in a well ventilated room, very quiet, and have only a very light diet. These means will gradually relieve the oppression, allay the fever, induce free perspiration. Patient must avoid exposure until quite recovered. Fresh air is most important. Add lemon juice to all drinking water.

The Herb Doctor's choice of botanical expectorants are: Pleurisy Root, Lungwort, Coughwort, Honey, Wild Cherry.

Preparation for Pneumonia—Use one ounce of the following: Skunk Cabbage, Comfrey, Elecampane, Spikenard, Horehound, Wild Cherry. Pour boiling water over herbs and let steep for 6 hours. This will make a gallon. Then strain, add a pint of honey, and it is ready for use. Wineglass every 3 hours is the dose. The lady that gave me this recipe, said it was used back in 1700. An old Herb Doctor gave it to her grandfather. She said it was known to cure when everything else failed. Writes W. P. D., Springville, Utah.

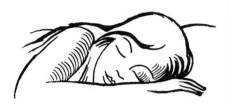

Pneumonia—Holy herbs made into a tea and drunk hot 30 minutes apart will break up a bad case of pneumonia, cold or la grippe. I have used this for years with unfailing success. Writes D. O. L., Memphis, Tenn.

Take Life Everlasting, 2 or 3 large handfuls and fry in lard, strain and use this salve by applying on hot flannel cloths as warm as can be borne. It is a simple remedy that has been long used with good results for pneumonia. Writes Mrs. K. P., Bauxite, Ark.

In case of lung fever or pneumonia, to open the lungs, etc., just pour boiling water on Turpentine and inhale it. I have tried this and it is very good. Writes M. J. H., Knoxville, Tenn.

Make a poultice of Horseradish, and lay on the chest, for pneumonia, and you will find it very good. Writes F. A. W., Tremont, Pa.

A good recipe for pneumonia: Make a salve of the following and put on the affected lungs, keep warmed up. I know of cases cured with this where doctors gave up. We always keep in house for colds on chest and sore throat: White Rosin, six ounces; Beeswax, six ounces; Camphor Gum, four ounces; Lard, twelve ounces; Balsam Peru, four drams; Oil Turpentine, four drams; Oil Cedar, four drams, and Oil of Eucalyptus, one ounce. Writes D. A. Y., Topeka, Ind.

My wife and two children were down with the flu, and one little girl had pneumonia. I gave her Boneset until the doctor came, and he just advised a mustard plaster, and quinine in the morning, but next morning the fever was broken with the Boneset. Writes J. C., Girard, Ala.

Editor's Note—Boneset is excellent for fevers. Its action is similar to quinine.

Recipe for Pneumonia—Take Lobelia Herb (ground) and put on a greased cloth and cover one with another greased cloth. Heat and place on the chest. Writes B. J. H., Brookville, Ohio.

—Jesuits Fever Bark
    Compound.....
Jesuits Fever Bark
Jamaica Ginger
Clove Buds
Cascara
Licorice Root
A useful substitute for quinine. Try it for colds, etc.

Make a tea of Butterfly Root, sweeten and drink one-half cup every two hours for pneumonia. Writes Miss M. P., Lexington, N. C.

For Pneumonia—Take a quart of red onions and 1 quart of vinegar. Cut up the onions in the vinegar and let come to boil. Make a poultice of this with corn meal. Put on chest and it will relieve in short time. Keep it up until not needed any more.

I will send you a tried remedy for all kinds of boils, bruises, etc. Take Dogwood Bark and boil. Then make a poultice of it, and it will draw to a head. I tried it in my own family many a time. Writes Mrs. T. T. H., Sharon, S. C.

My sons both had pneumonia and the doctor said one had T. B. and the other had heart trouble, and he swelled up from head to foot, so I ordered Black Root at 25c per box and it did the work when the doctor gave him up. I just made a tea of it and gave it to him. For the other, I gave him Holy Herbs at 25c per box, and now I would never be without these articles. Writes B. B., Robbins, Ill.

Editor's Note—This is good news for the suffering—but bad for the doctors.

Here is a remedy for pneumonia:
  1 tablespoonful Ground Cloves
  1 tablespoonful Ground Allspice
  1 tablespoonful Ground Nutmeg
  1 tablespoonful Ground Ginger
  1 tablespoonful Ground Mustard
  1 tablespoonful Corn Starch
White of one egg, and then add enough Olive Oil to make a thin poultice. Apply hot. Be very careful to keep patient well covered and give plenty of fresh air. A never-failing recipe as I have used it in many cases. Writes Mrs. F. H., Omaha, Neb.

For Pneumonia and Fever—Mix Sweet Oil and Camphor Gum. Dissolve the gum in the oil, and take cotton and saturate with the mixture. Place cotton around the chest and under the arms, or clear around the body. Put onion poultice on the feet. It will break up the worst case of fever. Writes L. B., Alligator, Miss.

A pneumonia remedy which was published in the ''Hartford Times'' and which was used by a nurse there in many cases with best results. It gave instant relief when massaged across the chest and back rubbed in thoroughly. Take one pound Pure Lard, one ounce Gum Camphor, one ounce Turpentine, and one ounce Aqua Ammonia. Melt the lard, camphor gum together, then add the rest and put in jars to cool. Writes Mrs. C. H., Wethersfield, Conn.

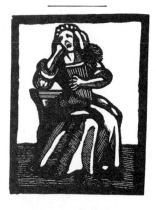

POISONINGS

Ivy Poisoning—A very simple remedy is to make a strong tea of Plantain Leaves by boiling them down. Allow the liquid to cool, then bathe the parts with this solution often and liberally.
Editor's Note—Ivy Poisoning affects different individuals in a different manner. That has been my experience.

One handful of Spearmint Leaves fried in one tablespoonful of lard until crisp, then apply freely to Dew Poison or Poison Ivy, and it will have a very soothing, healing effect. Writes Mrs. A. O., Opus, Fla.

For Poison Ivy—Make tea of Sassafras by using 2 ounces to a pint of boiling water, let it soak in that a few hours, then bathe the affected parts while tea is warm. This is particularly good after the blisters are formed. Write S. N. T., Worcester, Mass.

Ivy Poisoning—Plain Plantain Leaves steeped strong and soak the parts where the poison is. I have cured others as well as myself with this. Writes G. E. M., Freedom, Me.

For most cases of Blood Poison, burnt Alum is good. Pound a piece of Alum on the stove and let it burn. Make it into a fine powder, then it is ready to apply to all kinds of sores that don't heal. Writes G. B., Michigan City, Ind.

Sweet Fern steeped into a tea and used as a wash helped both myself and neighbors for Poison Ivy. There were also so many children around the neighborhood in bad shape from it when I helped them with this solution. Writes Mrs. L. F., North Oxford, Mass.
Editor's Note—That's an old Indian Remedy.

To Cure Blood Poison—Make a poultice of Flax Seed, ground, stir up with warm water. Change every hour. Keep poultice as hot as can be borne. Writes E. McD., St. John, N. D.

For Poison Ivy—Rub Golden Rod Leaves in cold water and wash hands and face or wherever you have it, allow it to dry by itself. Do this every time it itches. Writes Mrs. F. K., Valders, Wis.

For Ivy Poisoning, apply wet Epsom Salts, and note wonderful results. Writes I. S., St. Petersburg, Fla.

A wash from Spotted Alders, more commonly called Witch Hazel, is highly recommended for Ivy Poisoning. Writes S. S., North Garden, Va.

Here is a Good Recipe for Poison Ivy —Make a strong tea of Catnip and put in Sweet Oil or Olive Oil and put on the poison rash; be sure to mix well. If you know that you have been in contact with the ivy, wash the touched place with Apple Vinegar and it will keep it from breaking out. Writes Mrs. R. R., Springport, Mich.

For Poison Oak—This is a sure and tried remedy which I have used with very good results. Take Cedar Twigs and put them on the live coals and smoke the place where it is poisoned. Writes Mrs. J. H. D., Cana, Va.

Red Oak is good to use when one has had several teeth pulled at once. Keeps down blood poisoning, make like tea and hold in mouth. Writes G. W., New Sheffield, Pa.

Recipe for Blood Poison—Take Peach Tree Leaves and place in a bowl. Pour boiling water over them. Allow them to cool for about 10 minutes. Apply the leaves to the poison parts. This has done wonders. Writes Mrs. B. J., Oldfield, Mo.

Blood Poison—Use ground Slippery Elm, a 25c size box, and a bottle of Vaseline. Make a poultice of the Elm, the same as you would any other poultice. Then place the Elm in a cloth and have it as hot as you can bear, spread some Vaseline on the top of the poultice to keep it from sticking to the sore, and apply. Three applications will cure the worst case of poison. Writes G. E. M., Freedom, Me.

My uncle used Slippery Elm Poultice, which he made like Flax Seed Poultice for Blood Poisoning in his hand, and it cured him.

At one time I had a sliver cause Blood Poison, and I made a poultice of dried Plantain Leaves and in 3 hours the pain had disappeared, and in one week after the soreness had all left. I took one handful of the dried leaves to make a thick poultice. Writes J. V., Ann Arbor, Mich.

Take the Root of the Bear Grass, steep in just a little hot water to soften, then strain, mix with enough Vinegar to make a soft poultice, bind to the affected parts for Ground Itch or Dew Poison, and it will cure the worst cases. Writes Mrs. J. M., Richlands, N. C.

This is a simple remedy for Boils or Sores and Blood Poisoning, which we have always used. A hot poultice of the ground Flax Seed. Apply as warm as possible, and always keep it warm. Writes Mrs. J. B. G., Drummond, Wis.

Poultice for Blood Poisoning—One tablespoonful Flax Seed Meal and same amount of powdered Slippery Elm Bark, and make it black with the powdered Charcoal. Mix with enough boiling water to make a paste. Cook slowly for about 5 minutes. Apply hot to affected part.

Fry the leaves and tops of Yarrow in Lard, and then use this to grease any poisoned parts, and it will cure the worst cases. Writes D. A. B., Vandalia, Ohio.

Make a poultice of Cheese Plant Leaves by boiling them a little, then bind on sores for Blood Poison. Writes Mrs. H. D., Galena, Ill.

Make a salve of dried Catnip Leaves and fresh Butter. Pulverize the leaves and mix well. Apply fresh one an hour for Blood Poisoning. The wound will heal from the bone out. Writes I. S., St. Petersburg, Fla.

I am sending a recipe that cured my father of Blood Poisoning. This helped when the doctors failed. Take a pound of Epsom Salts to a gallon of water as hot as can be borne, and bathe the affected parts ½ hour, adding hot water as needed. Writes Mrs. H. W., Albany, Ore.

Rusty Nail Wound—Bacon wrapped around a wound from rusty nail is very good; the Bacon should be raw. Writes R. B., New York City.

Here is a sure cure for Poison Ivy, also for the Painter's Poison. Take Wild Cherry Bark, steep and make a rather strong tea, bathe the afflicted parts as often as it irritates one, and be sure to bathe just before going to bed. I have used this and know it is very good. Writes H. Z., Baraboo, Wis.

I would like to give you a cure for Poison Ivy to put in the "Almanac." A tea made of Sweet Fern if taken in swallow doses during the day will cure Poison Ivy in 1 or 2 days. Writes A. G., Paterson, N. J.

Blood Poisoning—I have a friend who has Blood Poisoning in his arm, which started from a sore finger. The doctors advised taking his arm off, as it was black to the shoulder. An old friend of his, however, asked him to bathe the arm in a hot tea of Cheese Plant. He did this and after 12 hours the black disappeared. The second day he soaked his arm in hot tea again for about six hours, and the skin pealed off, and the arm and fingers were well. Writes D. N. K., Allentown, Pa.

For Sores or Poison Ivy—Take Celandine Leaves and put in pan with some Lard and fry out together, then pour the grease off in a jar and cool. Then apply to sores or poison. It is very, very good for Ivy Poison and other Poisons as well. Writes Mrs. C. K., Benton, Pa.

Rattle Snake Root is a present cure for Blood Poison. Make a tea of it, and drink. It grows in rich places in the mountains here, and it will cure any snake bite, and is good for most any kind of ailments, stomach, etc. Writes J. B., Tellico Plains, Tenn.

Ivy Poison—Take the herb Lobelia and steep. After steeping, put in a tablespoonful of fine salt and bathe the parts poisoned with it. I never knew it to fail yet. It is also great on horse flesh when being cut with shoes, as no proud flesh will grow where it is used. Writes C. M., Londonderry, Vt.

Poison Ivy—Take Milkweed Root, and apply a tea prepared from it to the poisoned place, also drink freely of the tea. It certainly should be of service for this purpose. Writes L. B., Roxbury, Vt.

Take Poke Root and fry in fresh Lard and make a salve. This will cure most cases of Poison Oak. Writes L. E. N., West Union, Ill.

Take Tansy, boil the strength out of it, then take the juice and fry with Lard, then use this to rub on for Poison Oak. Writes P. C. S., Hackleburg, Ala.

For poison ivy steep a handful of Ground Ivy in sweet cream and apply as a salve. Writes Mrs. G. G. D., Coldwater, Mo.

For Blood Poisoning—One cup of Cornmeal, 1 tablespoonful Baking Soda, 1 teaspoonful Salt, a large handful Peach Tree Leaves. Place these leaves in a pint of boiling water, and bring to boiling point, strain and add the liquid to the dry ingredients and apply. Writes Mrs. O. C. P., Keokuk, Iowa.

Here is a recipe which I did not see in the Almanac. I have tried it and it does the work, for Poison Ivy. When it is in the eyes or ears or a tender place where you have to be careful what you use, take common Epsom Salts and wet and rub on and it does fine. Writes L. C., Lucas, Ia.

For Ivy Poisoning. Use a paste or salve made by mixing a spoonful of Rochelle Salts with thick sour milk. Writes Miss A. W., Londonville, Ohio.

Poison Ivy—Go on a fruit and vegetable diet.

Hives or Nettle Rash—Cleansing foods hasten recovery. Plenty of fresh fruits and green leafy vegetables. Better cut out all animal foods, tobacco and condiments.

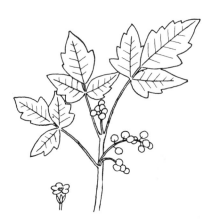

POISON IVY

For Poison Ivy—Take roots of the Rattle Weed, which is Black Cohosh, fry in bacon gravy and rub on the poison. One application is sufficient in most cases. Writes Miss G. N., Whiting, N. J.

I am writing a recipe for Poisons from Canned Vegetables and Meats. I have tried this remedy in emergencies with great success. Take a few Mayapple Roots and pour boiling water over them. Let cool and take ½ teaspoonful every 10 to 15 minutes until relieved. Writes H. L. P., Norfolk, Ark.
Editor's Note—Mayapple is a cathartic—call a doctor also.

Will send you another use for Golden Seal. Use the powder on any poison, it is good for I have used it. Cranberries bound on a sore will cure Blood Poison. Writes D. S., Howard, Kan.

PROSTATE TROUBLES

In severe agonizing cases of Prostatic troubles, the following gave a marvelous relief. This was evolved by great research by one who suffered almost intermittently for 10 years and I feel it has cured. One-half teaspoonful of powdered Slippery Elm. Mix with warm water to make a lumpless paste, then add half a glassful warm water and drink it both morning and evening. Cut out all stimulants and including meat. Writes F. J., San Diego, Calif.

Editor's Note—Absolutely harmless.

—Palmetto Damiana Compound.........
Palmetto Berries
Mexican Damiana
Sandalwood
Juniper Berries
Blue Mallow
Bearberry
German Cheese Plant
Corn Silk
Althea

more tonic and diuretic properties. The main ingredients of this formula are Saw Palmetto Berries and Damiana.

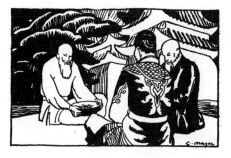

Tonic—The ingredients of this formula while of Indian origin, are now the main component parts of most of the modern so-called "Weak Men" tonics.

1 ounce Ground Palmetto Berries
2 ounces Ground Archangel Root
1 ounce Ground Gentian
1 ounce Ground Juniper Berries
1 ounce Ground Herb of the Sun

Steep a heaping teaspoonful into a cupful of boiling water. Use during day.

PROUD FLESH

For Proud Flesh cover the afflicted parts with burnt Alum. Writes G. P., Kirmansville, Ky.

Princess Pine has done more for me than the doctors have in 15 years. My face is almost healed except one spot and that is something that looked like proud flesh, now it begins to look like a wart but the pain has all stopped. I feel so thankful to think after 20 years suffering I have found something that at last really has given relief. Writes Mrs. E. P., Chatham, N. Y.

Editor's Note—I am not surprised.

QUINSY

Begins with redness, swelling of the throat and tonsils, difficult and painful swallowing, there is a fever and great prostration, and the disease may terminate in ulceration of the tonsils.

Treatment—
Goose Grease around the throat, covering with a flannel bandage, renewing as often as necessary.

The diet should be easily digestible and nourishing food: farina or other gruel, milk and beef tea. Lemon juice is also good.

Oil Peppermint applied externally around the neck and throat is a never-failing cure for Quinsy. Writes Mrs. F. S., Fiatt, Ill.

I am sending a recipe for Quinsy which I know is fine. Simmer Hops in Vinegar for a few minutes until the strength is extracted, strain the liquid, sweetening it with Sugar and give it frequently to the child or patient in small quantities until relieved. Writes Miss M. B. F., Harrisburg, Pa.

Quinsy—Take 4 ounces each of Hops and Blue Flag Root, and steep in 1 quart of water until it is boiled down one-half. Strain and sweeten with Honey. Use a gargle every half hour. This remedy has been known to give relief in less than 2 hours when the patient was not able to speak above a whisper. Writes J. T. F., Beaver Falls, Penn.

For Quinsy—An aged lady told my uncle to make a tea of Burdock Roots and gargle throat often and swallow a little each time. This cured him. Writes Mrs. J. A. B., Arcola, Ind.

A cure for Quinsy, use extract of
Witch Hazel. Bathe the throat well with
this extract and gargle with it on going
to bed. Anyone subject to Quinsy should
use the extract when they shave. Will
never have it after that. I used to
have it every winter until I tried this.
Writes T. C. D., Sharon, Pa.

RHEUMATISM

Rheumatism is an ailment that is frequently complicated by other affections.
Lumbago and Sciatica are forms of this
disease, and should be treated according
to its location.

Muscular Rheumatism—Muscular
Rheumatism is mostly due to exposure
to damp, cold weather. There is usually
fever, painful tenderness, soreness, lame-
ness and swelling of the affected part
and the disease may shift from one part
to another. It is generally confined to
the joints and extremities of the arms
and legs, but may involve any part of
the body.

Treatment—Take 1 or 2 Aspirin Tablets to relieve the pain if too severe.
Rest, in bed or easy chair, is essential.
Eat only plain food, avoiding acids,
sweets, meats and pastries and other
rich foods. Drink plenty of lemon juice
and water and take a good alterative or
anti-rheumatic remedy, and keep bowels
open.

The Herb Doctor's choice of mild Al-
teratives are: Virginia Snake Root,
Black Snake Root, Rheumatism Root,
Seven Barks, Rocky Mountain Grape
Root, Prickly Ash Bark, Burdock Root
and Seed, Yellow Dock Root, Angelica,
Celery Seed, Horse Radish, Yarrow,
White Bryony, Asparagus, Juniper Ber-
ries, Bayberry Bark, Bogbean, Centaury,
Wintergreen Leaves, Sweetfern and Bull
Nettle Root.

I am sending you recipe for Rheumatic Pains: Take four tablespoonful
of Wintergreen Leaves, two tablespoonsful of curled Yellow Dock Root.
Steep in a pint of boiling water, allow
the tea to cool for about half hour.
Dose—Two tablespoonsful of the liquid
one hour before and after meals. Writes
Mrs. M. S., Seattle, Wash.

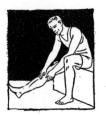

—Snake Root Compound

Snake Root
Sweet Fern
Kidney Liver Leaf
Juniper Berries
Mayapple
Wintergreen Leaves
Wild Yam
Fennel Seed
Wahoo, bark of root
German Cheese Plant

The main ingredient of this remarkable formula is Virginia Snake Root,
long used as an anti-rheumatic. While
rather bitter, it has an agreeable aroma.
A combination that will be hard to beat.

**—Queen of the Meadow
Compound........**
Queen of the Meadow
Black Cohosh
Wintergreen
Corn Silk
Juniper Berries
Gentian
Cheese Plant
Sassafras, bark of root

Black Cohosh is the most active botanical of this formula. Unlike Black
Cohosh when taken alone, this tea is
very mild and agreeable.

Virginia Snake Root we used with
Iron Weed Root, crushed them after
drying and covered with boiling water
and used with good results for Rheumatic Pains. Writes Mrs. J. S., Abilene,
Kan.

I have a treatment for rheumatic
pains which I find very good and in
my case and several others has given
relief. Make a tea from the bark of
Elder Roots and take a tablespoonful
after each meal. Writes F. S. F., New
Albany, Kan.

For those suffering with Rheumatic
Pains, try a pound of Sulphur mixed
with a pound of honey, making a paste,
and take it daily. Writes Mrs. C. L.
B., Headwaters, Ga.

Here is a remedy that I stumbled upon recently. I had been having rheumatic pains in my right side all summer, at about the waistline. My aunt sent me some Sweet Flag Root and I began nibbling on the roots for I had always liked them, and behold, the pain was relieved. I wondered what did it and one day I didn't eat any of the root, being busy outside, and I had the pain again. I came into the house and happened to think of my Sweet Flag Root, so I ate a tiny piece and the pain was lessened again so then I knew it must be that. If I eat a small piece of this each day I have no pain. Writes Mrs. L. G. B., Jefferson, Maine.

Not anywhere in your books do you recommend Angelica for rheumatic attacks. I have already ordered eight boxes for various people, and in every case where they chew the root and swallow the juice several times during the day, their pains vanishes. I gave Mrs. R. a box—she had pains for years—and before she used one 25c box all her aches were gone. She came to me for your address two days ago, and sent in her order for five boxes. Writes Mrs. L. M., Gold Hill, N. C.

I am sending you a good relief for Rheumatic Pains:
½ pint Epsom Salts
2 tablespoonsful Ginger
2 Lemons, cut fine
1 quart boiling water
Pour the water over the things and when cold shake well, and take a wineglassful before breakfast. Writes Mrs. E. B., Eau Galle, Wis.

For relief of pain in rheumatic attacks: One package of Black Cohosh steeped in a pint of Holland Gin. Let stand for one week. Dose: a teaspoonful after meals. Writes E. J. M., Oil City, Pa.

PRICKLY ASH—HANTOLA

The western tribes of American Indians, since time immemorial, have used Prickly Ash, or Hantola, with excellent results in the treatment of rheumatism, colics, cramps and allied complaints. Prickly Ash, or Hantola, blooms in April and May, before the appearance of leaves. It is a reliable diaphoretic, producing sweating in profusion.

Its value was fully recognized by Dr. King in 1849. He stated that Prickly Ash generally proved of immediate relief in Cholera and Typhoid conditions also. For rheumatism, I advise using Prickly Ash in a tea, with a mixture of Burdock, Black Cohosh and Poke-Root in equal parts. This mixture has proven to be the most effective remedy for rheumatism, lumbago, gout and backache. It has brought speedy relief so many times that I do not hesitate recommending it to the sufferers of these maladies.

It is made by mixing equal parts of Prickly Ash, Burdock, Black Cohosh and Poke-Root together, placing a heaping teaspoonful of the mixture into a teacupful of boiling water and allowing it to stand until cool. Strain and drink a mouthful of the tea several times a day.

I use a mixture of Boneset, Trailing Arbutus, Wintergreen and Peppermint for my Aches and Pains in my arms and throughout my body. I use the Horehound for my husband's Itching Piles and it helps him. Writes Mrs. E. M. S., Reynoldsville, Pa.

I would like to contribute a little for your herb booklet so I am enclosing a simple remedy or tea for the relief of Joint Rheumatic Pains. Just take the leaves of Canada Thistle and use one teaspoonful to every cup of tea. Pour boiling water over the leaves and let stand a little while, then drink but do not sweeten it. Writes T. H. L., Goodrich, Wis.

I want to tell you of the wonderful relief your herbs gave us. My husband and I had rheumatism for many years and now we seldom get any pains. We have been using Yarrow nearly every day, and also Red Clover and Elder Blossom Tea. Writes Mrs. P. H., Milwaukee, Wis.

To make a quart of liniment for muscular pains, mix one ounce each of Canada Snake Root, Capsicum, Mayapple Root and Indian Turnip and add two quarts of water to above mixture, boil down to one quart, add two ounces Camphor, strain and it is ready to rub on the parts. Writes A. J. F., Jersey City, N. J.

I am sending you recipe for Rheumatic Pains: Take four tablespoonfuls of Wintergreen Leaves, two tablespoonfuls of curled Yellow Dock Root. Steep in a pint of boiling water, allow the tea to cool for about half hour. Dose— Two tablespoonfuls of the liquid one hour before and after meals. Writes Mrs. M. S., Seattle, Wash.

This is a sure help for it helped my mother who suffered with Rheumatism, and was in bed for 13 weeks, and never sat up until she took this. Use equal parts Epsom Salts, and Cream of Tartar, and 3 Lemons. Put in quart of boiling water, and take a tablespoonful 2 or 3 times a day. Writes S. F., Akron, Ohio.

As a child I knew two old ladies who said common ground Red Pepper was a sure preventative of Rheumatism, and every night at bed time they would take a small amount, perhaps as much as a pea, mix with ½ cup of milk. They would drink a cup of milk after to wash it down. These two ladies lived to be nearly 80 years of age and never had a trace of Rheumatism or Stiffness, so common in elderly people. Whether it was due to the Pepper or just good fortune I cannot say, but it is such a simple remedy no one need fear while giving it a trial. Writes Mrs. C. C. B., Grand Island, Neb.

Here is a remedy that cured my father of Rheumatism. He was so crippled he couldn't lift his arms to put on his coat, which my mother had to do for him. He used Oil of Wintergreen taken inwardly beginning with 1 drop in a teaspoon of Sugar 3 times a day and increasing the dose to 2 drops the following day and increasing a drop every day until he was taking 9 drops and on the tenth day 8 drops and decreasing a drop every day until he was back to 1 drop again. It cured him and he has never had another attack of Rheumatism since and that has been over 25 years. Trusting that this may help someone I'm passing it along. Writes Mrs. D. W., Viola, Ill.

Editor's Note—It is very difficult to get the true Oil of Wintergreen-

Send me a box of Colombo, Peruvian Bark, and Quassia. We have only used this about 4 months and we really think it is helping my husband. He could not walk, had no use of his hands when he started, but now he can use his hands and walked about a half-mile up the street and back for the first time in 2 years. Hope he gains as much the next 4 months. I was told he would never get better. Writes Mrs. A. C. A., Akron, Ohio.

Editor's Note—Surely these letters prove that herb teas contain some mysterious substance— probably some vitamin not yet discovered.

I want to tell you what Mormon Plant has done for us. It got my husband so he could eat well and sleep well, and the Rheumatism left his legs, so I am sending for 8 more boxes of it. Writes L. F., New River, Va.

Here is my recipe for Poke Berries for Rheumatism. Take a pint of the Cider Vinegar and a pint of the Poke Berries, put them in a quart jar and bottle, let stand 12 hours and take a tablespoonful 3 times a day. It surely helped me. Writes Mrs. E. C., Claremore, Okla.

Take 3 drops of Oil of Wintergreen on a little Sugar 3 times a day, and it cannot be beat for Rheumatism. Writes G. M., Belle Center, Ohio.

Editor's Note—

Genuine Oil Wintergreen is very expensive and there are substitutes that are cheap and cannot be detected except by an expert.

For Rheumatism try chewing plenty of Ginger Root. Writes M. W., Louisville, Ky.

Here is a tested recipe for Rheumatism: Put a teaspoonful of Sulphur in each shoe and it will cure Rheumatism. Writes R. N. M., Thomas, Okla.

Editor's Note—I have nothing to add.

For Rheumatism—Take the Poke Root, boil until tender, mash and make into a poultice, then bind this on the bottom of the feet if the Rheumatism is in the back or lower limbs, but to the hands if in the upper part of the body, and you will find very good. Writes M. F., Pulaski, Va.

Prince's Pine Leaves, that have been cut up fine and steeped as tea is a fine tonic, makes one hungry and cures Rheumatism, and Lumbago. Acts as a mild physic and cleans the blood of impurities. Writes Mrs. L. S., Cocolalla, Idaho.

I wish to tell you that my sister has used the Oil of Wintergreen for Lumbago with good results, by using 10 drops on Sugar and a glass of water with it every 4 hours, when a doctor could not help her. (Of course it must be the genuine Oil of Wintergreen.) She got relief in 2 days in using this. Writes Miss J. D., Belle Plaine, Iowa.

Spanish Rheumatism Remedy—Always on the alert for new and strange remedies I have found what I am certain is a very good treatment for Rheumatism. The information came to me through a Greek Herbalist and his American associate who reside in a section of California that was formerly entirely Spanish. The Spaniards, as we all know, were very efficient in herbal treatments. The herb is Yerba Del Pasmo, a favorite Rheumatism remedy of the Spaniards. This herb, as my investigations have proven, is very rich in organic minerals. The herb tea is made by placing a teaspoonful of Yerba Del Pasmo in a cup of boiling hot water and when cool, strain and drink 1 or 2 cupfuls a day.

Sciatica—Sciatica is a form of Neuritis. The leading symptom is a pain along the track of nerve. The pain is felt behind the thigh, from the hip down, towards the knee and sometimes down to the heel.
Treatment—Most cases are very obstinate and require long treatment; the same as for Neuritis. Hot applications and hot liniments

Lumbago—Lumbago is characterized by a crick in the back or painful rheumatic stiffness across the loins and back.

Gout—The symptoms are a severe sharp shooting pain in the joint of the big toe preceded by various disturbances such as headache, neuralgic pains, drowsiness, tender sore throat, etc.

This is a remedy that my grandmother used for Rheumatism: Take Mullein, make a strong tea, and soak the parts with this. Put on as hot as can be borne and allow to remain on until cold. Also make a salve of the tea by adding Lard and boiling the water out. Rub on the affected parts after you have used the tea mentioned above. This cured Inflammatory Rheumatism. Writes Mrs. R. E. B., Georgetown, Ga.

Euca Leaves Compound—This is a combination of leaves from California that have given such good results in some forms of rheumatism that we were urged to add it to our list. These leaves are placed in a vessel containing two gallons of water and the feet are bathed in this every evening for seven nights as hot as it can be borne. The same herb liquid is used over and over again. In most cases the rheumatic pains, or lumbago, have flown before the seventh day. If not, the treatment is repeated with a fresh package of herbs.

—Cohosh Wild Root Compound.....
Black Cohosh Root
Sweet Fern Twgs. and Lvs.
German Cheese Plant
Juniper Berries
Wintergreen Leaves
Fennel Seed
Mayapple Root
Rosemary Leaves
Marshmallow Root
The first ingredient of this formula—Black Cohosh is often one of the main ingredients of remedies for Muscular Rheumatism.

—Rocky Mountain Tea..........
Rocky Mtn. Grape Root
Kidney Wort
Yellow Dock Root
Button Snake Root
Rosemary Leaves
Skunk Cabbage
Juniper Berries
German Cheese Plant
Black Mallow
Fennel Seed
The ingredients of this tea speak for themselves. Most of them can be found in Rheumatic Remedies of some sort or other.

Here is a recipe that gave my father and me relief from rheumatic pains:
2 oz. Yellow Dock Root
2 oz. Dandelion Root
1 oz. Burdock Root
½ oz. Blackberry Leaves
½ oz. Raspberry Leaves
4 oz. Elder Berries
1 oz. of Bull Nettle
Mix these together and use 1 teaspoonful of the mixture to a cup of boiling water, let cool, strain and drink. Writes H. P. K., New Palestine, Ind.

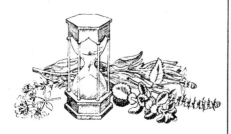

For rheumatic pains:
   2 oz. Prickly Ash Bark
   2 oz. Burdock Root
   2 oz. Buchu Leaves
   2 oz. Sassafras Root
Steep in two quarts of water and boil down to one quart; take one tablespoonful three times a day. It will be necessary to put something in it to keep it from spoiling. Writes Mrs. L. M. V., Glens Falls, N. Y.

Editor's Note—May be effective in some cases, but certainly not in all.

Rheumatism—3 oz. Virginia Snake Root, 3 oz. Indian Turnip, 3 oz. Prickly Ash Berries, 3 oz. Nettle Root, 3 oz. Juniper Berries, 1 oz. Blood Root. Place all in a gallon of boiling water and steep until cool. Take from 1 teaspoonful to a tablespoonful 3 times a day after meals. It cured me when everything else failed. Writes Rev. J. E. C., Cly, Pa.

Virginia Snake Root—An excellent blood purifier, much used in cases of skin diseases and fevers. Often combined with Yellow Dock and Sarsaparilla as a spring tonic. Produces perspiration, strengthens the stomach, and increases the appetite; also good in rheumatic complaints.

For Inflammatory Rheumatism—Take as much Choke Cherry Bark as you can pick up at two large handfuls, steep in 2 quarts of water, add whiskey to keep from souring. Dose: 1 teaspoonful 4 or 5 times a day. Writes L. E. McD., Rock Island, Tex.

For Rheumatism—Take 9 pods of Red Pepper, and a small cupful of Lard, and boil together. Then rub on the afflicted parts at night. Writes Miss E. B., Rocky Mount, Va.

Here is a recipe my father told about. An old slave in slave time had Rheumatism, and he was really past the going or working age, and his master was always on him trying to make him do when he couldn't, so the slave thought he would get out of the way so he crawled behind the barn in a patch of Poke Berries and ate a lot, which he thought would kill him. Next morning he could walk very well. My father uses them now, 12 or 15 berries at a time, like pills, 3 or 4 times a day. Writes R. H. W., Richlands, Va.

Editor's Note—Poke Berries and Poke Roots are old Indian remedies for rheumatism. This incident reminds me of that old song of our childhood, "If God So Loved the Little Birds, I Know He Loves Me Too." If we have faith in the Good Lord he will not desert us in the hour of need.

For Rheumatism — Take Mandrake, Culvers Root, Boneset, Black Cohosh, Canada Snake Root, Prickly Ash Berries, Lobelia, Pleurisy Root, Wild Yam, all equal parts, and mix thoroughly. Take 2 heaping tablespoonfuls of this, place in a vessel that will hold a quart of soft boiling water, let steep an hour (must not boil), sweeten, keep warm and strain only as used. As long as there is any pain, give patient 2 tablespoonfuls every hour until there are yellow discharges from the bowels. After that, 3 tablespoonfuls every 2 hours as long as there is a vestige of Rheumatism pain left in the body.

This specific can be prepared into syrup but we think the infusion is the best. This has cured a man in 48 hours who had to be turned over in his bed by four men who lifted the corners of the bed sheet.

During the treatment there must be no milk or meat taken. The diet must be toast, baked apple, lemonade, and gruels and lots of fruit, canned peaches, pears, pineapple and one can vary the meals during the treatment, but starvation is a part of the cure. When the yellow discharges from the bowels appear the pains will be gone and will not come back if you conquer your stomach and mind what you eat and drink.

In the morning before you eat anything drink as many glasses of milk or warm water as you can, if this starts you to vomit so much the better.

If the patient has never used any of the "Potashes" that crowd the shelves of the drug store, the Iodides and the Bromides, his chances to get well are more and more sure. Writes Mrs. K. R., Oakland, Md.

Here is one of the greatest liniments ever used. Use 50c worth Gum Camphor to a pint of Turpentine. Writes Mrs. C. R., Steedman, Mo.

Here is a recipe for a Liniment that sure is fine:
    1 ounce Oil of Cedar
    1 ounce Oil Spike
    1 ounce Oil Wintergreen
    ½ ounce Camphor Gum
    1 tablespoonful Turpentine
    3 eggs
Mi· all together, then add a quart of Cider Vinegar. Let set for a week, shake up every day, and it will be almost white when ready to use. It was given me by an old Gypsy woman and it is hard to beat. It of course is for external use only. Writes S. G., Stanberry, Mo.

Rheumatism—This is an old time remedy which never fails to cure if given a thorough test. I know a lady who had not walked in 16 years, and after taking this simple remedy for 3 months she began to walk a little and with a year's time, she regained the full use of her limbs, and restored to health.
    ½ ounce Colombo
    ½ ounce Peruvian Bark
    ½ ounce Quassia
To this add a half pint of Alcohol or Whiskey, let stand one day, then add ½ pint of water. Dose: One tablespoonful 4 times daily before each meal and at bedtime. Writes Mrs. C. A. E., Bangor, Calif.

My brother and another man was completely cured of Rheumatism in 24 hours by drinking a strong tea made from Witch Hazel Bark. When you use this drink no water. Doctors gave everything but it did no good. Writes J. F., St. Martinsville, La.

For Rheumatism—Use a quart of water, a d a package of Yellow Dock. Boil about an hour, then put in 3 slices of Lemon, an ounce of Epsom Salts, strain and take a wineglassful every morning. We tried it time and time again and it has never failed us. Writes A. Y., Moosup, Conn.

For Inflammatory Rheumatism—Take a teaspoonful of powdered Sulphur in an ordinary glass of milk every night for 11 nights, then stop. This has helped where doctors failed.
Editor's Note—I would prefer an herb tea.

A splendid liniment, which is very penetrating. Take Oil of Origanum 1 ounce, Oil Sassafras 1 ounce, Oil Rosemary 1 ounce, Tincture of Capsicum 1 ounce, Gum Camphor 1 ounce, and 12 ounces of Alcohol. Mix well. Serviceable for Sciatica Rheumatism, etc. I always keep this on hand. Writes Mrs. K., Ottawa, Ont., Canada.

A Recipe for the Cure of Rheumatism—Take Birch Bark and Yarrow Tea in equal parts, and boil 3 to 5 minutes, let this stand 30 minutes, strain and take 3 to 4 cupfuls a day. This will positively cure Rheumatism, Neuritis, etc. Writes H. W. F., Mill Hall, Pa.

Am. Poplar is a good tonic and a good remedy for Chronic Rheumatism, Dyspepsia and General Debility. A heaping teaspoonful 3 or 4 times a day is the dose. Writes L. W., Coldwater, Miss.

For Arthritis—Take a pint jar. In it put 3 tablespoonfuls of Rochelle Salts and juice of 1 Lemon. Put in jar and fill jar with water. Take a wineglassful 3 times a day before meals. Writes N. W., West Palm Beach, Fla.

A Sure Shot for Rheumatism—Take a large handful of Mayapple Root and boil down very slow, strain, and put the ooze in a frying pan with a small quantity of pure Hog Lard. Heat until the water is all removed. Apply this ointment freely to affected parts. Three applications will cure the ordinary case. Neither does it return. Writes W. L. C., Yarnaby, Okla.
Editor's Note—Any case of Rheumatism can return.

Black Cohosh is a very active and useful remedy in many diseases. It is slightly narcotic, sedative, antispasmodic, and exerts a marked influence over the nervous system. Valuable in all cases of inflammation of the nerves, tic douloureux, crick in the back or sides, rheumatism.

This is Col. Birch's recipe for Rheumatic Gout or Acute Rheumatism. Take half ounce of Saltpetre, half ounce of Sulphur, half ounce of Flowers of Mustard, half ounce of Turkey Rhubarb, fourth ounce of powdered Guaiacum. Mix and take a teaspoonful every other night for 3 nights and omit for 3 nights. Take it in a wineglassful of cold water, which has been previously boiled. Writes D. J. D., Corfu, N. Y.

For Rheumatism—Take leaves of Mullein and steep, drink 3 or 4 wineglassfuls daily. I know a party who cured himself in this manner. Writes Jno. P. J., Spooner, Wis.

Oil Wintergreen, used in coffee in this manner is also very helpful if you have Rheumatism. Writes Mrs. E. M., Willow Springs, Mo.

Editor's Note—Be sure you get the true Oil Wintergreen and not methyl salicylate—they both smell alike but are not the same.

Inflammatory Rheumatism and Gout—

The following is a very good remedy for Inflammatory Rheumatism and Gout and has a good reputation in Australia. In 3 quarts of water place 1 ounce Blue Flag Root, 1 ounce Buck Bean, 1 ounce Sassafras. Boil 1 hour. Strain and add ½ pound Sugar. Dose: a wineglassful 4 times daily. Writes C. M., Flemmington, Victoria, Australia.

Rheumatism—The following is a very excellent remedy for Rheumatism. I have used this recipe and know it is good. Take 1 ounce Wahoo Bark, 1 ounce Golden Seal, 1 ounce Wild Cherry Bark, 2 ounces Sarsaparilla, 1 ounce Yellow Dock, ½ Mandrake Root. Put all in ½ gallon of whiskey. Let it stand a few days. Dose: 1 tablespoonful before going to bed. Shake well before using. Writes J. N. H.

This is an excellent remedy for Rheumatism:

 1 handful Choke Cherry Bark
 1 handful Tamarack Bark
 1 handful Burdock Root
 1 handful Blackberry Root

Boil all together and get ½ pint from them. Strain, add a cup of Sugar, boil again; when luke warm add ½ pint of good Brandy. Dose: One tablespoonful after meals. Writes E. A. C., New Brunswick, Canada.

I am sending you a good relief for Rheumatic Pains:

 ½ pint Epsom Salts
 2 tablespoonfuls Ginger
 2 Lemons, cut fine
 1 quart boiling water

Pour the water over the things and when cold shake well, and take a wineglassful before breakfast. Writes Mrs. E. B., Eau Galle, Wis.

Rheumatism—Take about 8 heaping teaspoonsful of Tansy. Steep in a pint of water for 30 minutes. Strain. Add ½ pint of best Whiskey or Brandy. Sweeten to taste. Dose: 2 tablespoonsful 3 times daily. Writes N. A. J., Johnsburg, Ind.

For Rheumatism—Use the root of the Milkweed Plant which has been washed and dried thoroughly, also cut into pieces. Chew these pieces and swallow the juice, and this will cure within 3 weeks. I know of a woman who had been bedfast for 3 months and was entirely cured and doing her own work within 3 weeks after she tried this remedy. Writes H. W. L., Youngstown, Ohio.

Editor's Note—This is the Milkweed with the orange colored flowers, also called Pleurisy Root.

Here is a recipe my father told about. An old slave in slave time had Rheumatism, and he was really past the going or working age, and his master was always on him trying to make him do when he couldn't, so the slave thought he would get out of the way so he crawled behind the barn in a patch of Poke Berries and ate a lot, which he thought would kill him. Next morning he could walk very well. My father uses them now, 12 or 15 berries at a time, like pills, 3 or 4 times a day. Writes R. H. W., Richlands, Va.

Editor's Note—Poke Berries and Poke Roots are old Indian remedies for rheumatism. This incident reminds me of that old song of our childhood, "If God So Loved the Little Birds, I Know He Loves Me Too." If we have faith in the Good Lord he will not desert us in the hour of need.

A Rheumatism medicine and Tonic. Use ½ ounce Poke Root, Queen of the Meadow, and Gum Guaiac. Place in a quart of water, boil down to a pint, add 6 ounces of Glycerine to preserve and it is ready for use. One teaspoonful should be taken as the case requires, 2 to 4 times daily, and some people use even 1 tablespoonful at a time. Poke Root is known to most people here as "Skoke." A poultice will cure Salt Rheum, and is good for Carbuncles, Quinsy, and many other things. Writes P. M. B., Perry, Pa.

A Slow But Good Cure for Rheumatism—Dissolve a teaspoonful of powdered Rhubarb, a teaspoonful of Sugar and teaspoonful of Soda in a half-pint of boiling water and add a drop or two of pure Wintergreen Oil and bottle for use. The dose is a teaspoonful 4 times a day before meals and at bedtime. Shake well before using. Writes Mrs. R. R., Ashtabula, Ohio.

I had Sciatic Rheumatism and found the recipe calling for Poke Root. I used it both internally and as a poultice and I have not had a pain since. Writes A. U. M., Edwards, Mo.

Take 1 tablespoonful Prickly Ash Berries to a pint of good Whiskey or Brandy, 3 times a day, 1 tablespoonful at a time. This is fine for Rheumatism. Writes Mrs. C. D., Mapleton Depot, Pa.

For Rheumatism—Take 4 handfuls of Poke Berries, 4 handfuls of Elder Berries, 1 handful of Sumach Berries and 2 handfuls of Powdered Wild Blackberry Root. Add 2 quarts water and sufficient Sugar to taste, boil to Syrup and take teaspoonful 3 times daily. This is also good for Tonsilitis. Writes R. E. B., Princeton, W. Va.

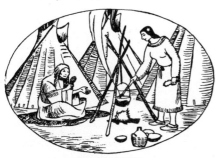

I have tried several of your herbal remedies and they surely were fine. I had a friend down with Rheumatism and I told him one of your remedies was to use a Poke Root Poultice and place on the feet and hands, and he did so. He was relieved from Rheumatism. Writes W. L. R., Goin, Tenn.

A lady advised me to try Yarrow for Rheumatism which I had, and I am getting results. Take what you can hold in your hand and steep it in a quart of water, drink all in one day, next day do it over until you are cured. She said her husband used this when he was 77 years old and was cured. You can publish this to help some one else if you desire. Writes Mrs. C. L., Louisville, Ohio.

the Pure Oil Wintergreen. This has done me more good for Rheumatism caused from an excess of uric acid than anything I have ever tried or used for it. Writes Mrs. H. C., Romeo, Mich.

Editor's Note—The true Oil of Wintergreen may be used as a liniment and also internally—just a few drops on sugar or in milk or water.

For Rheumatism—Make the patient drink tea of Wintergreen Leaves. Keep very warm so as to get a good sweat, and rub all over with Vaseline. Writes H. L., Tyler Hill, Pa.

I want to say how quickly I have been cured of Rheumatism with Poke Root. I have taken a glassful for 8 days, omitting one day, the fourth day, and only once during that period have I suffered. Let me remind you your Poke Root has been a sure shot in just 8 doses. The only remedy I have ever had that gave me relief from Rheumatism. Writes Mrs. M. J. Z., Waynesboro, Va.

Just a few lines today to let you know how good your herbs are. Last spring I had Rheumatism so bad that it was very hard for me to get around and I hardly was able to do anything. I sent for a package each of Rocky Mountain Grape Root, Skunk Cabbage and Black Cohosh and in a week's time I surely could notice a great difference. I have been rid of my Rheumatism long ago. Writes Mrs. H. F. E., Lytton, Ia.

Editor's Note—I was exceedingly glad to hear from you and of the good my herbs have done.

Rheumatism—It is always evidence of poor elimination, imperfect drainage of the system, of gluttony regarding foods which give a decidedly acid reaction. Uric acid is an end product of meat, fish, poultry. It would be well also to omit from the diet eggs, old cheese, dried peas and beans, white flour, white bread and all demineralized cereals.

RINGWORM

Bathe the afflicted parts with Medicated Witch Hazel. If of long standing apply Skin Paint or Sulphur Tar Salve after bathing.

Ringworm Recipe—Take a handful of Gold Thread Roots, put hot water on them and let them steep. Make good and strong, and paint the affected spot 3 or 4 times a day. Have the liquid as hot as you can bear. Writes F. W. V., Nehma, Mich.

I once saw a girl about 14 who had a ringworm on her head, so bad, and I asked why someone didn't do something for it, but they had done everything they could, so I got a bottle of Castor Oil and used plenty of it. It went away without further trouble. Writes Mrs. R. T., Appleton, Minn.

A cure for Ringworm is Yellow Dock Root steeped in Vinegar. This should be applied locally to affected parts. Writes C. M. A., Burke, S. D.

RUPTURE

I am sending you a recipe for Rupture cure:

1 quart or White Oak
1 quart of Wild Blackberry Roots

Boil to a thick liquid and apply 3 times a day externally. Writes L. D. Y., Lomira, Wis.

Editor's Note—May be good, but certainly cannot be called a cure for every case; however, it is entirely harmless.

White Oak

An infusion of White Oak Bark is often of service in Ruptures as it has a tendency to tighten the muscles. For this purpose it must be made very strong; about an ounce of the bark is placed in a pint of water and boiled down to measure 2 ounces. For internal use 1 teaspoonful is used to a cupful of boiling water.

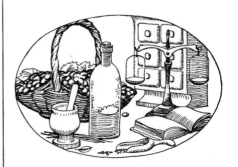

SCARLET FEVER

An acute, eruptive and infectious fever. The first symptom is usually vomiting, soon succeeded by violent heat, very rapid pulse and sore throat, which may be known by the pain on swallowing. Then a rash or reddish blush spreads over the body, commencing on the arms, neck, breast and face until the disease has reached its height, when later it becomes faintly yellowish and the outer skin flakes off in patches or in small, bran-like scales. Such is the course of a mild case, but it may become complicated with ulcerated throat or other symptoms.

Treatment—In suspected cases the patient should be immediately put to bed and kept warm and quiet. Call a doctor and give plenty of lemon juice in water.

The Herb Doctor's choice of diaphoretics and aromatics are: Lady Slipper, Borage, Chamomile, Elder Berries, Elder Flowers, Frostwort, Dandelion and Sweet Balm.

For Scarlet Fever—Make a tea of Saffron. This recipe was given me by an old German lady. Writes W. A. H., Portage, Wis.

Oats thoroughly sorted and washed, steep for an hour, then take warm. It will bring out very stubborn cases of scarlet fever. Writes Mrs. R. W., West Webster, N. Y.

I cured my grandson of Scarlet Fever without a doctor with Dittany, Oldfield Balsam, Golden Seal and Catnip with the best results. Writes J. J., Raby, Mo.

SKIN DISEASES

The botanicals listed are mostly of a mild alterative nature. Here again proper diet, fresh air and sunlight build up resistance to disease, and medicine and drugs, except for local application are quite useless.

The skin is an index to health. It is like a barometer, indicating the state of our body and certain organs. It demands scrupulous cleanliness. The pores should be kept open. There is no better tonic for the whole system than bathing in cold water followed by a vigorous rubbing.

It is common practice to treat eruptions of the skin by means of external applications, but eruptions rarely form upon the surface of the skin unless there is something wrong with the system. Therefore, there is the necessity of treating all such eruptions with internal remedies in addition to the external applications.

Tetter—Take Mullein Leaves, put in water, boil down to a strong solution. Bathe the hands or whatever part is afflicted. An old lady told me this recipe. It is very good. Writes G. B., Pavo, Ga.

Take one-half pound each Inner Bark of Prickly Ash, Walnut, and Dogwood, put in 3 gallons of water, boil down to one gallon or three quarts. Bathe parts in same three times a day and will cure any case of tetter. This is a never-failing cure. Writes C. N. D., Epworth, S. C.

A certain remedy for winter itch: Blood Root pulverized and steeped in a strong apple vinegar applied 3 or 4 times a day, cures the disease. Writes J. L. B., Remus, Mich.

I will tell you that I have found Quack Grass Roots very good for itch. Take a handful of the dry roots and steep for a few minutes in one pint of water. Drink several times a day. Writes O. C., Cadillac, Mich.

For Skin Eruptions—Half ounce Yellow Dock, Figwort, and Burdock, one ounce Sarsaparilla and one-fourth teaspoonful Cayenne, boil in one and one-half pints of water, down to one and one-fourth pints, and take wineglassful three times a day.

For Skin Eruptions or Rash—Take Red Willow, and steep and wash the affected parts with this. **Writes J. F. W.**, Sullivan, Mich.

—Clover Blue Flag Compound...
Red Clover Flowers
Blue Flag Root
Juniper Berries
Rocky Mountain Grape
Tinn. Senna Leaves
Alex. Senna Leaves
German Cheese Plant
Gentian
Wintergreen
Alfalfa

Mild alterative and only slightly laxative. A fine tea.

—Yellow Dock Clover Compound...
Yellow Dock Root
Red Clover Flowers
Stillingia Root
Poke Root
Prickly Ash Bark
Rocky Mt. Grape Root
Elder Flowers
Marshmallow Root
German Cheese Plant
Tinn. Senna Leaves
Sassafras, Bark of Root
Am. Sarsaparilla Root

A mild alterative. A scientific blend of twelve different botanicals in which Yellow Dock predominates. A very fine tea. All patent so-called "Blood Purifiers" are composed of one or more of these various botanicals. Yellow Dock is one of the botanicals richest in organic iron.

—Mormon Valley Herb Compound...
Mormon Valley Plant
Black Cohosh
Licorice
Gentian
Fennel Seed
Bluets
Wild Cherry Bark

A powerful astringent with tonic properties, a tea of hundreds of uses. May be used internally or externally as a wash for sores and ulcers. A book could be written on the varied usefulness of this remarkable compound. Look up the various ingredients in any good book on medicinal botany.

Add to a quart of water, three handfuls of Witch Hazel, White Oak Bark, and Apple Tree Bark. Boil down to a pint and strain. Add half a pound of lard, and simmer till the water disappears. This is very good for piles. Writes Mrs. J. C. E., Jovele, Utah.

Fry a handful of Catnip in half cup pure hog's lard, making a salve. Strain and use any time you have an itching skin. My husband's legs were covered with an itching rash, and we used this and the rash disappeared like magic. Writes Mrs. G. S. H., Auburn, N. Y.

Balm Gilead Buds are wonderful for healing. I had a red rash of some kind on my forehead. It had been there for some time but doctors did not help it. I took a Balm Gilead Bud and broke it apart and rubbed the gummy substance from the center of bud on my forehead. It smarted severely but nearly killed the rash in one application. Then I cooked the rest of the buds in lard, but the salve was not as strong as the buds alone. Writes Mrs. K. H., Sawyer, Mich.

Cocklebur Tea will kill the itch if from poison oak or other conditions. Writes M. F., Oronago, Mo.

For Tetter, take Catnip, boil and strain. Mix with pure lard and boil the water out and apply grease to the tetter, for it is a sure cure and has been tested. Writes R. W. O., Pisgah, Ala.

I have tried almost everything to cure my hives and Bull Nettle, price 25c per box, is the only thing that cured them. I will always recommend it for hives to my friends or whomever I hear that has them. Writes Miss M. S., Topeka, Kan.

Take Powdered Blood Root, mix with pure apple vinegar and paint your hands if you have Tetter and it will cure it if used regularly. Writes J. T. C., Quincy, Miss.
Editor's Note—This must be painful, and I cannot recommend it.

Use a strong tea of Twigs of Alder as a remedy for pimples and skin rash.

This is for Salt Rheum: Wash clean the bark from Bitter Sweet Roots and put in sweet butter (without salt) and let simmer on back of stove all day. This makes a good salve to be applied locally. Also make a tea of the bark and drink. This is an absolutely sure cure. Writes Mrs. D. M., Toledo, Ohio.

For Itch or Eczema—Prince's Pine made by steeping a teaspoonful to a cup of water, drinking 3 cups a day, half cup at a time. Bathe affected parts with the same kind of tea also 3 times daily. This will cure many a case. Writes S. H. J., Woodville, Wis.

Steep a tablespoonful of Bull Nettle Root in a teacupful of boiling water, sweeten and give 1 teaspoonful every two hours to children up to one year. This is good for any kind of a skin disease and for boils and hives. Writes E. E. P., Shelbyville, Texas.

Will say that Bull Nettle Root is the best of anything I ever used for skin troubles. Writes Mrs. R. B., Los Angeles, Calif.
Editor's Note—I have had so many remarkable reports on this root that I am constrained to print them.

Take Dogwood Bark and make a strong tea, then make a poultice and put on the feet. This has cured the worst cases of ground itch. Writes Mrs. M. B., Sylvarena, Miss.

For tetter, on hands or ankles, take the roots of Burdock, and string like beads and wear around the affected parts, and also drink tea made from same. This cured a lady friend of mine who had tried everything. Writes Mrs. H. B. A., Walled Lake, Mich.
Editor's Note—Our Burdock cut probably would not be suitable for stringing into beads as it is cut too finely, but why not use as a wash, as well as taken internally?

Make a tea of the root of Burdock and drink several times a day. Drink it instead of water. This recipe cured my sister of scrofula when the doctors failed. Writes Mrs. H., Cincinnati, Ohio.

Here is a Recipe for Scrofula—Use ½ pound Poke Root, ½ pound Burdock Root, 1½ pounds Sassafras, and ¾ pound Mayapple, and ¼ pound Red Puccoon Root. Boiled down this will make 2 gallons of medicine, and only a teaspoonful should be used 3 times a day. Writes T. H. P., Waverly, Ky.
Editor's Note—This is sure to spoil if not kept on ice. You could add a little good liquor to preserve this.

Itch Cured in 36 Hours—Rub the parts with a mixture of two parts liquid Storax (priced at 25c), and one part Sweet Oil and a teaspoonful of Sulphur. Writes Mrs. W. M., Berlin, Wis.

For Prickly Heat—Bathe the affected part with hot water, and while the flesh is still wet, sprinkle dry pulverized Sulphur on the affected part until the flesh can not be seen. If one application does not give the desired relief, repeat again. Writes D. M., Mapleville, Md.

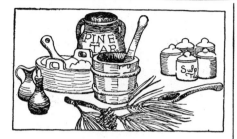

Take Tar run from the rich pine wood, and common lard, and mix together. Heat it, and allow to cool. It will cure skin troubles such as itch, etc. Writes I. D., Brookland, Texas.

Take Marigold Flowers when dried and boil down to an ooze, then add pure hog's lard and make a salve. This is very healing and soothing to Tetter on the hands. Writes Miss G. W., Livingston, Tenn.

Eczema—Is an inflammation of the skin and may be acute or chronic. It may appear on the face, around the mouth, or on the ears, cheeks or forehead, or any part of the body, with rough, scaly chapped skin, attended with itching and burning: the crusts fall off, leaving an angry, sore surface, upon which the crusts form anew.

Treatment—During the first course of this disease, it is most important to keep the bowels open.

Diet is of extreme importance. All salty, greasy and fried food, also pastry and cheese, should be avoided. The affected parts should be cleansed with Medicated Witch Hazel, avoiding the use of water.

The Herb Doctor's choice of mild botanical alteratives and astringents are: Sweet Fern Leaves and Twigs, Goose Grass, Huckleberry Leaves, Yellow Dock, Red Clover Flowers, Seven Barks, Queen's Delight, Rocky Mountain Grape, Bittersweet Twigs.

For Nettle Rash—Take Horsemint Weed, make a tea of it and drink it cold. This cured my daughter after having a doctor fail. Writes Mrs. L. K., Stamps, Ark.

Prickly Heat—Take more exercise in the great outdoors.

Prickly Heat—Is very annoying. It consists of small vesicles filled with a watery fluid and producing a continuous redness or inflammatory blush of the skin. These vesicles break, forming small, thin scales. They are attended with itching, burning and often with fever. Prickly heat is the result of excessive heat, or living in unwholesome air and eating improper food.

Treatment—Bathe the affected parts with Medicated Witch Hazel. Keep the bowels open.   Drink plenty of lemonade.

The Herb Doctor's choice of mild botanical alteratives are: Yellow Dock, Blue Flag, Queen's Delight, Prickly Ash Bark, Sweet Fern, Red Clover Flowers.

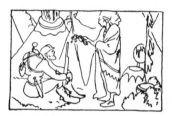

SCROFULA

Tea made from dried Whortle Berries and drunk in place of water, tea or coffee cures scrofulous difficulty no matter how bad. Writes K. R. R., Oakland, Md.

Scrofula Remedy

2 ounces of Sarsaparilla
1 ounce of Licorice
1 ounce of Sassafras
4 ounces of Guaiac Wood

Mix and divide into eight equal parts, to one part add six cups of water and boil until there are four cups of liquid, drink a cupful a day. Writes Mrs. J. H. E., Ballston, Va.

For Blood or Skin Disease—Use 2 drams Sassafras Bark, ½ ounce Queens Delight Root, ½ ounce Sarsaparilla, 3 drams Burdock, ½ ounce Mezereon, ½ ounce Guaiacum, 1 ounce Licorice Root. Boil in quart of water, slow for 15 minutes, strain, boil second time in 3 half pints of water 15 minutes, strain, and shake before using. Take a wineglassful 4 times a day. Keep in cool place. Writes G. G., Providence, R. I.

Scrofula—Make a decoction of Walnut Leaves, one ounce to a pint of boiling water and give one tablespoonful three times a day. Writes M. F. B.,

—Sage-Mullein Clover

Italian Sage Leaves
Low Mullein Leaves
Red Clover Flowers
Bearberry Leaves
Palmetto Berries
Bluets
Gentian Root

Properties, Mild Tonic and Carminative.

___

SHINGLES

Is a form of eruption composed of small sac-like bodies, which come out in blisters on the breast or sides, extending partly around the body like a belt.

___

For the disease called shingles, use common Epsom Salts, making a paste of it by adding water to the right consistency, then apply frequently to the affected parts until one gets relief which will be in a short time. I know of two neighbors that tried this just recently. Writes Mrs. H. M. B., Rock Falls, Ill.

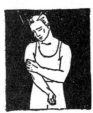

SMALLPOX

Smallpox comes on with a severe pain in the back, chills occur with intense headache, followed by fever. The rash comes on about the third day and at first looks very much like measles or scarlet fever. About the eighth day the postules appear on the face and arms and these are gradually covered with thick crusts which drop off, leaving well-known "pits" or scars. Various internal organs may become affected and the patient may have bronchitis, pneumonia or inflammation of the kidneys.
    Treatment—
            Call a doctor. Give lemon juice diluted a little with water.

I just learned another way of curing smallpox. A friend was working on the railroad at Athens, Ohio. Being warned by the foreman that a very virulent case of smallpox was in the vicinity, a member of an extra gang made an uncomplimentary remark about the doctors. He then went to a grocery and got a bushel of onions. He took them to the house and tramped them to a pulp on the floor. Selecting the nicest and strongest of them, he placed a heavy bunch in a towel and laid it across the patient's chest. Next day the smallpox had practically ceased and the patient was working. The doctors had said that death must ensue within two days. Writes L. J. F., Chillicothe, Ohio.

For Prevention and Cure of Smallpox.—One ounce of Cream of Tartar, dissolved in a pint of boiling water to be drank when cold at short intervals. It is a sure and never-failing remedy, cures in about 3 days. Has been found so by many who have tried it. It never leaves a mark, never causes blindness and always prevents tedious lingering. Can do no harm. This is copied from a newspaper article. Writes I. S., St. Petersburg, Fla.

___

SOCIAL DISEASES

Gonorrhea and Gleet—A purulent inflammation of the mucous membrane of the genitals of both sexes. It may be acute, subacute or chronic.
    Treatment—Consult only a specialist of high repute. Much harm can be done by quacks and inexperienced doctors. Tea to keep the bowels open. Use soothing demulcent herb teas. Keep the organs clean by frequent bathing; and douches for females. Destroy or thoroughly sterilize all bandages and clothing.
    The Herb Doctor's choice of botanical demulcents are: Sweet Fern, Golden Seal, Sandalwood, Cubeb Berries, Marshmallow Root, German Cheese Plant, Juniper Berries.

___

For Gonorrhea—Take a handful of Red Shank Root and the same amount of Bull Nettle and Watermelon Seeds. Boil 30 minutes, strain and drink a mouthful night and morning. You can even add a little Golden Seal to this tea. Writes I. M., Vienna, La.

Bull Nettle—I have found much to interest me in your herb book, but was surprised to find one of the greatest of all herbs not mentioned. This is Bull Nettle. Make a strong tea by boiling an ounce of the root into a quart of water. Boil down to 1 pint or less. Drink the entire pint during the day. This cures Syphilis within a month without anything else. It is just as good for any similar troubles, such as Scrofula and Necrosis. Have used it in my practice for many years without a single failure when correctly made. Writes Dr. R. M. J., Oklahoma City, Okla.

Editor's Note—The above is reproduced as we received it. We have had no opportunity to try this root for this purpose, and can only state that it is harmless and beneficial as a mild alterative.

Dr. S....... begs to inform you that he has cured the gonorrhea with an injection of the juice of the lime and Balsam Copaiba. Here is the recipe:

Lime Juice—10 to 15 drops
Copaiba—20 drops
Water—1 tablespoonful
Inject—Thrice daily

Writes N. T., Corozol, B. H.

Editor's Note—This may be all right but I fear the lime juice would be very painful to use. I would think more water should be used. Better take it under a doctor's supervision.

We sent to you a little over a year ago and got a supply of Bull Nettle for a case of syphilis, for had heard of it being used. I am glad to say that after six weeks' steady use of this Bull Nettle Tea it seemed completely driven out of the system and without any signs of it showing at this date—a year later. Writes J. W. T., Seattle, Wash.

Editor's Note—I doubt if this was real syphilis. Would like to hear from others who have used Bull Nettle for this purpose. No names will be mentioned.

—U. U. Tea...
Palmetto Berries
Bearberry Leaves
Pipsissewa
Cubeb Berries
Juniper Berries
Althea Root
Sweet Fern
Cheese Plant
Fennel Seed
Bluets

The experienced herbal physician will recognize this as a very valuable formula. It is a mild diuretic and tonic with emollient and soothing properties to the urinary passages.

—Echinecea
Compound...
Echinecea
Prickly Ash Bark
Poke Root
Bluets
Rocky Mt. Grape Root
Marshmallow

Mild Alterative. Most of the highly touted and advertised blood tonics and blood purifiers are composed mainly of one or more of these simple ingredients.

For Blood Poisoning—Pulverize Slippery Elm Bark and Sassafras Bark. Mix in equal parts. This is to be put into a pan with enough water to be absorbed. Put into a gauze bag and apply to the affected area. It is the finest remedy I know of for blood poisoning from spiders, insects, snake bites and injuries. Writes Dr. F. W. C., Newark, N. J.

Here is a home remedy which is fine for the blood:

3 teaspoonsful Cream of Tartar
3 teaspoonsful Sugar
3 teaspoonsful Sulphur

Mix these and take 1 teaspoonful for adults at bedtime for nine nights. Children according to age. Writes K. H., Carmine, Tex.

I want to write you about Bull Nettle Root for Syphilis. My husband contracted same and gave it to me. He took treatments without my knowledge and then I had it 8 months and did not know it. Five years ago last May it caused me to have a blood clot on the brain, bringing on a paralytic stroke and my whole right side was paralyzed, and for 4 months my doctor, not knowing the cause of my illness, then called in another doctor from the city and he pronounced it syphilis. I took $600 worth of treatments and was told that I would have to take them the rest of my days or go insane. I saw about Bull Nettle, and took the tea every day for 30 days, and then went to a doctor in another city for a blood test and the answer came back negative, O. K., fine. That was last May and I have not a trace of it in my system today, neither my husband. Writes Mrs. J. E. F., Ramsey, Ill.

Editor's Note—This is the most sensational letter I have yet received on the value of Bull Nettle. Will others who try it kindly give me the results, so I can complete my investigations of this root, as I am still a Doubting Thomas.

Bull Nettle is just fine and is doing just wonderful with the case of Syphilis I had. I can recommend it to be the very medicine for Syphilis. I am almost well and am sending for four more boxes of Bull Nettle. Writes G. P., Betsy Layne, Ky.

SORE MOUTH AND THROAT

For Sore Mouth—Chew Golden Seal Root. I have tried this many times, with results. Writes Miss A. L. B., Toccoa, Ga.

Sore Throat—Take Hard Cider as hot as you can drink, with as much Red Pepper as the patient can stand. Will cure in one evening. Drink a little, often. Writes O. P. M., Moline, Mich.

Here is a Cure for Tonsillitis—Make a strong tea of Persimmon Bark and Blackberry Roots, then add Alum and Brown Sugar and boil down until it begins to make a syrup. Gargle this in the throat while warm. Writes Mrs. I. S., Savoy, Ky.

Take about a quart of Red Oak Bark and put in 1½ quarts of water, boiled down to a cupful, then add a cup of clear boiling water to it, and let it steep ½ hour. Strain, and gargle the throat. I had tonsillitis last week and that is what I used and it brought it out in 48 hours. Writes Mrs. C. C., Olanta, S. C.

Sore Throat—Take a tablespoonful of Pineapple juice, as it is a wonderful remedy for sore throat. Take as often as necessary according to the seriousness of the trouble. Writes M. A. M., Atlanta, Mich.
Editor's Note—Yes, Pineapple juice is fine in throat affections of children, and is pleasant to take.

Blue Cohosh is also good for sore throat and mouth combined with equal parts of Golden Seal made into a tea and sweetened with Honey. Writes Mrs. D. R. G., Leon, W. Va.

For Sore Throat—A very good remedy for Swollen Glands, and Sore Throat is Bitter Sweet. Take the roots and steep well, drain off liquid, and add as much Mutton or Beef Tallow as you want to make a salve, cook down to that amount or until it quits frying like grease, put away, let get cold and apply to the throat on the outside every 2 or 3 hours and it will reduce swelling and soreness. Writes G. L. M., Odin.

Make a tea by placing Yellow Root and Persimmon Bark in water. Makes an excellent mouth wash, and Alum often makes it better.

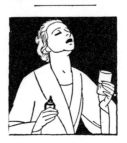

One of the Best Remedies for Tonsillitis or Sore Throat—Take White Oak Bark and White Pine Bark and make a strong tea of equal parts, then add a small lump of Alum, a little Red Pepper and Table Salt and a tablespoonful of Epsom Salts and gargle every half hour. Writes Mrs. C. W. G., Copper Hill, Tenn.

For Tonsillitis—Gargle the throat several times a day with a tea made of Red Oak Bark and a pinch of Alum. Writes W. H. F., La Fayette, Ga.

Alum is the best thing for sore mouth and sore throat that you can find. Writes F. A., Ritner, Ky.

Witch Hazel is very good for Cold Sores. You can open them, then apply the Witch Hazel solution, and continue doing this every 5 minutes and the sore will dry up. Writes Mrs. L. D., Wakeman, Ohio.

A Remedy for Tonsillitis—A lady told me she had tried it and it would almost cure in one night. Crush leaves and stalks of Catnip, with the hands, make a poultice of it with hot water and Flour, and bind on the throat, just enough Flour to make it hold together. You sure should find this fine. Writes D. W., Duhring, W. Va.

For Enlarged Tonsils—Boil Red Root in a quart of water, and gargle 3 times a day and it will take them down and will not give any more trouble. Writes L. S., Swannona, N. C.

Tonsillitis, Quinsy, Sore Throat—Make a tea of 8 parts Sage and 1 part of Blood Root. Add the juice of a half of a Lemon. Sweeten with Honey. Drink before retiring a small teacupful while hot. Writes Miss L. G., Ann Arbor, Mich.

For Sore Throat or Ulcerated Throat —Make a strong tea of Red Pepper, put in a small lump of Alum, and use as a gargle. Writes Mrs. E. L., Costelow, Ky.

I am sending a simple recipe which has proven its merits and in hopes it will help many. For Sore Throat, take a very small pinch of powdered Golden Seal. Put on tongue as far back as possible. It will dissolve and cover throat. Do this 3 times a day or at night on retiring. Also good for bad tonsils, and especially good for babies and children as it is almost impossible to get to the inside of their little throats. Of course, the bowels must be kept open. Writes Mrs. G. W. L., Bentonville, Ark.

Editor's Note—I fear Golden Seal is too bitter for babies.

I have tried this for Sore Throat, Tonsillitis, etc. Use a tea of Sage and Alum, as a gargle, and mop the throat if you have an Ulcer. Writes F. L. A., Huntsville, Texas.

I cured myself and have cured others when doctors failed with the following recipe and wish to pass it on to other Tonsilitis sufferers. Take equal amounts: Apple Tree Bark, Persimmon Tree Bark, Red Shank and Sage Leaves. Boil until a very strong tea is made, then strain, and to each pint of tea add a piece of Alum the size of the thumb, and a cup of Honey. Boil to about a cough syrup consistency, use as a gargle every 30 minutes until relieved. This is also very good in cases of Cold or Whooping Cough. Take one teaspoonful when cough appears and at bed time. Writes Mrs. F. H., Yulee, Fla.

A Sure Cure for Tonsilitis—To 2 tablespoonfuls of Pine Tar add 2 tablespoonfuls of Salt and the Yolk of an Egg. Mix all together, bind on the throat and leave it on until it loosens of its own accord. To remove the stain grease the throat with fresh Lard. Writes Mrs. N. M. D., Tolono, Ill.

I see where you would like to have remedies. Here is one I have tried for enlarged Glands inside of the Throat, also Quinsy. Use the dried Smart Weed, put a handful in a pan, cover with boiling water, and leave on the back of the stove for 5 minutes, then put this in a thin cloth sack and have it large enough to go around the neck. Place on warm and allow it to remain on all night. In one night the soreness is all gone. Writes Mrs. McF., Peoria, Ill.

Editor's Note—Would advise also to gargle with a hot tea of Pimpinella Anisum.

Golden Seal Root will cure Sores in the mouth. Writes N. R., Rammer, Tenn.

Here is a Sure Cure for Tonsilitis—I was given up and went to an Herb Doctor who gave me a handful of Sage and some Sumach Berries. I made a strong tea of these and gargled the throat with it, making 2 teas and using 1 an hour after the other. After using this 10 hours, bathe the throat with Sassafras Oil to take the swelling down. I have told several about it, and they laughed and thought it foolish but it did the work. Writes J. E. G., Redlands, Calif.

Try This Remedy for Tonsilitis—A teaspoonful Persimmon Bark, Red Oak Bark and Golden Seal and just a pinch of powdered Alum. Make a tea and then gargle the throat 3 to 5 times, and you will find a sure cure. Writes J. W. B., Mount Clemens, Mich.

Editor's Note—If you purchase herbs that have been on the shelves of some drug store for years —you will be disappointed. Herbs lose their value after one year.

Take 1 tablespoonful of pulverized Rhubarb and a cube of Sugar, dissolve in a teacup of boiling water, and stir until all is well dissolved. Use as gargle for Sore Throat for it is excellent. Writes H. E., Kansas City, Mo.

Rhubarb Roots is a sure cure for Sore Throat. Slice roots thin and dry. Chew it and swallow the juice. It cured me of a blood raw Sore Throat. Writes L. S., Wilbar, N. C.

Take 2 parts of White Oak Bark, 2 parts of Sweet Gum Bark, 2 parts of Sage, and 1 part of Borax, and a little Honey. This is a fine remedy for Sore Throat. Writes M. S., Huntsville, Ky.

Mix Pine Tar 2 ounces with pure Hog's Lard and put on flannel cloth, tie around the neck and it is a sure cure for Sore Throat.

Sore Throat—Boil Persimmon Bark and Sage leaves together, strain, cool and use as a gargle. Writes Mrs. E. B., Greencastle, Ind.

For Tonsillitis—Make a weak tea of Red Pepper, not strong enough to burn, but just to tickle the throat and gargle often. Will cure the worst cases. Remedy was given me by a retired physician. Writes J. P. C., Rufus, N. C.

White Oak Bark is good for Tonsillitis and Coughs. Boil the bark and gargle or drink it. It is harmless. Writes Mrs. L. E., Poresknob, N. C.

Canker or Sore Mouth—Take the root of the Wild Oregon Grape and chew it good. Writes Mrs. D. E., Jackson, Wyo.

Your Almanac is sure handy to have around. My oldest boy got up with Tonsillitis one morning and I looked up a recipe in the Almanac—it was for Sage and Alum—and I fixed him some and had him gargle with it several times that day and the next day he was rid of it, where other times he would suffer for weeks and could not eat or sleep. Writes Mrs. J. C. R., Asher, Okla.

Editor's Note—Quick action—or in other words "a stitch in time saves nine."

For Sore Throat—Mix dry Sulphur and White Sugar, equal parts, take a teaspoonful, hold in the mouth until dissolved, then let it run down the throat slowly, repeat several times a day. Writes H. B. E., Lewiston, Mont.

Mix 2 teaspoonfuls of powdered Borax with an ounce of Glycerine; hold a half spoonful in mouth at a time for Canker Sores. Writes G. W., New Sheffield, Pa.

Several years ago I had a Raw, Sore Throat. There was 10 weeks I was confined to the house. Every time I stepped out, the cold wind would make me worse. I tried everything I could think of, when finally my husband suggested smoking the dried Life Everlasting, which I did. I held the smoke in my throat as long as I could retain it, 3 smokings cured me. My father smoked it for Asthma for years, getting relief when expensive remedies failed. Writes Mrs. S. W., Norborne, Mo.

For Sore Throat—Take a teaspoonful of Tincture of Myrrh in as hot a water as you can stand to gargle the throat. It is sure to help it if taken in time. Writes B. K., Logan, W. Va.

For a Sore Mouth Yellow Root is Excellent—Boil and make a tea and wash the mouth with it several times a day. Writes D. S. R., McMechen, W. Va.

Blue Cohosh is also good for sore throat and mouth combined with equal parts of Golden Seal made into a tea and sweetened with Honey. Writes Mrs. D. R. G., Leon, W. Va.

I have tried your White Oak Bark as a gargle in simple sore throat and find it is wonderful. My husband always had trouble with his bowels but he saw in the Almanac to use Senna leaves and now he is getting along fine. He is also taking Yellow Dock and he says he has a lot more pep. We have spent so much money for medicine at the drug store, but now we find that this stuff is so much better. Writes Mrs. I. M. S., Hollidaysburg, Pa.

Take a handful of Peach Tree Leaves and make a tea and drink it. It is a sure cure for Sore Throat. Writes W. S., Winslow, Ark.

Salt is good for Sore Mouth, also for washing Sores, and for bathing where one has been vaccinated, as it will take soreness and swelling out. It has many uses. Writes C. K. P., Milford, Dela.

Take a few Mullein Leaves, put in Vinegar, boil until the virtues are extracted, say 10 minutes or more, and bind on neck, good for any kind of Sore Throat. Don't put the leaves next to the skin but between cloths. Writes Mrs. W. H., O'Fallon, Ill.

Put pure Peppermint Oil on the finger and down the throat for Sore Throat. Writes C. O., Bloomingdale, Mich.

I am sending you a remedy for Sore Throat. Take a handful of Persimmon Bark and a heaping teaspoonful of powdered Sage, a lump of Alum. Boil Sage and bark into a tea, then put in the Alum. Sweeten with Molasses or Honey. Gargle 3 times a day and at bedtime. This will cure a severe Sore Throat. Writes Mrs. C. M., Access, Ky.

Yellow Root is the best treatment for Sore Mouth that I have ever tried. Writes Mrs. R. P. C., Gastonia, N. C.

A very good gargle for Quinsy or Sore Throat is made as follows: Make a strong tea of old fashioned Chamomile and gargle as hot as you can, every hour. Writes Mrs. S. B. R., Milwaukee, Wis.

Tonsillitis—Cut Loveage Root, fry in Lard and apply as a poultice. Writes Mrs. C. H., Pilger, Neb.

For Sore Throat—Gargle the throat several times a day with pure Glycerine. It is a sure cure. Writes M. E. T., Burlington, Vt.

Tonsillitis—Make a poultice of the inner bark of Sassafras for it has been known to cure where the throat was almost closed up.

A Sure Remedy for Sore Mouth in Infants—Take Poke Berries, put them in a clean bag, bruise and rub the gums with the juice, or if you use the dried berries, steep them, and then use the infusion in the same manner. Hope this will help others as it has me. Writes Mrs. F. A. H., Los Angeles, Calif.

Editor's Note—But do not let the little one drink this.

This Is a Good Gargle for Bad Sore Throat—One cup water, or a half cupful would be better, ½ cup Vinegar, and a pinch of Sage; let boil good. Then add a piece of Alum, size of a Hazel Nut, till dissolved. Gargle every little while. Do not swallow any. Writes Mrs. J. T. D., Cedar Rapids, Ia.

Powdered Alum used as a gargle will cure the worst cases of Ulcerated Tonsils and Sore Throat, when ulcerated all over.

For small Sores in the mouth, apply ground Cloves or Clove Spice, and repeat until cured. Writes Mrs. H. B. E., Lewiston, Mont.

Take Golden Seal and make a tea out of it for the Sore Mouth. It surely is fine. Wash the mouth several times a day. Writes Mrs. A. C. M., Acworth, Ga.

Take off the outside bark of the Pussy Willow and take the inside bark and let it stand overnight in water—then steep and gargle the throat a number of times through the day. A sure cure for Canker in the mouth. Writes Mrs. L., Bernardston, Mass.

SORES AND ULCERS

My father had Running Sores on both his legs, and he spent over $500 and also crossed the ocean twice, and all the doctors have done him no good. He went to a doctor in England, and when he came back to America, and got these herbs, and I saw him cured sound with them. Here is the formula: Burdock, Yellow Dock, Ground Ivy and make one good gallon of each, put in 4 gallon jar, while hot, mix them up stirring them while hot too, and put in 3 or 4 pounds of unslacked lime, let cool for 24 hours, then take wineglassful 3 times a day. In less than a year this cured him. He also used Plantain Leaves on the sores every morning and evening so as to keep his clothes from touching the sores, and so help heal them. Writes T. T., Salisbury, Pa.

Salve for old sores that refuse to heal. Bitter Sweet fried in pure Hog's Lard. This is an old recipe in our family. Writes M. E. P., Cedar Rapids, Ia.

Take a large handful of Jimson Weed, put in a stewer, with fresh Lard, and enough water to boil the juice out of the leaves. Let it cook down to a salve, then take some Poke Root and boil the substance out of it, and use it as a wash just as hot as possible. Then apply the Jimson Weed as a salve and it is a sure cure for all sores. Writes E. W., Wilson, Ark.

Concerning the Sheep Sorrel Leaves made into a salve, I prepared it myself and can recommend it. I paid a visit to a cousin of mine last spring, and she had a very sore finger on the right hand. It was the forefinger and there seemed to be a lump on it. I made her some salve, and now lately having the pleasure of meeting her again, she said the salve had healed her finger. Writes Mrs. L. L. F., Gap, Pa.

Sores, Boils, Cuts and Corns—There is nothing better than White Pine Pitch or Balsam, it takes the soreness out and draws all poison out of the flesh. Also good for scratches on horses. Writes V. H. R., Brewer, Me.

For Running Sores—Soak Bay Leaves in cup of hot water for ½ hour, then bathe the sores with the water, when somewhat cooled off. Apply the soaked leaves to the running leg sores over night or keep Bay Leaves on for 24 hours, do this every night until cured. A tried and true remedy. Writes M. S. C., Chicago, Ill.

For Nail Wounds, etc.—Use Peach Tree Leaves. Beat them up and warm them, then apply. It will draw all swelling and soreness out. Writes Mrs. O. C. B., Greenville, Texas.

For Healing Salve—Use 4 ounces Canadian Pine Pitch, 3 ounces Lard, and 2 ounces of Beeswax. Mix Lard and Wax and then add the Pine Pitch while hot, and stir until cool. This is to be applied after the formula given above. Writes T. H. P., Waverly, Ky.

Salve for Healing Purposes—Use ¼ part Resin and ¾ parts Hog Lard. Writes Mrs. W. H. T., Ingersoll, Ont., Canada.

Here is a formula of a home-made salve my father used to make to cure old or dry sores. Melt together equal parts of soft Pine Rosin, Tallow and Beeswax, strain into a tin box. When this salve hardens, take a little on the end of a knife and work into the palm of the hand until salve is white. Spread on cloth, cover sore. This will soften sores, draws out corruption, etc. After using this, apply another plaster with Sulphur worked into this salve. Writes Mrs. I. B., Laneville, Tex.

My mother had a running sore on her limb caused by typhoid fever, she had it for many years. I read about using Clover Blossoms Tea made as follows: One-half ounce of flowers and 1 pint of water boiled together for 30 minutes. So I thought that I would give it a trial. It was supposed to be used 3 or 4 times daily, but she only used it once daily and in a very short time it was healed up, which has been about 16 months ago. She said it did not burn.

SPRAINS

A tested and tried remedy for sprains, bruises and swellings. I had a big iron bar drop on my foot and it took the swelling down like magic. It has been used extensively by coal miners in England. Take 4 ounces of Comfrey to a quart and a half of water, boil to a quart and bathe the affected parts. Writes S. L., Muskegon, Mich.

I am sending you a remedy for a sprain which proved valuable to my husband when his ankle was sprained. Dip Mullein Leaves in hot Salt Vinegar, and place on sprain, and place towel over this. Writes A. J. G., Aberdeen, Wash.

For Sprains—Steep for 5 minutes or so a generous supply of Smart Weed, bathe the part with the warm tea and, if convenient, bind the weed on the sprained part. This has been found very good for man or beast. Writes A. B., Lincoln, Kan.

Take Deers Tongue Leaves and Mullein and steep together into boiling water, and then bathe the limbs in same. This is very good for swelling limbs. Writes Mrs. J. H., Tunis, N. C.

I wish to tell about my sore foot. I needed something for immediate relief. I had a box of Buchu Leaves in the house, and I knew it was good for taking down swelling, as I had used it before when my legs were swollen. I drank 2 cupsful of the tea as directed on the box, and got a common Onion from the garden, cut it into slices as round as the Onion and put it right on the sore. Bandaged and changed the Onion morning, noon and night, and it took the poison out and healed my leg. Writes Mrs. M. P., Goderich, Ont., Canada.

Use Red Oak Bark, boil good, and then make a poultice with corn meal and apple vinegar, and you will find a sure cure for any kind of sprains. Writes T. P., Flowery Branch, Ga.

Life Everlasting is good for any Sore. Make a poultice and apply to the affected part. Writes Mrs. L. T., Maud, Ala.

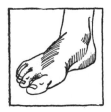

For Sprains—Take St. Johnswort, make a poultice of it. It is just as good for boils and bruises too. Writes S. B., Conehatta, Miss.

To take down swelling of legs and arms, get Smart Weed and make a tea out of it, and bathe the swollen part. Writes E. P., Fort Dodge, Iowa.

For Badly Sprained Ankles—Take Epsom Salts and bind on with a cloth and keep wet with water. It will draw all of the swelling and soreness out. Writes Mrs. A. V. W., Kennard, Tex.

STOMACH AND BOWEL DISORDERS
(See Dyspepsia)

These are almost entirely due to improper diet. The botanicals mentioned are not held out as specifics for these disorders. They are recommended merely for their bitter tonic effect, improving and increasing the gastric juice, or, as is the case with demulcents, to soothe or lubricate the organs or passage. They are in the main mild tonics, laxatives and demulcents.

Stomach Ulcers—This ailment is commonly due to acidity, indiscretion in food, alcohol, etc. The symptoms are: Indigestion and loss of weight; hyperacidity; constant pain in the pit of the stomach, which is increased by taking food; vomiting soon after eating; the vomited matter is mixed with red blood. The disease is liable to terminate in perforation of the stomach and death.

Treatment—Diet of milk, eggs, and light foods, excluding meats, sweets, etc.; perfect rest in bed; give Bismuth Subnitrate, two grains every 3 hours (price 50c), and one-half teaspoonful of Soda Bicarbonate in half a glass of water 1 hour after meals; regulate the bowels; for severe pain take one or two Aspirin Tablets. Soothing Emollients or Demulcents are excellent in this ailment.

The Herb Doctor's choice of botanical Demulcents and Emollients are: Golden Seal, Marshmallow Root, Strawberry Leaves, Red Raspberry Leaves, Elm Bark, Flax Seed, Wallwort, German Cheese Plant, Linden Flowers.

Bowel Ulcers
Treatment—Same as Stomach Ulcers.

This is a recipe that has been in our family for many years. In this age of youth and beauty this recipe should be welcomed by all the ladies. Take a tablespoonful of Chamomile Flowers in a glass of boiling water. Let stand a while, drink every night for several weeks and one will have a complexion that one can be proud of. The tea acts as a mild tonic and keeps one in tip-top condition. Writes A. W., Mead, Colo.

Editor's Note—Here you are girls—A secret I know you have been looking for. The true Chamomile Flowers are absolutely harmless

Stomach Remedy—Gives prompt relief. Steep three teaspoonfuls Wild Sage, one teaspoonful Colic Root, one teaspoonful Wormwood in a pint of boiling water for 30 minutes. Dose—Two tablespoonfuls, cold, after meals.

Use the Pipsissewa Leaves as a tea or just chew the leaves, swallowing the juice and it will cure cramps in the stomach without fail. Writes J. W. M., Smithville, W. Va.

Here is a recipe that I have never known to fail. Blackberry Root for stomach troubles. Take a handful of the cut roots to a quart of water and boil down to a pint, and take a wineglassful, one at night, and one the next morning, and you are well. Writes J. H., Holly Grove, Ark.

Gas on the Stomach—Make a tea of Caraway Seeds. This is one of the very best cures for gas on the stomach, and anyone so suffering will sure find quick relief. Writes E. G. W., San Francisco, Calif.

Here is a recipe for stomach trouble that is wonderful. Take Black Oak Bark, either chew and swallow the juice or steep into a tea. It is a wonderful tea as a man right here in this community was cured of a severe stomach trouble when doctors failed. Writes Mrs. C. H., Altoona, Pa.

Take a handful of Peppermint and put in a glass of cold water and drink it. It is very good for sick stomach. Writes H. W., Waltersville, Ky.
Editor's Note—I'll say it is. But use only fresh —this season's crop.

I am herewith enclosing a formula for ulcerated stomach. Take five tablespoonfuls of Gentian and Lungwort, each, and two tablespoonfuls each of Golden Seal and Ginseng, and mix the whole together. Then place a teaspoonful of the mixture into a teacupful of boiling water and steep for 30 minutes, then strain through a tea strainer and set aside to cool. When cold, drink a cupful 20 minutes after each meal. This has cured some of the worst cases of catarrh of the stomach. Writes Mrs. S. S., Verda, Ky.

I am sending you a sure cure for ulcers of the stomach if taken freely. This is it: Take Fever Bush or what some call Spice Wood, steep and drink it before meals. This will cure the worst case if followed out. I hope you will print this as I have given it a test many times with good results. Writes W. M. M., Haverhill, Mass.

Chew a few Pine Needles and swallow the juice and it will give immediate relief for heartburn or sour stomach. Writes M. P. H., Waters, Ark.

This is my recipe for taking Cod Liver Oil. Use one-half glass real warm milk, 1 tablespoonful Cod Liver Oil, and salt and pepper to taste, take before meals. It is so much easier to get down this way. Writes Mrs. H. V., Caldwell, Kan.

Soak Peppermint in cold water 15 or 20 minutes and take and it will settle a sick stomach. Writes L. S., Swannona, N. C.

For Stomach Troubles—Mix equal parts of Golden Seal Root, Yellow Parilla, Cheese Plant and Peppermint. Place these herbs in a pint of water and boil for 30 minutes. Drink cold, one tablespoonful one hour after each meal. Writes C. D. F., Buena Vista, Pa.

Below is a good household remedy for your columns. Apply Smartweed poultice as hot as can be borne to the abdomen. This will cure inflammation of the bowels. Writes Miss E. G. H., Grand Rapids, Ohio.

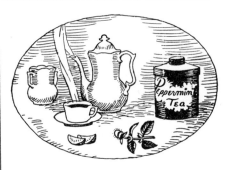

—Father John's Stomach
    Tea...........
    Thousand Seal
    Juniper Berries
    Milk Weed
    Gentian
    Wormwood Leaves
    German Cheese Plant
    Rose Pink
An old fashioned carminative and tonic. Useful in gastritis, belching, etc.

—Father Bernard's Stomach
    Tea...........
    Italian Sage Leaves
    Stone Root
    Colic Root
    Fennel Seed
    Wormwood Leaves
    Genetian Root
    Juniper Berries
    Wild Strawberry Leaves
    German Cheese Plant
A combination of valuable stomachics. Gives tone to the stomach and improves the gastric juice.

Use Broken Root of Golden Seal and Boneset, mixed. A teaspoonful of the mixture to a cupful of boiling water for it will cure ulcerated stomach and mouth. This is a recipe from an old Indian doctor here, and my wife used it to cure her stomach. Writes L. M. A., Bangor, Me.

This recipe was used by mother for pains in the stomach. Take Yellow Root, make into tea and, when luke warm, strain and take it, for it certainly is fine for the stomach. Writes N. U., Indianapolis, Ind.

Gentian Root—This is a root that gives one an appetite. Boy, but one surely can eat after drinking a tea of this root. Writes S. R., Milwaukee, Wis.

Editor's Note—Yes, I have noticed that.

Marvel Internal Emollient—whenever the stomach becomes too acid, as it frequently does in these days of unbalanced diets and hastily eaten meals, in conditions of mental strain and stress, we suffer from what is commonly known as Hyperacidity. This condition naturally has a tendency to irritate the stomach and intestines and thus to cause much discomfort.

In connection with the correction of this condition, through change of diet and use of an alkaline medicine, it also may be desired to employ a medicine that will exert a soothing influence or act as an emollient to the irritation.

Diet—It is advisable to abstain from meat, pastries and sweets. Eat vegetables—cooked or raw. Drink at least one cupful of milk each day.

Stomach Remedy—For children and very weak persons. Steep two teaspoonfuls Wild Strawberry Leaves and one teaspoonful Fennel Seed in a pint of boiling water for thirty minutes. Dose —Two tablespoonfuls after each meal.

For Stomach Cramps—Take strong vinegar, one-half wineglassful and if not relieved in half an hour repeat the dose for it is a sure cure. Writes I. W. W., Easton, Pa.

Editor's Note—A strong tea of Sweetflag I am sure would be much better.

For Gas on Stomach—A teaspoonful of Caraway Seed in a cup of water and boiled for a few minutes is good. Drink as hot as you can stand it. Writes Mrs. J. F., Bonnie, Ill.

I received an Almanac a few days ago in which I found the recipe for Peach Tree Leaves as a tea for stomach trouble. I made a tea for my fifteen months old baby. He was sick with summer complaint and cutting teeth. It did the work I wanted it to do. I could ask no more of it. I really was surprised in what it did. I sure prize Peach Tree Leaves highly and also thank you for publishing the recipe. Writes Mrs. J. S., Paris, Tenn.

Editor's Note—Now you Michiganders get busy —and gather a few handfuls for future use.

I am sending you a recipe for stomach and blood. It is the best I ever saw. Take 2 parts Wild Alum Root, 2 parts Blackberry Root, 1 part Golden Seal Root, 1 Burdock, 1 Sarsaparilla, ½ part Mayapple and 1 part Rhubarb. Powder all together and take a tablespoonful and place in a half pint of water, let steep 30 minutes, strain and sweeten. Drink 3 times a day. Writes G. L. D., Idal, Tenn.

A recipe for the stomach which I used myself and is very good. An old German gave it to me and it may help someone else if you care to print it. Colombo Root, Powdered Rhubarb, Ginger Root, Baking Soda, Fennel Seed. Use twice as much Fennel Seed as you do of Colombo and Powdered Rhubarb, and only a small pinch of the other two. Writes Mrs. H. E. B., Royersford, Pa.

Here are some recipes my old dad used, and surely are good: Take a handful of Burdock Root and put in a large cupful of water and boil for a few minutes, when cooked, drink a tablespoonful every half-hour until relieved and you should find it very good for colic. Writes M. B., Gilmore, Ky.

A Remedy for Stomach Trouble— Take 1 teaspoonful Golden Seal Root, add to 1½ glass of boiling water, and let cool. Drink through the day. It done me good when our doctors failed. Writes W. L. W., Leoma, Tenn.

—Golden Seal Marigold Clover Compound....
Golden Seal Root
Marigold Flowers
Red Clover Flowers
Strawberry Leaves
Linden Flowers
Colic Root
Marshmallow Root
Solomon Seal Root
Fennel Seed
Bluets
Wild Cherry Bark

A stomach tea. Mild tonic and soothing demulcent. Very few botanic formulas can beat this. Golden Seal, one of the main ingredients, is used by physicians of every country to this day. It is considered antiseptic and tonic.

Use 1 part Yellow Root, 1 part Colic Root, 3 parts Red Raspberry Leaves, 2 parts Fennel Seed and 4 of Wild Cherry Bark. Mix well, and take 1 teaspoonful in a cup of hot water, let stand for half a day, strain and drink in 3 equal doses in 24 hours. This I have used with good results as I am a doctor of Naturopathy and we use all natural means to cure disease. This remedy is for catarrh of the stomach. Writes Dr. L. T. E., New Lexington, Ohio.

I was troubled with a very bad stomach and the doctor did me no good, so I took a tablespoonful of Senna Leaves, and a half teaspoonful of ground Golden Seal, put it in a pint of boiling water and allowed it to cool. I took a teaspoonful of this in a wine glass with a little water for 3 days, then stopped 3 days. I took this 3 times a day. I kept it up until I felt better, and now I dont' have any more pain in the stomach or heart. However, one has to be careful of eating too much, and of eating things which do not agree with one. I am sending this recipe in the hope that it will help someone. Writes Mrs. F. A., Spartanburg, Pa.

I am sending a formula for ulcer of the stomach, for I use this to treat that affection and give chiropractic adjustments to correct the cause: Mix thoroughly 1½ teaspoonfuls of powdered Slippery Elm, and a teaspoonful of Sugar to a paste with cold water. Beat out all lumps. Have a pint of rich milk on stove and as milk reaches the boiling point stir in Elm mixture, and keep stirring from 5 to 10 seconds. Pour off and drink warm. A dash of powdered Cinnamon or Nutmeg may be added if patient desires. Take 3 times daily. Writes Dr. E. H., Imperial, Neb.
Editor's Note—This would be more helpful without the sugar.

A remedy for gas, indigestion, constipation and other stomach trouble. Mix well equal parts of Gentian, Burdock Root and Sarsaparilla with half the amount of Senna, Dandelion, and Anise Seed. Steep generous teaspoonful in a cup of boiling water and take this tea during the day. Writes R. M., Gideon, Mo.
Editor's Note—These roots and herbs are all harmless and may be eaten freely or used as a tea.

Boil Elder Berries down, and take juice 2 or 3 times daily, never fails for cramps in stomach. Writes W. B., Pittsfield, Wis.

A good remedy for acid stomach: Take ½ teaspoonful Soda and same amount of Ginger, in ½ glass of water after meals. Writes Mr. H. M., North Canton, Ohio.
Editor's Note—A remedy like this is alright to take for occasional acid stomach, but will do more harm than good if used persistently. Better to go back to Natures Roots and Barks and get at the *cause* of the ailment.

Yellow Dock Tea will stop vomiting and will settle the stomach. Writes Mrs. W. H. B., Albright, W. Va.

When cooking turnips, navy beans or sweet potatoes, if a teaspoonful of powdered Ginger is added it will avoid gas forming on the stomach. Writes Mrs. H. W., Omaha, Neb.

Dried Red Clover Blossoms steeped are fine for anyone that has stomach troubles. Writes E. K., Gloucester, Mass.

I had a son who had been in two hospitals and given up to die. He had stomach troubles, and vomited when he would drink even water, and could eat nothing. Doctors did no good, but as soon as he took this tea, he began to get better, after all doctors failed:
    1 ounce Wild Cherry Bark
    1 ounce Prickly Ash Bark
    1 ounce Peruvian Bark
    1 ounce Gentian Root
    1 ounce Wahoo Chips
Mix all together and grind up fine ready for use. Dose: One-eighth teaspoonful 3 times a day. Put the doses in capsules for they are very bitter, but good for almost any stomach trouble and will stop vomiting. Writes Mrs. T. J. C., Piedmont, Kan.

Stomach Troubles or Run Down Condition—Take 1 tablespoonful of Oregon Grape Root, German Chamomile, 1 teaspoonful Golden Seal and Elder Flowers. Place all the ingredients into a vessel of earth or stone, pour over it 1 quart of boiling water, cover well with china plate (avoid tin or iron), let remain until cool and take a small wine glassful 3 or 4 times a day. I used this remedy for years and never had it fail. It can be sweetened to taste. This remedy may also be made use of in cases of cancer of the stomach, but instead of 1 quart of water, only use 1 pint and make application of poultices over the stomach with: Black Oak Bark and Chamomile. Massage bowels gently with downward motion. In case of cancer do not sweeten the drink, avoid alcoholic or strong drinks. Writes Rev. J. S., Akron, Ohio.

Here is a Remedy for Ulcers of the Stomach—Take 1 tablespoonful of Flaxseed, place in a cup and pour boiling water over. Cover the cup and let it steep. Can be taken hot or cold. Use 1 tablespoonful each day and drink seeds and liquid. Writes C. H., St. Cloud, Minn.

Sometime ago I sent for one of your "Herbalist Almanacs" and found it full of good recipes and want to add one more to your list for bad cases of stomach troubles. Take a box of Worm Wood to a pint of boiling water and make a tea, then add a stick of Licorice, dissolve in a pint of water. If constipated you can add Cascara, ½ ounce, to this mixture. The dose is a wineglassful 3 times a day. This has done wonders for my stomach. Writes C. T., Broomley, Ky.

This medicine will cure any stomach trouble in the world. It has never failed me for the last 26 years:
  1 tablespoonful Golden Seal Root
  1 tablespoonful Yellow Parilla
  1 tablespoonful Boneset
  1 tablespoonful Cheese Plant
  1 tablespoonful Peppermint
Put all these herbs in 1 pint of boiling water. Simmer 30 minutes, cover, let stand till cold. Strain. Dose: 1 tablespoonful 1 hour after each meal. Writes C. D. F., Buena Vista, Pa.

Canker of Stomach—This prescription was given me by a leading Herb Doctor in Worcester, Mass., several years ago:
  1 oz. Golden Seal
  ½ oz. Upland Cranberry
  ½ oz. Juniper Berries
  ½ oz. Red Peruvian Bark
  ½ oz. Celery Seeds
  ½ oz. Senna Leaves
Steep in 3 pints of water, down to 1 quart. Strain. Dose: 1 tablespoonful before eating. Writes E. L. M., Oxford, Mass.

I have cured a bad case of stomach trouble with Linden Bark or Basswood Bark, by taking the bark and charring it over a fire, and while hot or burning, quenching it in water and drinking the water. Writes A. P., Cleveland, Ohio.

For Stomach Troubles, Ulcers, etc.—This is very good. Equal parts of Soda, Ginger powdered, Golden Seal powdered. Fill 3 grain capsules, take 1 at each meal. Writes Mrs. C. W. J., Ozark, Mo.
Editor's Note—This would be better without the Soda. You could add powdered Elm Bark or any other demulcent. These are soothing and emollient.

Boil 1 quart of Chestnut Bark in a gallon of water, drain out the bark and thicken with Bran, put in sack and use as a poultice. Very good for inflammation of the stomach.

For Stomach and Liver—Use the Tansy Leaves, crush and steep in a cup of boiling water and drink during the day instead of water. Writes J. K., Summerville, Pa.

For Cramps in the Stomach and Diarrhoea with Cramps—Try Ginger made into a syrup. Dose: One-third spoonful in glass of water. Writes R. P., Minden, Neb.

Powdered Charcoal made from burning most any kind of soft wood, especially Willow is excellent for gas on the stomach or most any kind of stomach troubles. Writes M. McN., Dennis, Miss.

Here is a positive remedy for Colitis, having cured any number of cases troubled with it. Steep what you can hold in your double hands of Sweet Gum Bark, Slippery Elm Bark and Blackberry Roots, equal parts. Steep by placing enough boiling water over to cover, and set on the back of the stove until it becomes dark and bitter, then strain, sweeten, and give as often as necessary. It is perfectly harmless. One teaspoonful is the amount for the baby or smaller children while for the adult one to three tablespoonfuls is used. It is a cure, for it was used in my husband's father's practice and he was a physician and a very successful one, too. Writes Mrs. R. E. C., Henderson, Ky.
Editor's Note—I fear this is rather strong for babies.

Stomach Tonic—A very excellent stomach tonic or stomach bitters can be made of the following: One-half oz. of each: Gentian, Angelica, Strawberry, Wild Cherry Bark and Fennel Seed, all ground fine except Fennel. Place these articles in a quart of boiling water, when cool, drink ½ cupful a day, a large mouthful at a time, or same may be placed in a pint of good whiskey and it makes an excellent bitters.

Stomach and Bowel Disorders—Avoid all animal foods. They give acid reaction. Fruits, nuts and fresh vegetables help to give tone to the stomach and bring the blood back to its normal alkaline condition.

Some time ago a friend got me some Comfrey Root from you and I want to tell you that it helped me more than half a dozen doctors did. About a year and one-half ago I was taken with a very bad pain in my back and it went right through to the pit of my stomach. Some times I could not lay down and other times I could not get up, the pain would shut my breath off, and many a night I laid all night on a heating pad with an ice pack on my stomach and all the doctor would give me was dope for the pain. Finally I decided to leave everything else alone and take only Comfrey and before I took it one week steady I got relief.

Writes Mrs. E. B., Rochester, N. Y.

For ulcers in the stomach make a tea of Flax Seed Meal and drink ½ cupful 3 times a day. Writes G. W. A., Omaha, Neb.

Here is a new one to cure or heal a bad stomach: Hops steeped in boiling water, and taken morning, noon and night, also at bedtime before retiring, and it should work wonders in a short time. It is tried and tested for results. Writes H. P., Muscatine, Iowa.

For Ulcerated Sore Throat and Stomach
—One teaspoonful Boneset and same amount of the broken Golden Seal Root to a pint of boiling water, let stand until cold, and the dose is 3 to 6 teaspoonfuls in 24 hours. This is an Indian remedy I got from Ellsworth, Me. Writes L. M. A., Bangor, Me.

Devil's Shoestring is a good stomach tonic, and may be used alone by steeping a teaspoonful of the crushed root into a cupful of boiling water, and drinking cold during the day a large mouthful at a time, half cupful after each meal. Or it may be mixed with other stomach remedies in the usual way. Writes Mrs. E. E., Cincinnati, Ohio.

Make a strong tea of Golden Seal Root and take a teaspoonful 3 times a day for stomach troubles. Also good as a gargle for sore throat or mouth. The powdered root is also good for all kinds of sores, bathing the affected parts first in warm water and then applying the powder. Writes Mrs. M. L. G., Camargo, Okla.

TONICS

—Ladies Floral Beauty Tea...........
German Cheese Plant
Bluets
Sassafras Pith
Sassafras Bark
Juniper Berries
Althea Root
American Sarsaparilla
Marigold Flowers
Rosemary Leaves
Fennel Seed
Yellow Root
Bearberry Leaves
A nice, clean and beautiful looking tea. Properties: Mild Diuretic. Demulcent and Carminative.

—Spring Tonic....
Sassafras Bark of Root
Red Clover Flowers
Turtlebloom Leaves
Tinn. Senna Leaves
Fennel Seed
Anise Seed
This is one of the old fashioned Spring Tonics. It has been handed down from generation to generation and is without doubt a valuable formula. Its action is slightly laxative.

—Mormon Valley Herb Compound.......
Mormon Valley Plant
Black Cohosh
Licorice
Gentian
Fennel Seed
Bluets
Wild Cherry Bark
A powerful astringent with tonic properties, a tea of hundreds of uses. May be used internally or externally as a wash for sores and ulcers. A book could be written on the varied usefulness of this remarkable compound. Look up the various ingredients in any good book on medicinal botany.

—American Sarsaparilla Compound.....
Am. Sarsaparilla
Mex. Sarsaparilla
Hon. Sarsaparilla
Sassafras Bark
This is a pleasant aromatic compound of Sarsaparilla. A formula that every Herbalist will recognize.

—Celery Compound.
Celery Seed
Angelica Root
Gentian Root
Sacred Bark
Marshmallow Root
Bearberry Leaves
Juniper Berries
German Cheese Plant

A well known compound. Advertised so extensively it needs no comment. Properties: Carminative, Tonic and Demulcent.

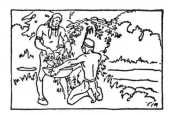

—Buffalo Herb Tea
. . . .
Buffalo Herb
Gentian
Juniper Berries
Corn Silk
Wild Yam
Boneset
Rocky Mountain Grape
Mullein Leaves
German Cheese Plant
Hop Flowers
Foenugreek Seed
Chicory Blue Malva

This tea is composed of Nature's Leaves, Seeds, Berries and Flowers, etc. Nutritive, Tonic and Carminative.

—Old Chieftain Bitters.
These bitters are composed of the following powdered roots and herbs: Gentian Root, Wahoo Bark, Wild Cherry Bark, Prickly Ash Bark and Peruvian Bark. Valuable as a stomach bitters and general tonic.

Take Wormwood, German Chamomile, Rhubarb Root, Dandelion Root, and American Sarsaparilla, of equal measure, and a little Cinnamon and Cloves. Pour over water to make a tea, and st ep 5 or 6 hours, set it away to cool, then strain, add Sugar if desired. Take a mouthful at mealtime and this will build up the stomach and nerves and is very good for all old people. Can be made up fresh every day, or the entire lot at a time just as you desire. Writes Mrs. E. L., Chatfield, Ohio.

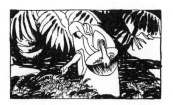

Boteka Leaves—This is the finest substitute for ordinary tea or coffee that we have been able to discover in the entire herbal kingdom.
Boteka is a real household tea.
Superior to ordinary tea in aroma and flavor, and far more healthful. It has a more decided flavor than the Central American Mate. Sold at 25c and $1 a box. Many people love it more. This, however, appears to be a matter of taste.
It is beneficial in many ailments where ordinary tea is prohibited. It is often used externally as a wash for sores and ulcers. The reports of the wonderful benefits derived from the use of this tea read like fairy tales.
We are certain that eventually this tea will become a household necessity—more popular than ordinary tea.
We have imported thousands of pounds of this delicious tea and are confident that every user above 40 years of age will never be without it. It appears to be the health tea of the aged and middle aged.

I must say a few words about Yellow Dock. It is just wonderful. I feel better now than I have in 16 years. Writes Mrs. M. E., Belleville, Tex.

I have taken the Yellow Dock tonic as recommended in your Almanac and found it wonderful. Writes Mrs. L. C., Waverly, Ohio.

I supposed every one knows that White Ask Bark, Poplar Bark, Cherry Bark as well as Sassafras is a good Spring Tonic.
Editor's Note—They should—but they don't—but you're telling them.

Spice Bitters—Use Golden Seal, Poplar Bark, Bayberry and Sassafras, Unicorn, Cloves, Capsicum, 4 ounces of each and 4 pounds of Sugar. Put to 1 ounce of this powder, 1 quart of Sweet Wine, let it stand a week or two before using it. Dose: One wineglassful 2 or 3 times a day. Writes Mrs. M. H. McG., Los Angeles, Calif.

Medicine Beer—Here is a medicinal beer or Spring medicine. Use 1 gallon of water, and an ounce of Burdock, Yellow Dock, Sarsaparilla, Dandelion, and Spikenard. Boil 20 minutes, and then you can add Oil Spruce ¼ teaspoonful if desired, and a little Sassafras. When cool, add 1 cake of Yeast, tie cloth over jar, let stand until fermentation is nearly over, then bottle. Keep cool. Writes Sallie C. L., Baxter Springs, Kan.

Last year in Rochester, N. Y., I ordered some Buffalo Herb. It was necessary for us to stay up late and copy work for graduation thesis and I do not know what we would have done had it not been for the Buffalo Herb. One time we did not retire until 4 a. m., but the tea surely did give us pep—we did not even feel sleepy. So I want you to send us some more. Our little girl has been having bad teeth and we are going to try her on the Buffalo Herb to see if it makes strong teeth and brings up her resistance to colds. Writes Mrs. J. S. W., Logansport, Ind.

One ounce of Wild Cherry Bark, 1 Lemon, and 2 tablespoonfuls of whole Flax Seed to a quart of water, sweetened with either Honey or Brown Sugar, the dose being small glassful twice a day will build up the whole body. Writes F. C., Montreal, Que., Canada.

General Tonic—Four cloves of Garlic, ground fine mixed with 1 ounce of Pecans ground fine, eat a teaspoonful several times daily. Pint glass of strong Lemonade made with juice of 3 or 4 Lemons, 1 tablespoonful pure Honey and balance pure water, at meal time or during the meal, and it would be well to add a good pinch of ground fine Red Pepper to this Lemonade too. Sauerkraut juice at meal is fine, also ground Cranberries sweetened to taste with good Honey, but don't take too heavy of this last. Avoid practically all starches and sweets for many days, until results are noticed, then use lightly. Plenty of potlicker, old southern turnip green potlicker without meat, plenty of celery, and Irish potato peeling soup to alkalinize the blood and feed the nerves, plenty of leafy vegetables, especially lettuce, cabbage, spinach, tomatoes. Avoid meats and animal fats, use vegetable oils, keep the bowels open freely. Writes Dr. W. C. H., Paducah, Ky.

American Poplar Bark is a mild but valuable tonic for domestic use. Writes Mrs. C. B., Crisco, Ia.

When one gets cross and worn out, take a warm bath with Epsom Salts added to the water. This is refreshing. As a foot bath it never fails to relieve. Writes R. N., Shreveport, La.

For Correcting the Bile and Creating an Appetite—The following preparation will be found useful to those who are bilious:

       2 ounces American Centaury
       2 ounces Bayberry Bark
       2 ounces Poplar Bark
       2 ounces Balmony
       1 ounce Ginger
       ½ ounce Licorice Root

Simmer in 2 quarts of water, down to 3 pints, strain, add 4 ounces of spirits, and take a wineglassful 3 times a day. Writes Mrs. F. A. P., Willand, Ont., Canada.

Here is a recipe from Nature's Medicine Chest, that I know to be good. Nettle tea is used as a strengthening tonic by many of my friends and by myself. I also learned later that Nettles have formic acid with much prized tonic qualities. Take a handful of Nettle Leaves and a quart of water. Bring to boiling point, strain and take a wineglassful before breakfast. This is also good for nettle-rash too. Writes M. M., Stephentown Centre, N. Y.

Here is an old tonic that a friend gave me. It is a general tonic and very easily made: Three parts Red Oak Bark, 2 parts Persimmons Bark, 2 parts Sweet Gum Bark. Place cupful in hot water and let steep until cool, take by mouthfuls any time during the day. Writes B. H. S., Ochlocknee, Ga.

During my 3 years stay in the Dutch East Indies, I have noticed the natives massage each other with Cajeput Oil, and while there I have had many a massage myself with that oil and must say it takes that tired feeling out of the bones. What I mean by that is that after a day's work is done and one is given a massage with Cajeput Oil, it is just like new life pouring into your body. Writes J. O., Bakersfield, Calif.
Editor's Note— I believe it is too strong to use undiluted. Better mix 1 ounce with 16 ounces of Olive Oil or any other bland oil.

A Good Tonic. Take Burdock and Red Alder and make a tea. It is surely a fine medicine. Writes Mrs. A. C., Allardt, Tenn.

I have also found to increase or restore one's appetite one should take Valerian Root 4 ounces of it, which has been ground coarsely and make into a tea by steeping a round tablespoonful in a pint of water, and take 1 or 2 tablespoonfuls just before meals and half a wineglassful at bedtime. It is supposed to cleanse the blood, too. Writes Mrs. D. H., Hoquiam, Wash.

TEETH

For Toothache—Boil Red Oak Bark into a strong tea and apply hot to the teeth. Writes B. M. H., Johnetta, Ky.

Here is a recipe for sore gums when you have caught cold in your face and teeth: Take dry Sage Leaves and lay on the gums over the affected parts. Apply these twice during the day and upon retiring at night. I used this when nothing else helped. Writes G. B. S., Denton, Md.

For the Teeth and Bones—I wish to contribute a formula that will supply the blood with Calcium and other minerals and is an ideal combination for softening of the bones and for the teeth. Almost any infection of the bones and teeth will be benefited by this tea. Take a handful of each of these herbs, Buffalo Herb Leaves, Mormon Valley Plant, Horsetail Grass and Sassafras Root and mix. Of this take a heaping teaspoonful and bring to boiling point in a cup of water, strain and drink a cupful of this tea during the day a large mouthful at a time. This tea has also a marked influence on weak men. It is very astringent and will pucker the mouth, but it is good. May also be used as a wash for old sores, varicose veins and rupture. For these latter purposes make it extra strong. It is harmless.

I tried the Wild Cherry Bark for toothache and the first time I used it, it stopped and I have not been bothered since. Writes J. W. D., Blakesburg, Iowa.

After 3 days of suffering with the toothache my grandmother made a poultice of Horehound and it was applied to my jaw. The swelling ceased immediately and I was relieved of the pain. Writes Mrs. J. W. E., Gladys, Va.

Charcoal beat up fine with Salt is good for bleeding gums and to clean the teeth. Writes Mrs. F. E., Munday, Texas.

Take the Bark of Wild Cherry, make a strong tea and hold in the mouth as hot as you can bear it. This is good for toothache and early stages of pyorrhea. Writes S. W., Cowan, Tenn.

The Toothache Herb, or Crawl Grass, received from you is great. It has hardened my teeth and gums to a great extent. Writes R. B., Grand Rapids, Mich.

A good cure for toothache is to chew the root of Bull Nettle on the tooth that is hurting. This is said to stop a toothache no matter how bad. Writes B. H., Macdoel, Calif.

I will give you this tried and true honest remedy for babies: During the teething period give a teaspoonful of Cod Liver Oil every morning after breakfast, as this supplies extra bone food and keeps up the appetite, also the correct weight, where otherwise most babies' vitality is lowered during the teething time, causing no end of sickness and trouble. Writes Mrs. D. B., Anoka, Minn.

Take a handful of Red Oak Bark, boil in a quart of water, and hold on the aching tooth, and it will relieve it at once. Do not swallow. Writes Mrs. L. E. L., Newport, Va.

Chew Sassafras Bark 3 times a day, and it will cure gum boils. Writes M. L., Gilmer, Texas.

In slight cases of toothache, chewing unbleached Jamaica Ginger will often do in slight cases, while good Pellitory Root often gives good results in severe cases. Writes Mrs. H. W., Omaha, Neb.

To ease toothache, take Asafoetida, and mix with whiskey if obtainable and will relieve toothache quickly. Writes J. H., Wildwood, Fla.

Take a small amount of the dried Holly Leaves, burn them, then take the ashes, mix with Honey and apply to affected gums. Is a sure cure and a good treatment in the early stages of pyorrhea. It is said to be an Indian remedy. Writes T. B., Holloday, Tenn.

My grandmother was part Indian and I am sending a recipe she used for thrush in baby's mouth. Take Yellow Root, Sage Leaves, and Alum and make a tea, then mix with Honey and use as a mouth wash. Writes Mrs. R. M. P., Gastonia, N. C.

THRUSH

Simple Cure for Thrush—Make a tea of the second bark (next to the wood) of a Black Jack Tree or Persimmon Bark; add a pinch of Alum, swab the sore mouth a few times and you will be wonderfully surprised at the quick results. Writes Mrs. I. W., Drumwright, Okla.

Mix pure Hog's Lard with powdered Sulphur, rub it in baby's mouth a little at a time, and you will find it a sure cure for thrush. Writes S. B., Conehatta, Miss.

Take a small handful of the inside of Bark of Persimmon and put in a pint of water; boil down to half pint. Strain, add Sugar or Honey, boil down to a syrup to which add a small piece of Alum, while cooking. This will cure the thrush in baby's mouth.

For Yellow Thrush in the Mouth—Take a little of the Persimmon Bark, and put in water, let stand a few minutes, and wash the mouth twice daily with it, and it is a sure cure. Writes J. H., Wildwood, Fla.

As a mouth wash for Thrush, make a wash of a little honey and borax. Wash every three or four hours, and it is good and you will find it a very old-time remedy. Writes Mrs. J. F. A.,

A Cure for Typhoid Fever—I have seen this tried and have broke up fever four different times myself and know it to be a sure cure. After the bowels are working right, take Fever Weed, and drink of the tea freely. Writes A. T., Speedwell, Tenn.

I wish also to say my youngest daughter had Typhoid Fever and we had a physician, but she seemed to grow worse instead of better. An old colored lady told me to give her Boneset Tea, which I did, and she commenced to get better right away. She was soon up and around. The doctor was certainly surprised the way she gained. Writes Mrs. E. C., Tulsa, Okla.

Editor's Note—So was I—but one can never tell what wonders some of these herbs perform.

VARICOSE VEINS

An old French lady in this town had varicose veins so bad she could scarcely get around the house and they were very painful, too. She had a lot of what we call Sheep Sorrel gathered and she made a tea and drank it and soon she was able to walk way down town, some 14 blocks. I have never tried this, as I am thankful that I do not have varicose veins, but this might help many others that do have them. Writes Mrs. C. B., Bicknell, Ind.

Editor's Note—Sure worth a trial—it is harmless.

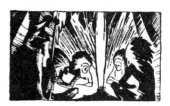

VOMITING

(See Stomach Disorders)

Timothy Seed is very good to stop vomiting. Writes A. C. B., Kokomo, Ind.

Yellow Dock Tea will stop vomiting and will settle the stomach. Writes Mrs. W. H. B., Albright, W. Va.

For Vomiting—Take Black Tar and smell it every 5 minutes until it relieves. Don't eat sweets. Will cure vomiting as I tried it many times and cured myself.

For Vomiting — Take Peach Tree Leaves and make a tea of them and drink it. It will stop any kind of vomiting even in pregnancy. It has been tried and proven. Writes Mrs. E .W. C., Centralia, Wash.

Editor's Note—Entirely harmless—and should interest mothers to be.

Indigestion, Acute—So many foods today are robbed of vital elements before they are offered for sale. White flour, polished rice, degerminated corn meal, pearled barley, white sugar are examples: thus they are insipid to the taste, and call for high seasoning and condiments which in turn do much to upset digestion. Starchy foods sweetened with sugar, starch and acid foods in combination cause fermentation to digestion sufferers.

WARTS

Apply Castor Oil twice daily to warts, that so often come on the hands, and watch the results. Writes Mrs. A. B., Monarch, Ark.

I had a black wart the size of a nickel on my right temple. I made a salve of Sulphur, Lard and a little Salt, and used it morning and evening for a few weeks and it removed the wart without a scar. Writes A. C., Jefferson, Ohio.

I am sending a sure cure for warts. I had a wart on my heel for two years. A friend told me to paint it with Poke Root. After painting the wart with same four or five times it came off. The roots of Poke Root should be fried in hot grease. Writes Mrs. R. W., Girard, Ala.

I have a remedy for warts that is infallible, which I am pleased to contribute to your columns. Take equal parts Bitter Sweet and Lard, add a pinch of salt and boil 15 minutes. When cool, apply 2 or 3 times during the day. Writes W. E. P., Stanford, Ky.
Editor's Note—If this fails try our "Vanishing Balm"

For Taking Off Warts and Corns— Take and burn the Willow Bark, take the ashes and mix with vinegar, so as to make a paste and apply it. Writes C. G., Powhatan Point, Ohio.

Warts—Sweet Oil will take off any kind. Persevere in using it. Writes O. L. M., Lathrop, Mich.

I find that warts disappear within a few weeks after being daubed with Iodine. I have had one for years until the Iodine treatment rid me of it. Writes R. L. K., Des Moines, Iowa.
Editor's Note—Warts are peculiar things, some yield to this, others defy everything. Mr........ of Lowell, Ind., came to my office recently with the largest wart I ever saw—over one-half inch thick and over an inch in diameter. He said several doctors tried to remove it but had failed. I recommended he use Sheep Sorrel Herb pounded to a pulp and apply it. He did and the wart fell off. Fresh Sheep Sorrel is the herb so often recommended for benign cancer.

WEAK LIMBS

Weak Limbs—Take Betony and St. Johnswort, and put them in good old rye whiskey, if obtainable. Drink this in the mornings before taking anything else, and it is a sure cure for weakness of the limbs. A tea made of the Acorns of the White Oak is also fine for weak limbs. Writes Mrs. P. J. M., Oklahoma City, Okla.
Editor's Note—The Acorns referred to are the sweet variety, and should be used locally only.

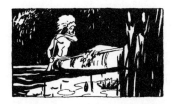

WHOOPING COUGH

I will give you a recipe that I have tried for whooping cough. Take Angelica Root, boil into a strong tea, cool, strain and take 4 ounces of white sugar, add to the Angelica tea and boil into a syrup. Give a swallow 6 or 8 times a day, and it will cause the phlegm to vomit up and cure the cough. Writes S. E. S., Woodbine, Ky.

Here is a good relief recipe which I have used on my children, and my grandchildren for whooping cough. Take one ounce Mouse Ear, boil from one quart to a pint, add Rock Sugar Candy and Honey, an ounce of each. It was the only remedy that gave relief. Give a spoonful when coughing spell has finished and it seems to heal same. Writes A. G., Bloomfield, N. J.

For Whooping Cough—Take Indian Turnip Root, put in sweet milk, steep 30 minutes, give tablespoonful every 4 hours. Writes G. B., Turley, Tenn.

Take a handful of Chestnut Leaves to a pint of water, strain and sweeten, drink for whooping cough. Writes Mrs. C. M., Verona, Pa.

For Whooping Cough—Take Garlic Bulbs and put them in a rag, beat with a hammer and rub between babies' shoulders. This will relieve the whooping cough, and is a remedy given us by an old doctor. Writes E. T., Talking Rock, Ga.

RECIPES FROM WALES
Contributed by W. W. J., Whiting, Ind.

Sir—I have heard from various parts that there is an epidemic of whooping-cough abroad. Sad to relate, quite a lot of people think that it must be left to take its course. This is the greatest mistake a parent can make. As soon as a child is noticed developing this disease it should be isolated from all other children, otherwise all children that come in contact will get it. There is no reason why any child should get whooping-cough; it never would if it did not get the germs of this disease from others. However, here is a certain remedy: Keep the child in a warm, well-ventilated room, if very cold; keep it away from other children, and get the following preparation: 1 oz. of Wild Thyme, 1 oz. Mouse-ear; pour over one pint of boiling water, and sweeten with a little honey or treacle. For young children, a half to one teaspoonful frequently; children over 2, one tablespoonful; 4 years, half a wineglassful. This will quickly control the cough. Rub the chest with the following: 2 oz. of Russian Tallow, or Mutton Fat; melt it; when hot, grate a little Ginger Root into it; also add six spots of Eucalyptus Oil, three spots of Oil of Pine, and place the mixture in a jar, which should be kept air-tight. Rub the child's chest and back once a day. A very young baby should only be rubbed with ointment every other day.

The above remedy will quickly cure this troublesome disease.

If anyone tells you whooping-cough is incurable get this remedy and tell them to watch the result. They will quickly change their view. In my opinion it is criminal to leave dear, innocent little children suffer. If people would only get back to Nature, there would be thousands living that are now gone to the happy hunting grounds. I say again—herbs will cure diseases when all other remedies have failed. There are thousands of people living today who can prove this. God sent these herbs for our use, and He knows best. He is the greatest physician of all.— Yours etc., H. G. Hereford, Wales.

Editor's Note—Any grease may be used in this ointment.

Dr. Loeffler, German botanist, valued Coughwort leaves highly for catarrhal conditions of mucous membrane of the bronchial tubes and lungs.

Whooping Cough—Take the sour Sumach Berries. Put about one cupful in a basin and cover with boiling water. Steep If you think this is too strong, dilute with water. Add a little sugar to help taste. Dose—Give children one or two teaspoonfuls when coughing hard. This is not a cure, but will ease the coughing very much. Writes G. B. S., Deferiet, N. Y.

Relief for Whooping Cough—Take enough Chestnut Leaves to make a strong cup of tea and add equal parts of Sweet Oil Give 1 teaspoonful every hour until relieved. Writes Mrs. S. S. K., Chelan, Wash.

For Whooping Cough—Take the juice of one Lemon and 1 ounce of Pure Glycerine. Add the glycerine to the lemon juice and give one teaspoonful every hour or two, depending upon how bad the cough is. Writes Mrs. A. B., Eufaula, Okla.

I know by my own experience that White Clover Flowers in tea is very good to use during whooping cough. Writes Mrs. L. B., Sullivan, Mo.

Give a tea of Red Clover Blossoms two or three times a day and the child will never whoop. Writes Mrs. L. W., Elmwood, Ill.

I cured my child in ten days from whooping cough with this remedy. Take the stems of Black Cherries, draw tea of them. For every drawing take four saucerfuls of water, and as many Cherry Stems as may be held between three fingers, boil like any other tea, and take this tea until the coughing ceases, and I am sure the most violent cough will be cured. Writes A. K., St. Louis, Mo.

A tried recipe for whooping cough which is very good. Mix one Lemon, sliced, half pint of Flax Seed, and 2 or 3 ounces of Honey and one quart of water, and simmer (not boil), strain, and if there is less than a pint of the mixture add water. Dose: One tablespoonful 4 times a day, and one after a spell of coughing. Warranted to cure in four days after child first whoops. Writes Mrs. J. B., Richland Center, Wis.

Take a handful of Chestnut Leaves to a pint of water, strain and sweeten, drink for whooping cough. Writes Mrs. C. M., Verona, Pa.

For Whooping Cough—Mix a fourth of a pound of ground Elecampane into a pint of strained Honey and a half a pint of water. Place in glazed earthen pot and place in stone oven if one is obtainable, and bake or use half the heat required to bake bread. Let bake until about the consistency of the honey and take it out. Give a teaspoonful before each meal if a child and double the dose if an adult. Writes A. H., Lafayette, Ind.

For Whooping Cough—Make a tea of Sunflower Seeds, strain, add granulated sugar and cook until rather thick and give same as any other cough medicine. Writes Mrs. J. A., Ft. Recovery, Ohio.

Take equal parts of Glycerine and strained Honey and give to a child with whooping cough whenever it coughs hard. About one teaspoonful at a time is the dose. This is very good. Writes B. A. G., Arkville, N. Y.

Take Garlic and fry in Bacon Grease and rub in neck and breast, then cover with warm flannel. This is sure relief for whooping cough.

Whooping Cough—Take one-half gallon Red Clover Blooms, put one quart of water over them and boil until all the strength is extracted, which is about an hour, then strain, and put back on fire and boil down half. Add enough granulated sugar to make a thick syrup and boil until it is about like an ordinary cough syrup. Give as often as necessary, according to the coughing spells, but no danger of giving too much as it is harmless. Writes Mrs. L. J., Drexel, Mo.

My children have just recovered from whooping cough. I was told to make a tea of Red Clover Blossoms, as this was both a cure and preventive. I gave them as much of the tea as they would drink each day. Although it did not prevent the disease, they had it much lighter than most children. Red Clover Blossoms in tea form is a very good blood medicine, too. Writes Mrs. P. S. C., Pringle, S. D.

—Wild Cherry Pectoral...
  Wild Cherry Bark
  Gum Plant
  White Pine Bark
  Coughwort Leaves
  Horehound Leaves
A very good combination of botanicals for coughs, colds, etc. May be used as a tea or thickened with honey for use as a cough syrup.

WORMS

WORMS, ROUND

Symptoms—Itching of the nose, foul breath, colicky pains, nausea, vomiting, diarrhoea, etc. Can be seen in stools.

Treatment—Abstain from all food for 12 to 16 hours.

The Herb Doctor's choice of botanicals are: Jerusalem Oak, Pomegranate, Pumpkin Seed, Chamomile, Mulberry Root, Nettle Leaves, Peach Leaves, Southernwood, Wormwood, Wood Betony, Gentian, Hops, Motherwort, Tansy, Calamus, Goatsrue, Worm Grass Root, St. Johnswort, Groundsel, Walnuts and Raw Carrots.

WORMS, SEAT

These inhabit the large intestines and especially the region of the rectum and may migrate to the sexual organs. They resemble a piece of white thread ¼ to ½ inch long.

Treatment — Same as for round worms. Apply Sulphur Tar Salve to the anus or bathe the external and private organs with warm water.

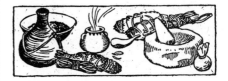

TAPE WORM

Symptoms—Segments of tape worm in stools, voracious appetite, does not put on flesh, digestive disturbances.

Treatment—Follow same directions as for round worms but take larger doses of the Vermifuge. Watch for the head of the worm in the stools. When it appears a cure is effected.

The Herb Doctor's choice of botanical vermifuges are: Jerusalem Oak, Pomegranate, Ailanthus, Wormgrass Root, Walnut Leaves, Pumpkin Seed, Mulberry Root.

For Worms in Children—Make molasses candy and stir thick with Jerusalem Oak Seed. Give this to the children every morning for three or four mornings. While giving this candy have the children on a light diet. Writes Mrs. E. W. P., Marion, N. C.

Tape Worm Remedy—Eat no food for 18 or 20 hours. Peel enough Pumpkin Seeds to make four ounces of kernel. Eat them at night on an empty stomach. Take a tea of Pumpkin Seeds the next morning. Eat nothing until noon. This treatment may have to be repeated but this is very seldom. Use a good laxative in connection. This is a sure remedy. Writes Mrs. H. R., Edgar, Wis.

I am sending the following recipe for worms in children. I have used nothing else for my own children and my mother also used it for her family. Take the bark from Poplar and steep, being careful not to get the tea too strong, as children don't like bitter medicine. Weaken and add sugar to make a syrup. Give one or two teaspoonfuls at night followed by a laxative in the morning. Writes Mrs. L. V. G., Spring Creek, Pa.

Garlic, chop fine and sprinkle sparingly on bread and butter sandwich, is a cure for pin worms. Writes F. G., Columbus, Ohio.

I am enclosing a remedy which I have tried in my own family as my husband had tape worm. An old aunt told me how to doctor it and in doing so I was successful, and hope it will benefit others. I got a pint of Pumpkin Seeds and 2 quarts of milk. He went without his supper, also his breakfast, and he would eat a few seeds now and then and drink a glass of milk. After he had used all the seeds, I fixed him a cathartic, and in an hour he had passed the worm. Writes Mrs. F. A., St. Louis, Mich.

For Worms in Children—Use equal parts of Sugar and powdered Sage. Give a teaspoonful before meals until relieved. This may be moistened with a few drops of water if the dry sage chokes the child. Writes Mrs. F. R., Milton, Ind.

Take the seeds of Jerusalem Oak and stir into the molasses when making candy and let the children eat it and you can say good-bye to worms. Writes Mrs. W. S., Sevierville, Tenn.

Worms—Take a cup of Pumpkin Seed, ground, 1 cup Raisins, ground, put in one-half gallon of water, and boil down to quart. Dose: One wineglassful four times a day.

Should the children be bothered with worms, just take a handful of Peach Tree Leaves and steep to make a tea. Drink either hot or cold. Writes D. B., Vanlue, Ohio.
Editor's Note—There seems to be no end to uses of Peach Tree Leaves.

Sage Tea is very good for worms in children. Drink with milk and sugar. This is not bad to the taste. Writes Mrs. J. S. P., Bowdoinham, Me.
Editor's Note—You cannot get results from herbs that have been on the shelves of drug stores for years.

For a Child with Pin Worms—Give a tea of Spearmint. This is known to have cured some of the worst cases. Writes Mrs. D. H., Hoquiam, Wash.

To Drive Out a Tape Worm—Take one-half pound of Pumpkin Seeds, peel them, and eat them in two days, taking nothing but that and some water. The third day when you arise, take a dose of Castor Oil and it will pass within a few hours. Writes Miss P. R., New Britain, Conn.

Sage is a good remedy for worms. Writes S. H., Vallejo, Calif.

Sweetened Alder Tea is just fine to rid children of worms.

A strong infusion made of seeds of Jerusalem Oak is very beneficial for worms. The dose should be one teaspoonful mixed with syrup three times a day. Writes Mrs. M. G., Texarkana, Tex.

Make any kind of candy and gather and clean Jerusalem Oak Seed and stir in candy while hot; let the children eat when they want it, and you will find valuable for worms. Writes Mrs. O. L., Rising Fawn, Ga.

For Worms in Children—In February make a paste of Molasses and Sulphur in equal parts and give one teaspoonful each morning for three mornings, then miss one morning. Repeat this until nine doses have been given. This is also excellent for thinning the blood. Writes L. E., Price, Utah.

Here is a Good Recipe for Expelling Worms—Take the seed of Jerusalem Oak and place in vessel with Sorghum Molasses and boil until it makes candy. Children eat this candy easily for it tastes delicious. Writes K. M. N., Good Springs, Tenn.

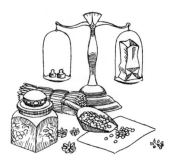

Anthelmintics—These are drugs which destroy or expel worms from the stomach and intestines.

Those in the first column are the best —Pomegranate, Pumpkin Seeds are the ones usually used for tape worms.

Jerusalem Oak	Flax Seed
Am. Worm Seed	Pomegranate Bark
Wormwood	Worm Grass Root
Elm Bark	Pink Root
Devil's Shoe String	

Any of the above drugs may be powdered and mixed with honey or with syrup in equal parts or made into candy.

The dose should be one teaspoonful of the syrup or one dram of the candy three times during the day upon an empty stomach. No food whatever, except water should be taken during this treatment. After the last dose at night a good dose of a cathartic should be taken.

For Worms in Children—Just get the dried Garden Rue, steep and give, or if you have the fresh Garden Rue, give juice. Writes Mrs. E. W., Rochester, Minn.

I am sending a recipe for tape worm: A pound of Pumpkin Seed, shelled and ground in a meat chopper and mixed in cold milk Eat it all and then take a laxative. Writes P. T., Reeder, N. D.

For a child with worms take Wormseed and make any kind of candy, adding the Wormseed and give it to them to eat. Writes Miss E. B., Rocky Mount, Va.

Tape Worm—It is generally considered that the frequent use of pork is one of the causes of tapeworm. Unquestionably a diet of fruit, nuts, vegetables will help considerably in bringing health back to normal.

For Worms—Tried and true. Steep one teaspoonful Spearmint in a cup of boiling water 10 minutes. Give one-half cupful 3 times a day. Writes Mrs. A. S., Cleveland, Ohio.

Equal parts of ground Sage, Saffron, mixed with Molasses and Sulphur will rid one of worms, too. Take one, or if for children only a half teaspoonful to a dose. Writes O. C. C., Marietta, Ohio.

Here is a good prescription for tape worms, or any other kind. Take Gentian Root, and steep 30 minutes, and drink one pint in the morning and one pint in the evening. Eat only little and it will come the next day. Need no physic. Sweeten if you cannot take it any other way. It's a good tonic to take all the time. Writes L. S. B., Buffalo, Mo.

Worm Remedy—Take Sage and Senna, boil together, strain and put in sugar or molasses and boil down to a syrup. Writes L. M., Seneca, S. C.

YELLOW JAUNDICE

A condition arising from derangement of the liver, with yellow hue of the skin and eyes. One cup of No. 99 Calumet Herb Laxative Tea will be beneficial. Those subject to jaundice should avoid rich foods, fats, pastries, sweets, and red meats.

The Herb Doctor's choice of botanicals are: Sacred Bark, May Apple, Dandelion, Parsley Herb, Peach Tree Leaves, Plantain Leaves, Black Root, Butternut Bark, Bayberry, Rocky Mountain Grape Root, Eye Bright, St. Johnswort, Toadflax.

For Yellow Jaundice—Make a tea of Saffron Flowers and drink two tablespoonfuls at a dose two or three times a day. Writes Mrs. J. A., Ft. Recovery, Ohio.

I was suffering greatly from catarrhal jaundice, when a friend of mine met me and noticed my condition. He told me he had a buddy that tramps the woods, trapping, etc., and he would order his buddy to get something for me. He did, for he came with Wild Cherry Bark and made me take two cupfuls a day, and in a week I was up and around. Writes F. S., Royal Oak, Mich.

Get Hickory Bark, boil into a strong tea, or until it is black and drink one cupful a day. It is a sure cure for jaundice. Writes H. M. J., Laurel, Miss.

When I had yellow jaundice they told me to take a pinch of Saffron to a cup of hot water three times a day and it cured me, when I was in pretty bad shape. Writes Mrs. E. T., Mesick, Mich.
Editor's Note—Yellow dock root is also very good in this ailment.

For Yellow Jaundice—Take the bark of Indian Arrow Wood, boil down to a strong tea, sweeten and give the child as much of the tea as it can drink 3 or 4 times a day. Writes J. L. D., Tanksley, Ky.

We also drank the water from Wild Cherry Bark for jaundice. Writes Miss E. F., Lancaster, Ohio.
Editor's Note—You are a very sensible Miss, and I predict that you will some day make a man very happy. Your family will save many doctor bills. I wish there were more like you in this ignorant world of dope users.

Try using Hickory Bark for yellow jaundice. Make into a tea and use. It has cured me and several others. Writes J. B. D., Carthage, Tex.

Yellow Jaundice—Take the bark of Elderberry, and make a tea of it. Drink cold, 3 or 4 cups during the day. Also make a tea of Dandelion Roots or just chew them. Writes Mrs. M. H. McG., Los Angeles, Calif.

For Yellow Jaundice—Turkish Rhubarb (Rheum Palmatum) either in the powdered or cut form. Chew a small quantity three times a day. This will tone up the most sluggish liver. Should the case prove obstinate, eat stewed carrots also. Writes H. W. M., Lykens, Pa.

Take Cinque-Foil Weed and boil down to a good color. Sweeten with sugar and give while luke warm, three or four teaspoonfuls twice a day, until baby bleaches. Writes Mrs. P. S., Boston, Tenn.

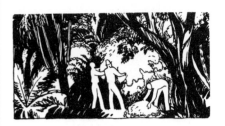

Jaundice — Liver Troubles — Quicker progress will be made towards health on a fruit, nut, cottage cheese and vegetable diet.

For Yellow Jaundice—I cured myself on this. Make a strong tea of Red Alder Bark that grows along branches. Use the Red Alder treatment for three days, drink more of a night than you do of a day. Drink half-pint each dose every five hours. If this seems too much reduce the dose. Don't make too strong. When your Red Alder treatment is out use the Sassafras Pith treatment, or the roots, either one will do.
Take Sassafras Bark from the roots or pith. Boil the roots or pith. Take one tablespoonful every three or four hours. Same at bedtime. Sassafras Bark Tea cleanses the bladder, restores weakness, throws the poison out of the body. Writes A. L. H., Cander, N. C.

Here is a Remedy for Yellow Jaundice—Take Mulberry Bark of root, and the bark of Wild Cherry. Steep them together in boiling water, but do not boil much. Drink reasonably plenty. I would not trade it for any doctor's medicine for jaundice. Writes J. A. K., Grahn, Ky.

—Fringe Tree Comp.
   Fringe Tree
   Master of the Woods
   Blue Vervain Flrs. and Lvs.
   Elecampane
   Wormwood Leaves
   Water Plantain
A fine combination of aromatics and tonics, that have a good influence on the liver.

DIETARY ADVICE IN ALL DISEASES

By the Noted English Naturopath, Dr. Maxwell

Anemia—The diet may include foods rich in iron and sodium as leaf lettuce, leeks, nettles, spinach, rice bran, strawberries, radishes, asparagus, onions, celery, Swiss chard, pumpkins, carrots, dandelions, cabbage, dried figs, milk, beets, apples, tu-nips and cauliflowers. Have one fresh fruit meal a day with raw milk. One salad meal, one meal of steamed or baked vegetables with cottage cheese or flaked nuts. Whole wheat or whole rye bread and sweet butter. Also take warm and thick vegetable soups with lima beans, soy beans or peas.

Appendicitis—It is advisable to abstain from food, other than hot lemonade until all pain, inflammation and fever have subsided. Then nothing but orange juice for a few days. Avoid foods which constipate: for example, meats, fried foods, tea and coffee, white bread, white sugar.

Arteriosclerosis—Among the causes are the constant use of high protein foods, meats, fish, poultry, etc., alcoholic beverages, tobacco, spices, condiments, tea, coffee demineralized foods, and even a diet too heavy in cereals and legumes. In its early stages relief can be obtained by a diet of fresh fruits and green leafy vegetables with a moderate amount of such proteins as nuts and cottage cheese. Eat freely of raw vegetable salads. As an extra, a cupful of freshly-expressed fruit juice and later a cupful of freshly-expressed vegetable juices may be taken daily.

Asthma—It is considered that the diet has been very faulty before such attacks can develop; too great a fondness for carbohydrate foods, starches and sugars. Discontinue the use of all carbohydrate foods for a while—white bread, pastry, potatoes, all cereals and refined white sugar. Eat freely of citrus fruits and green leafy vegetable salads.

Baby's Ailments—If at any time the child is feverish, stop feeding until temperature is again normal. Give only water flavored with lemon juice. If necessary, a small enema, if not too young, then a warm bath and put to bed. Much trouble is sometimes caused by over-feeding.

Bleeders' Disease—There is always a deficiency of calcium or lime in the diet when there is a tendency to hemorrhage. The foods which are richest in calcium are nettles, water cress, dill cabbage, lettuce, dandelions, spinach, Swiss chard, chives, radishes, cottage cheese, turnips, whey, milk, lemons, onions, and leeks. Squeeze out the fresh juices of any of the above and drink suitable quantities whenever desirable in addition to regular meals.

Boils—One should avoid high protein foods, meat, fish, poultry, etc., and feed largely on fresh fruits, fresh green vegetables and a moderate supply of nuts or cottage cheese.

Bright's Disease—All high protein foods should be avoided—meats, fish, poultry, eggs, cheese, dried peas and beans, lentils. All condiments, especially salt, pepper, mustard, vinegar should be abstained from. Patient should be put on an absolutely salt-free diet. Fresh fruits and fresh green vegetables are always to be recommended.

Bronchitis—In all bronchial troubles there is evidence that the sufferer has been eating too freely of carbohydrate foods, starches and sugars. Omit from the diet, bread, pastry, cereals, sugar, milk, coffee and tea, fried foods, potatoes and all starchy foods until the system is thoroughly cleared up. Fresh fruits, especially the citrus ones, and fresh vegetables are very acceptable.

Diabetes—In diabetes there is always hyperacidity—a very acid condition of the system, therefore, all decidedly acid-forming foods such as meats, fish, poultry, and all high protein foods should be avoided, as well as all the carbohydrates, starches and sugars. The green leafy vegetables are the diabetic's best friends among foods, especially when taken as raw salads.

Diphtheria and Croup—Foods rich in organic sodium are very useful, such as celery, spinach, and Swiss chard. Express and drink the fresh juices of these vegetables.

Dropsy—The frequent use of condiments, especially salt, is a contributing factor, also the general use of high protein foods which irritate the kidneys.

Incontinence of Urine—High protein foods, meats, fish, poultry, eggs, old cheese should be avoided, also all condiments such as salt, pepper, mustard and vinegar, which are irritants to the kidneys. Fruits and fresh vegetables, with a few flaked nuts or cottage cheese will be the most suitable foods. Drink soothing demulcent drinks with slight astringent properties.

Indigestion, Acute—So many foods today are robbed of vital elements before they are offered for sale. White flour, polished rice, degerminated corn meal, pearled barley, white sugar are examples: thus they are insipid to the taste, and call for high seasoning and condiments which in turn do much to upset digestion. Starchy foods sweetened with sugar, starch and acid foods in combination cause fermentation to digestion sufferers.

Fried foods are responsible for more trouble. A short fast, then a diet of fresh fruits and vegetables, careful mastication, eating only when hungry, choosing only foods that have not in any way been denatured by processing will help recovery from this condition.

Inflammation of the Bladder—All animal foods, or products of high protein foods such as meats, fish, poultry, heavy and continuous use of condiments, tobacco, coffee, tea and alcohol should be carefully avoided. Take nothing but soothing and cooling demulcents in tea form.

Inflammation of the Kidneys—It may be of more help to put a cool compress over the small of the back and feet in a hot foot bath with a tablespoonful of mustard added to the bath.

A few days' fast—no food but all the water thirst calls for—will give the kidneys a needed rest, and allow the natural recuperative powers of the body to do their repair work unhampered.

Then do not feed any animal food, but give fruit or vegetable meals, with a few nuts or cottage cheese. No white bread or white sugar, coffee, tea; no fried foods or eggs, no pickles or condiments. Absolutely nothing that has been salted.

Inflammation of the Womb—Take no foods save hot lemonade until system is perfectly at ease, even if fast lasts several days. Water whenever thirst calls for it. Bowels must be kept open. No animal food, but fresh fruits and vegetables when feeding is resumed.

Influenza or La Grippe—No food should be given while fever or temperature is above normal. The whole body needs absolute rest. Remain in bed until convalescent. Sweating should be induced by hot diaphoretic teas. Feet should be kept warm by hot water bottles or hot packs. Hot lemonade when thirsty. Give nothing but orange juice for 2 or 3 days, then fruit and vegetables; no meat or meat broths.

Itch or Scabies—Avoid all animal foods. Fruits and fresh vegetables with a few nuts and cottage cheese daily will bring blood back to normal alkaline condition.

Jaundice — Liver Troubles — Quicker progress will be made towards health on a fruit, nut, cottage cheese and vegetable diet.

Laryngitis — Sufferer has probably been rather too fond of starchy and sugary foods, taken more carbohydrates than the oxygen breathed can oxidize. Eat more fruits and salads. Avoid tobacco and constipation.

Leucorrhea or Whites—There is generally a run down condition before this trouble manifests itself. Cleansing and nutritive food is needed. Note diet offered under anemia.

Neuralgia—There is always an acid condition of the system, therefore the body needs foods that give an alkaline reaction, such as fruits, green leafy vegetables. The following foods should be avoided as they give a harmful acid reaction: meats, fish, poultry, fried foods, coffee and tea, eggs, white bread, white sugar and old cheese.

Neurasthenia — Alkaline foods are needed, as found in fruits and fresh green vegetables. All kinds of meat are acid forming. Vegetarian diet is corrective, especially vegetable salads.

Neuralgia of the Heart—The use of tobacco is one prominent cause. Inhalation of tobacco smoke will cause hardening of the large arteries, particularly where cigarettes are used. Patient should avoid excitement of every kind. Sponge down with warm water daily. Get plenty of rest and sunshine.

Obesity—Green vegetable salads and vegetable soups without meat, also fresh juicy fruit meals play a very important part also, in bringing one back to normal weight. Avoid constipation, white sugar, white bread and candies.

Eczema—Eczema and other skin diseases are evidence that the regular eliminatory channels have not been clearing out toxins as fast as they accumulate, and too much of high protein foods. A fruit, nut and fresh vegetable diet is recommended, especially green vegetable salads.

Epilepsy, Fits or Falling Disease—A deficient mineral supply in one's foods causes nerve depletion, nerve weakening. It interferes with muscular activity. The use of such denatured foods as meats, white flour, refined sugar, degerminated cereals, the use of coffee, tea, salt, pepper, mustard, vinegar and fried foods bring about such a very decided and harmful acid condition that the rhythm of the nervous system is disturbed and the system is unbalanced. Nothing but a fruit and vegetable diet until recovery is complete.

Erysipelas—Better avoid high protein meat diet. Use fresh fruits and fresh green vegetables freely.

Falling of the Womb—Avoid the use of demineralized foods. There is generally a lack of sufficient potassium in the diet when any of the muscular tissues are flabby. The regular, daily use of fresh green vegetables should improve conditions.

Flatulence—Eat less starchy foods and avoid rich gravies, pastries, coffee and teas with refined sugar. Use honey instead of sugar. Eat more fresh fruits. Avoid cabbage, Brussels sprouts, onions, dried beans, and peas. Use other green vegetables in salads or steamed.

Gall Stones—Gall bladder trouble may also come from a deficiency of sodium in the diet. The foods richest in sodium are celery, spinach, Swiss chard. A glass of lemon juice in a cup of water morning and night may be helpful. Make breakfast of fresh fruit only. Vegetable salads are very beneficial.

Goitre—We may be told there is a deficiency of iodine. If that is so, you may find a supply in sea lettuce, dulse, pineapple, green kidney beans and several green leafy vegetables. But gluttony is more frequently the cause of trouble than deficiency of iodine and a fast may do much to clear up the condition.

Gonorrhea and Gleet—Avoid all animal foods. There will be quicker recovery through a diet of fresh fruits, nuts and vegetable salads than if a more complicated diet were used.

Gravel—The diet should be without condiments; no salt, pepper, mustard or vinegar. No animal foods. Plenty of fresh fruit and green leafy vegetables. In addition, one or two cupfuls a day of the freshly expressed juice of raw vegetables, especially radishes.

Hay Fever—Take the juice of a lemon in a glass of water morning and evening. Eat four oranges for breakfast and four for supper. Have a large plateful of vegetable salad for lunch. Better abstain from milk until recovered.

Headaches—Headache usually indicates some disease or derangement of the system. If the headache is an indication of intestinal uncleanness, poisoning from the gases from toxins retained in the system, live for a while largely on fresh fruits and fresh vegetable salads.

Heart Diseases—Avoid all animal foods. Eat freely of fresh fruit and fresh green vegetables, with four ounces of nuts or cottage cheese per day. Do not drink during meals. Practice deep breathing. Avoid violent exercise, but get out in sunshine whenever possible. Walking is one of the best exercises. Lie down to rest, in fact stay in bed when acute trouble threatens.

No matter what may be the peculiar affection or form of heart trouble, such as palpitation of the heart, fatty heart disease, neuralgia of the heart (Angina Pectoris) or heart dropsy, foods rich in potassium may be especially helpful such as apples, apricots, blackberries, cherries, peaches, plums, prunes, raspberries, watermelons, bananas, figs, lemons, oranges, dried olives, every kind of green leafy vegetables, radishes with their green tops, rutabagas, tomatoes, turnips and water cress.

Hives or Nettle Rash—Cleansing foods hasten recovery. Plenty of fresh fruits and green leafy vegetables. Better cut out all animal foods, tobacco and condiments.

Hysteria—Food should consist of fresh fruits, nuts, fresh vegetables, vegetable soups, with no meat, fish or poultry. Avoid condiments, salt, pepper, mustard and vinegar. Nightly take a few laxative fruits such as figs, prunes, dates.

Painful Menses—Acid forming foods have a tendency to bring trouble at the monthly periods. Meats, fish, poultry, coffee and tea, fried foods, white bread and white sugar are all very acid-forming. Fruits and green vegetables have an opposite effect. Take these with a few nuts and some cottage cheese and vegetable soups made without meats.

Piles—A non-constipating diet will hasten recovery. Meats are constipating. Avoid all condiments. Eat freely of fresh fruits and figs, prunes and dates, also all fresh vegetables. Few nuts, and cottage cheese daily.

Pleurisy—No food, absolutely nothing to eat until all fever and inflammation has disappeared, save weak hot lemonade and all of that thirst calls for. No food even though recuperating and the patient clamours for something to eat through an awakened appetite, no matter if the fast lasts several days. When all danger has passed, pain and fever gone, and not until then, think about feeding. First day or two nothing but pure orange juice. Afterwards fresh fruit or fresh vegetable meals, with a few nuts or cottage cheese. No meats or meat broths.

Pneumonia—See information under Pleurisy. The smoker has a much harder time than the non-smoker if seized by this trouble.

Poison Ivy—Go on a fruit and vegetable diet.

Prickly Heat—Take more exercise in the great outdoors.

Profuse Menses—Correct the general diet. Try vegetarianism. Fresh vegetables will give your blood more needed calcium.

Rheumatism—It is always evidence of poor elimination, imperfect drainage of the system, of gluttony regarding foods which give a decidedly acid reaction. Uric acid is an end product of meat, fish, poultry. It would be well also to omit from the diet eggs, old cheese, dried peas and beans, white flour, white bread and all demineralized cereals.

Rickets—It is evidence of the lack of certain organic minerals in the diet, a lack of Vitamin A. Cod Liver Oil is said to supply this, but there are also foods where the supply of this vitamin is adequate as butter, yolk of egg, cabbage, carrots, spinach and raw milk. Oranges, tomatoes, parsnips and lettuce also furnish a share. Calcium is needed

and the best supplies of that are found in nettles, water cress, cabbage, lettuce, dandelions, spinach and swiss chard.

Sciatica—Diet needs careful attention. Plenty of alkaline foods as found in fruits and green leafy vegetables. No meats or tobacco.

Shingles—See information under "Prickly Heat."

Skin Diseases—See information under Eczema.

Smallpox—Smallpox must be given attention the same as other skin diseases. The cleansing must come from within. It must not be suppressed, it must not be driven back into the system. Avoid all animal foods, for their end products are putrefaction and would intensify the trouble. Copious sweats must help to clear up the skin. Deep breathing will bring more oxygen into the system. Scrupulous cleanliness must prevail. Diet should be composed entirely of fresh ripe fruits and fresh vegetables with a few nuts. Avoid all stimulants, all condiments. Give water with lemon juice added whenever needed to quench thirst.

Stomach and Bowel Disorders—Avoid all animal foods. They give acid reaction. Fruits, nuts and fresh vegetables help to give tone to the stomach and bring the blood back to its normal alkaline condition.

Stomach Ulcers—The raw juices of fresh green vegetables taken half a cupful at a time, 3 or 4 times a day, and a little freshly expressed fruit juice at other times, will be all the food needed at first. Afterwards fresh fruit for one meal and a finely chopped and well masticated green vegetable salad twice a day for awhile will be salutary. Later cooked vegetables.

Suppressed Menses—Try diet as mentioned under "Profuse Menses."

Tape Worm—It is generally considered that the frequent use of pork is one of the causes of tapeworm. Unquestionably a diet of fruit, nuts, vegetables will help considerably in bringing health back to normal.

Tonsillitis and Quinsy—No food whatever. Warm lemonade or water when thirsty, until fever has subsided and pain has gone. Then orange juice for two days. Afterwards a vegetarian diet, no meats or meat broths. Feeding will surely retard recovery.

INDEX

INDEX

Abscess, 29
Anemia, 9, 163
Animal Care, 10, 11
Ants, 96
Appendicitus, 11, 12, 163
Appetite, 13, 154
Arteries, hardening, 12
Arteriosclerosis, 163.
   See also Arteries, hardening
Arthritus, 133. See also Rheumatism
Asthma, 9, 14-18, 163

Baby care; colic, 18, 59; constipation,
   18; fever, 163; teeth, 156
Backache, 19, 101
Bedwetting, 20-23
Bee sting, 25
Bites; dog, 24-25; snake, 24-25
Bladder, 21-24, 163. See also Kidney
Blood; circulation, 9; purifiers, 26-28.
   See also Poisoning
Blood pressure, high, 12
Boils, 29-32, 94, 163
Brights Disease, 33, 163
Bronchial trouble, 34, 163. See also
   Lungs
Bronchitis, See Lungs, Bronchial
   trouble
Bruises, 35
Bunions, 37
Burns, 36, 37

Catarrh, 38-39
Chilblains, 82
Chills, 40-42
Cholera, 42
Colds, 43-55
Colic. See Baby
Colitis, 151
Constipation, 56-58. See also Baby
   care
Consumption, 106. See also Lungs
Convulsions, 58
Corns, 58
Cough, 43-55

Cramps, 59. See also Female
   disorders, Stomach disorders
Croup, 60, 163
Cuts, 60-62

Dandruff, 87
Diabetes, 67-68, 70, 163
Diarrhoea, 63-66, 102, 151
Diptheria, 163
Dropsy, 68-69, 163
Dysentery, 63, 66
Dyspepsia, 70

Earache, 71
Eczema, 165
Epilepsy, 104, 165
Erysipelas, 72-73, 165
Eyes, sore, 72-73

Feet, sore, 74, 146, 154. See also
   Bunions
Felons, 29, 74-75
Female disorders, 75-81, 163, 166
Fever, 40-42, 163
Flux, 102
Frostbite, 82

Gall stones, 82-83, 165
Goiter, 84, 165
Gonorrhea, 140
Gout, 131
Gravel, 85, 165

Hair, 87-88
Hay fever, 88. See also Asthma
Headache; bilious, 89; nervous, 90;
   sick, 89
Heartburn, 91. See also Dyspepsia,
   Stomach disorders
Heart disease, 90-91, 165; fatty, 90;
   neuralgia, 90, 164; palpitation, 90
Heart dropsy, 92
Hiccoughs, 92
Hives, 92-93, 165